Practice Guidelines

for

Family Nurse Practitioners

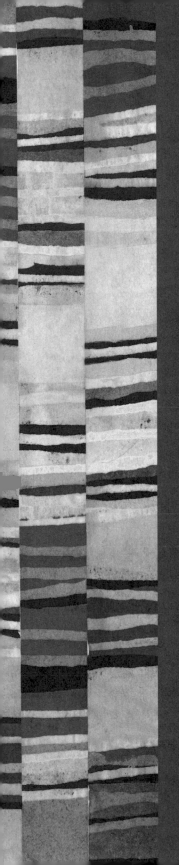

Practice Guidelines
for
Family Nurse
Practitioners

Third Edition
Revised Reprint

Karen Fenstermacher, MS, RN, CS
Family Nurse Practitioner
Freeman Professional Center
Carthage, Missouri

Barbara Toni Hudson, MSN, RN, CS
Family Nurse Practitioner
Ash Grove Family Care Clinic
Citizens Memorial Hospital
Ash Grove, Missouri

SAUNDERS
An Imprint of Elsevier

ELSEVIER
SAUNDERS

3251 Riverport Lane
St. Louis, Missouri 63043

PRACTICE GUIDELINES FOR FAMILY NURSE PRACTITIONERS,   ISBN: 978-0-323-24071-0
THIRD EDITION REVISED REPRINT

Notices

Previous editions copyrighted 2000, 1997

Library of Congress Cataloging-in-Publication Data

Fenstermacher, Karen, author.
   Practice guidelines for family nurse practitioners/Karen Fenstermacher, Barbara Toni Hudson.—
Third edition, revised reprint.
      p. ; cm.
   Includes bibliographical references and index.
   ISBN 978-0-323-24071-0 (spiral bound: alk. Paper)
   I.   Hudson, Barbara Toni, author. II.   Title.
   [DNLM: 1.   Nurse Practitioners. 2.   Family Nursing—methods. WY 128]
   RT120.F34
   610.73—dc23   2013020571

Acquisitions Editor: Lee Henderson
Developmental Editor: Rae Robertson
Publishing Services Manager: Deborah L. Vogel
Project Manager: Pat Costigan
Designer: Amy Buxton

Printed in the United States of America

Last digit is the print number: 9 8 7 6 5 4 3 2 1

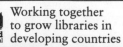

Working together
to grow libraries in
developing countries

www.elsevier.com • www.bookaid.org

Reviewers

Kathryn A. Blair, RN-CS, FNP, PhD
University of Northern Colorado
North Colorado Family Medicine
    Residency Training Program
Greeley, Colorado

Susan Harvey, MSN, RNC, FNP
Winslow Indian Health Center, USPHS
Winslow, Arizona

Judy Rogers, MSN, CRNP
Mercy Health Partners
Scranton, Wilkes-Barre, Pennsylvania

Catherine E. Turner, BSN, MSN, FNP-C
Cherry Point, North Carolina

Preface

Practice Guidelines for Family Nurse Practitioners is a quick reference book for practicing and student nurse practitioners in a variety of disciplines. Although not intended as a textbook, it is an excellent resource, providing protocols for treatment options for patients in varied settings and of varied ages.

Health maintenance guidelines are presented in a chart format. For ease of use, Unit I contains chapters about complete and detailed histories and physical examinations of adult, pediatric, and geriatric patients. Specialized physical examinations are included (e.g., sports and preemployment). Chapters are written in an easy-to-read and accessible format, according to body systems. Common diseases are covered, including signs and symptoms, diagnostic methods, drug therapies, and treatment and adjunctive therapies. There are also blank "notes" pages at the end of each chapter. Some conditions (e.g., asthma, fibromyalgia, menstrual conditions, and diabetes) have been expanded. National standard guidelines are used where available (e.g., asthma, diabetes, Pap smears).

Special chapters include geriatric evaluation, pediatrics, and physical conditions. There is also a section on the care of wounds resulting from vascular disease or peripheral pressure. Appendixes provide information about NSAIDs (comparison chart), dietary sources for different nutrients, and dietary supplement comparison charts. This edition includes multiple herbal therapies, including contraindicated preparations. Pain management guidelines have been expanded.

Karen Fenstermacher
Barbara Toni Hudson

Acknowledgments

My thanks first to God, without whose help I would not be where I am now. Thanks also to Greg Unruh, DO. The mutual respect and collegial relationship we have makes work enjoyable and rewarding. Thanks to last, but not least, my co-workers: Tammy, Kathy, Curtis, Sara, and Diana; you make my job not only easier but also fun.

Karen

My thanks go to my family, David and Cody, for all their support, encouragement, and understanding for all the lost time. My thanks to Shane Bennoch, MD, who never hesitates to help me grow and improve my practice; we make a great pair. I cannot forget my faithful friends Kim, Lynda, and Ann for their hours of help with reading and re-reading the chapters.

Toni

We also want to thank the people at Elsevier for all of their help: Julie Vitale and Claire Kramer. Our book would not be what it is without their input.

Contents

Practice Guidelines for

Family Nurse Practitioners

Unit I

History and Physical Examination

1

Adult Assessment

Guideline for Integrated, Comprehensive Physical Examination*

HISTORY

Biographic information (e.g., "facesheet information")

Chief complaint (CC)
- State in the patient's own words
- Note if the patient's actions agree with or contradict the stated CC

History of the present illness (HPI)
- Try to present a clear account of the patient's CC
- Question the patient regarding the following:
  □ Onset (e.g., when, where)
  □ Characteristics (e.g., description of the quality of discomfort, radiation, associated symptoms like N/V)
  □ Course (e.g., length of event, alleviating or aggravating factors)
  □ What does the patient think is wrong?
- Also note pertinent negative responses (e.g., absence of cough or fever)

Past medical history (PMH)
- This tells the nurse practitioner when to be more concerned (e.g., someone with an essentially negative PMH is not as worrisome as a patient with heart disease or an underlying chronic illness)
- Question the patient regarding significant childhood and adult illnesses, surgeries, and hospitalizations, including ED visits
- Ask about current medications and treatments, including OTC preparations, OCs, inhalers, eyedrops, herbs or vitamins, and customs
- Ask about immunization status, including influenza, pneumococcal vaccine (Pneumovax), and TB test

---

*The suggested format assumes the patient is in a stable condition. The order would be modified as the patient's condition warrants. In an acute illness, the initial focus is on the affected and related body systems with emphasis on the history of the present illness.

- Ask whether the patient has reactions (e.g., allergies, sensitivities) to any medicine and what occurs when patient is taking it (common side effects, such as nausea, are often perceived as an allergy)
- Ask about street drug, alcohol, and tobacco use (specific types, amounts, and routes)

Family history (FH)
- FH is important in the identification of risk factors; gather information about grandparents, parents, and siblings
- Focus on cardiovascular disease, diabetes, cancer, PVD, seizure disorders, asthma, and psychiatric disorder
- The phrase "significant FH" denotes when several members of the family, from different generations, have had a specific disease

Psychosocial history
- Living situation, including significant other in life
- Dietary and rest patterns
- Types of exercise in general
- Occupation
- Inquiry into an average day

Review of systems (ROS): offers the chance to systematically investigate the various body systems to obtain any additional information that would be helpful in arriving at an accurate diagnosis.

Recording the History

Record historical data in the above sequence, remembering to include pertinent negative responses and pertinent past laboratory data. Only positive responses are usually recorded in the ROS. (See p. 21 for a sample History and Physical Exam form.)

PHYSICAL EXAMINATION

General appearance and skin turgor

*Appears acutely ill**

Dehydration

Cyanosis or pallor

SOB or use of accessory muscles to breathe

Drooling (epiglottitis; see Table 15–4)

Vital signs: temperature, pulse, respirations, BP (including postural VS with dizziness or syncope), weight, height

Inspect skin

Fingernail clubbing

Suspicious lesions

---

*Italicized conditions are not to be missed.

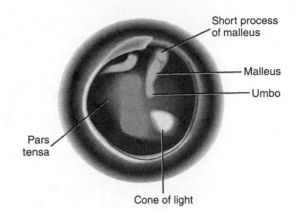

FIGURE I–I Right tympanic membrane.

Head, ears, eyes, nose, and throat (HEENT)
* Inspect face and head
* Palpate scalp and masseter muscles (have patient clench teeth)
* Eyes
  □ Check for visual acuity: OD, OS, and OU
  □ Test EOMs
  □ Inspect conjunctiva, sclera, and cornea
  □ Test pupillary reactions to light and accommodation
  □ Perform ophthalmoscopy

*Red eye** (see Table 5–1)

* Ears
  □ Palpate auricle and tragus
  □ Perform otoscopy (Figure 1–1)
  □ Administer appropriate hearing tests: Weber's test, Rinne test (Figure 1–2), and 2- to 3-foot whisper

Bulging, perforation, retraction, or decreased mobility of TM

Bullae on TM (mycoplasma infection)

* Examine nasal septum and nares for mucosal color and presence of swelling
* Inspect lips, gums, teeth, tongue, buccal mucosa, uvula, and pharynx
  □ Determine "grade" of tonsils
    1+ barely extend beyond tonsillar pillars

    2+ halfway to uvula

    3+ touch uvula

    4+ touch each other
  □ Determine presence of partial plates, full dentures, caries, if any

Peritonsillar abscess

Exudative pharyngitis

---

*Italicized conditions are not to be missed.

Rinne	Weber's	Hearing status
Air conduction > bone conduction	Sound equal to both ears	Either no hearing loss or symmetric hearing loss
Air conduction > bone conduction	Sound lateralizes to right ear	Sensorineural hearing loss in left ear
Bone conduction > air conduction	Sound lateralizes to left ear	Conductive hearing loss in left ear
Bone conduction > air conduction	Sound lateralizes to right ear	Severe sensorineural hearing loss in left ear

FIGURE 1–2 Rinne and Weber's tests.

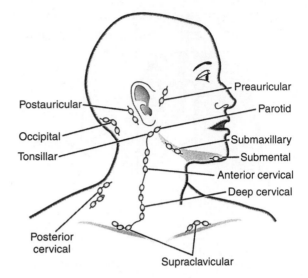

FIGURE I–3 Lymph nodes of the head and neck.

Preauricular
Postauricular
Parotid
Occipital
Submaxillary
Tonsillar
Submental
Anterior cervical
Deep cervical
Posterior cervical
Supraclavicular

*Palatine petechiae**

Postnasal drainage

- Palpation
  □ Over sinuses
  □ Neck

Lymphadenopathy with tenderness (Figure 1–3)

Thyroid abnormalities

Respiratory
- Observe chest for AP and lateral diameter and deformities
- Auscultate the anterior and posterior chest and right lateral chest (Figure 1–4)

Rales: fine, crackly sounds that can be associated with fluid in the airways or with fibrosis

Rhonchi: coarser sounds, as with someone who needs to cough; often clears with cough

Stridor: high-pitched inspiratory sound associated with laryngeal spasm

Wheeze: low-pitched inspiratory or expiratory sound associated with bronchospasm or pulmonary congestion

- Examine chest: respiratory excursion; perform bronchophony, egophony, and whispered pectoriloquy, if indicated
- Percuss posterior lung fields

Dullness = consolidation

Hyperresonance = emphysema

---

*Italicized conditions are not to be missed.

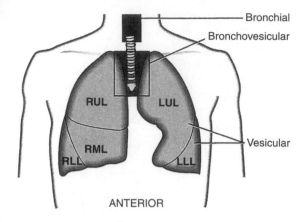

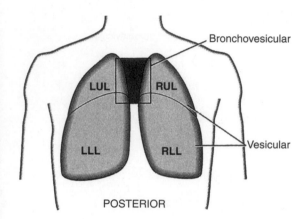

FIGURE I–4 Lung lobes and breath sounds.

- Percuss diaphragmatic excursion and palpate vocal fremitus if indicated
- Examine capillary refill of nailbeds

*Capillary refill >3 seconds**

Cardiovascular

- Palpate the precordium

Thrills, heaves, or lifts

Displacement of PMI

- Auscultation (Figure 1–5)
  - □ Listen over the precordium with the patient seated upright and leaning forward, in the supine position, and in the left lateral position

Murmurs (also see p. 161 and Table 6–1)

Clicks

---

*Italicized conditions are not to be missed.

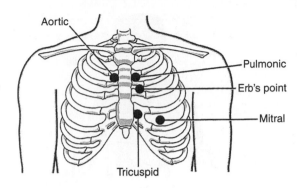

FIGURE I-5 Heart auscultatory sites.

Opening snap*

Friction rubs

S_3 *or* S_4 (see p. 161)

- Use both the bell and the diaphragm
- Listen for S_1 and S_2 (including splits); to identify S_1, time it with the carotid pulse

  Split S_1 is usually normal; best heard at tricuspid area

  Split S_2 is physiologic (normal) if it resolves with deep expiration (i.e., it is "blown away")

  Paradoxical split S_2: think left bundle branch block (LBBB) or aortic stenosis

  Fixed split S_2: think atrial septal defect
- Listen over the carotid arteries, abdominal aorta, and renal and femoral arteries

Bruits

Renal artery stenosis

Abdominal aortic aneurysm

- Inspect the neck (with the head of the bed at 45 degrees) for carotid and jugular pulsations and jugular venous pressure (JVP)

  JVP elevated >2 cm above clavicle (would mean a pressure of >7 cm because the clavicle is approximately 5 cm above the right atrium)
- Palpation
  - Check carotid pulses (individually)
  - Check abdomen for hepatojugular reflux and aortic pulsation

Widened aortic pulsation

  - Check peripheral pulses for rate, rhythm, and amplitude (Figure 1–6)

---

*Italicized conditions are not to be missed.

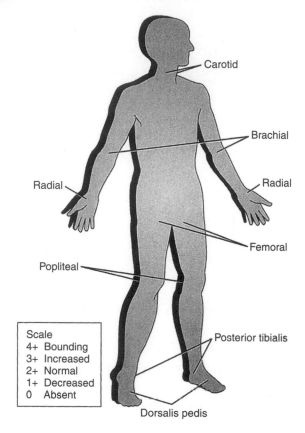

Carotid

Brachial

Radial

Radial

FIGURE 1-6 Peripheral pulses.

Femoral

Popliteal

Scale
4+ Bounding
3+ Increased
2+ Normal
1+ Decreased
0   Absent

Posterior tibialis

Dorsalis pedis

*Absence of pulse(s)**

Femoral aneurysm

  □ Check lower extremities for edema

Abdomen

  • Inspect for contour and scars

    □ Have the patient raise head and shoulders off the table

Hernia

Masses

  □ Scars and striae

Purple striae of Cushing's syndrome (see Table 13–2)

  □ Check for engorged veins

Hepatic cirrhosis

---

*Italicized conditions are not to be missed.

*Inferior vena cava obstruction**
  □ Inspect for distention
Ascites
Tumor
• Auscultate for bowel sounds
Intestinal obstruction
Paralytic ileus
Peritonitis
• Percussion
  □ Liver and splenic borders
Hepatosplenomegaly
  □ Other areas as necessary
  □ Costovertebral angle tenderness: the patient must sit for this test
Positive test (pain with examination)
• Palpation
  □ Light
Peritoneal irritation
  □ Deep
Liver or spleen palpable or tender
Masses
Aortic aneurysm
  □ Rebound tenderness
Peritoneal irritation
  □ Inguinal nodes
Infection
Malignancy
• Rectal (if indicated)
  □ Perform digital examination of prostate (if male >40 yr)
Rectal masses
Fecal retention
Abnormal prostate
  □ Stool for occult blood
Positive guaiac
• With possible rebound tenderness, also ascertain presence of the following:
  □ Iliopsoas sign: pain increases when the patient raises a leg and then resists against it being pushed down

---

*Italicized conditions are not to be missed.

- Obturator sign: have the patient flex and externally rotate hip ("froglegged" position); pain increases when the patient resists against further rotation of hip

*Peritoneal irritation**

Genitalia—male
- Check for inguinal hernia
- Check skin (including ventral side of penis) for any lesions
- Testicular examination (teach self-testicular examination)

Undescended testicle

Right testis lower than left (consider situs inversus or renal cell cancer; obtain renal sonogram)

Epispadias (refer to urologist)

Genitalia—female
- Inspect breasts for skin redness, dimpling, or puckering; to do this, inspect while having the woman (1) place her hands on her hips and shrug shoulders and (2) press palms together over her head
- Palpate breasts and axillary, clavicular, and epitrochlear nodes; teach breast self-examination

Abnormal skin changes

Nodules or lymphadenopathy

Nipple discharge

Supraclavicular nodes

- External genitalia
  - Inspect hair pattern
  - Observe for lesions
  - Determine presence and condition of hymen
  - Perineal support: spread labia and have patient "bear down"; inspect for drainage and rectocele or cystocele
  - Palpate Bartholin's, urethral, and Skene's glands for pain, swelling, drainage

Lesions

Abnormal discharge

- Urethra: check for discharge and erythema
- Perform vaginal examination
  - Inspect by inserting speculum to visualize cervix and vaginal walls (do not lubricate with anything but warm water, if needed)
  - Inspect vaginal walls for color, discharge, rugae, and lesions
  - Inspect cervix for color, parity, lesions, discharge, friability; note cervical os size and position and lesions

---

*Italicized conditions are not to be missed.

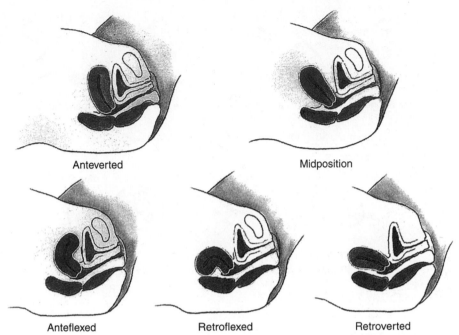

Anteverted   Midposition

Anteflexed   Retroflexed   Retroverted

FIGURE 1-7 Cervix and uterus positions. (From Jarvis C. [2002]. *Physical examination and health assessment* [3rd ed.]. Philadelphia: W.B. Saunders.)

□ Obtain indicated cultures and Pap smear (GC and *Chlamydia* cultures must be obtained before a Pap smear); perform a wet mount if indicated (see following section, "How to Do a Wet Prep")

*Vaginal or cervical infection**

• Bimanual examination
   □ Palpate cervix for contour, smoothness, cervical motion tenderness
   □ Palpate uterus for size and shape, position, and consistency (Figure 1-7)
   □ Palpate adnexa for size, presence of masses, and tenderness; if unable to palpate, document such; it is often difficult to palpate adnexa on larger women

Cervical motion tenderness (may indicate pelvic infection or inflammation)

Enlarged or tender uterus

Adnexal fullness or tenderness

HOW TO DO A WET PREP

Need:

Pap smear spatula, two cotton-tipped applicators, and two capped test tubes, one with 1 to 2 ml of saline and one with 1 to 2 ml of potassium hydroxide (KOH)

---

*Italicized conditions are not to be missed.

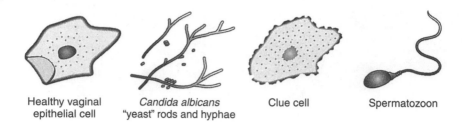

Healthy vaginal epithelial cell   *Candida albicans* "yeast" rods and hyphae   Clue cell   Spermatozoon

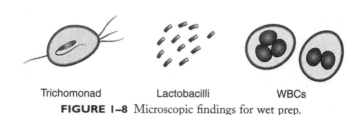

Trichomonad   Lactobacilli   WBCs

FIGURE 1–8 Microscopic findings for wet prep.

Nitrazine paper

Two slides with slide covers

- Obtain specimens from the lateral wall of the vagina; place one of the applicators in each of the test tubes
- Use the specimen on the spatula to check vaginal pH with nitrazine paper
- Perform a "whiff" test by smelling the applicator in the KOH tube; the result is considered positive if there is an "amine" or fishy odor
- If pH is normal and whiff is negative, no further testing may be needed for bacterial vaginosis (BV) or trichomoniasis
- To check for BV, trichomoniasis, or *Candida* infection (yeast) using the applicator, place a few drops from the saline tube on one slide and top with a slide cover; repeat with the KOH tube applicator on the other slide
- View under high power looking for epithelial cells, WBCs, clue cells, lactobacilli, or other cells on saline-prepared slide; view for yeast bud and hyphae on KOH-prepared slide (Figure 1–8).

Musculoskeletal (also see Chapter 12)
- Observe gait

*Abnormal gait**

- Inspect joints for redness, increased heat, painful ROM
- Examine back

---

*Italicized conditions are not to be missed.

Table I–I Speech Disturbances: Characteristics and Pattern

SPEECH DISTURBANCE	CHARACTERISTICS
Fluent aphasia (Wernicke's area)	Lacks content Unable to comprehend spoken words and phrases Unable to repeat or name objects
Nonfluent aphasia (Broca's area)	Slow, scanning speech Intact comprehension Impaired writing ability Inability to verbally express thoughts
Global aphasia (combined Broca's and Wernicke's areas)	Nonfluent speech Unable to comprehend, read, or write Unable to name objects

*Scoliosis**

Kyphosis

Neurologic system (may be integrated with rest of examination)
- For cognitive status, refer to Mini-Mental State Examination
  - Test for intellectual ability
  - Determine judgment and problem-solving ability: ask, "If you smell smoke in the house, what do you do?"
  - Test cognition of abstract thought: ask the patient to explain a proverb like, "A stitch in time saves nine."
  - Evaluate affect: behaviors that may signify depression or lability of mood
- Language
  - Test verbal abilities, namely speech patterns, fluency, and content
  - Test ability to write and copy
  - Check gestures and the ability to follow serial and three-step commands; for example, ask the patient: "Hold up your right hand, stick out your tongue, and close your eyes."
  - Does patient have appropriate recognition skills, that is, the ability to name common objects?
  - Check reading ability and comprehension

Agraphia (inability to write)

Alexia (inability to read, when patient has been able to read)
- Speech disturbances (Table 1–1)
- Ophthalmologic examination (Tables 1–2 and 1–3)

---

*Italicized conditions are not to be missed.

Table 1–2 Ophthalmologic Examination

FINDING	CHARACTERISTICS	POSSIBLE CAUSES
Normal	Yellow-white disc Well-defined disc margins Arteries (smaller) enter and veins (larger) leave at optic disc	
Papilledema	Edema of optic disc: unilateral if inflammatory (may have sudden loss of vision in inflammatory state); usually bilateral if noninflammatory Impaired visual acuity in chronic stage	Lesions that increase intracranial pressure Encephalopathy Optic artery aneurysm or cavernous sinus thrombosis Guillain-Barré syndrome
Optic atrophy	Decreased vision Optic disc white or gray-white May have absent cup	Optic neuritis Neurosyphilis Trauma to orbit Toxins or poisons Diabetes

Table 1–3 Eye Signs

EYE SIGN	CHARACTERISTICS	PATHOLOGY
Normal findings	Pupils 3–4 mm, symmetric, round, and reactive to light and accommodation Palpebral fissure 8–12 mm and symmetric	
Adie's pupil	Unilateral, large pupil Sluggish constriction to prolonged light exposure Direct light reflex absent	Postviral infection Loss of parasympathetic reactions
Anisocoria	Unequal pupil size Reactive to light and accommodation	May be normal variant Compression of CN III
Argyll Robertson pupil	Pupils smaller than normal in dim light Minimal dilation, often unequal Pupils may appear irregular Visual disturbance	Neurosyphilis, viral encephalitis Lesion in midbrain Diabetes

Table 1–3 Eye Signs—cont'd

EYE SIGN	CHARACTERISTICS	PATHOLOGY
Dysconjugate gaze	Inability to follow moving finger to all eye fields Deviation of eye Lack of gaze coordination	Space-occupying lesion Neuromuscular disorders Frontal lobe dysfunction (dementia or trauma) Diabetes mellitus
Hippus	Pupil with brisk light constriction Slowly rhythmic relaxation and constriction when direct light held in place	May be normal variant Midbrain lesion Barbiturate toxicity
Marcus Gunn pupil	Pupils equal, with positive direct light reflex Pupil dilates when direct light is moved from intact eye to eye with abnormal pupil	Optic nerve involved Retinal diseases
Nystagmus	Involuntary, oscillating eye movements May occur at rest or during eye field examination May be vertical or lateral	May be associated with strain secondary to poor lighting Side effect of certain drugs (phenytoin, alcohol, barbiturates) Bilateral nystagmus may indicate myasthenia gravis
Ptosis	Palpebral fissure <5 mm Asymmetric	CN III palsy Myopathy Neuromuscular disorders (e.g., myasthenia gravis) Atonic eyelid muscles Inflammatory lesion of eyelid

- Sensory: head and neck
  - Always test right and left separately
  - Check tactile ability: ask patient to identify the body part being touched
  - Test for auditory ability: Rinne and Weber's tests (see Figure 1–2) and comprehension of sound
- Motor
  - Always test right and left separately
    Ataxia*: test with tandem gait (walk in a straight line)
    Apraxia: inability to execute volitional activity
- Cranial nerve examination (Table 1–4)

---

*Italicized conditions are not to be missed.

Table 1–4 Cranial Nerve Examination

CRANIAL NERVE	FUNCTION	TYPE*	TESTS	ABNORMAL FINDINGS
I. Olfactory	Smell	S	*Do not* use ammonia Test each nostril separately with alcohol preparation, mint, and coffee	Obstructive nasal passage Lesions of the frontal lobe, pituitary uncus, or hippocampal gyrus
II. Optic	Central and peripheral vision	S	Snellen's chart Newspaper print Color vision Count fingers in peripheral fields Ophthalmoscopic examination	Amaurosis (loss of vision); *refer immediately* Cataracts Cortical blindness Papilledema Optic atrophy
III. Oculomotor	Pupillary constriction Eyelid elevation	M	Pupil size, symmetry, shape, and accommodation	Ptosis Nonreactive pupil Anisocoria Optic nerve lesions
IV. Trochlear	Eye movements	M	Follow finger or object in all planes (EOMs)	Nystagmus Diplopia Dysconjugate gaze
V. Trigeminal	Tongue and facial sensation Corneal reflex	B	Pinprick to face with eyes closed Have the patient open and close jaw Corneal reflex (use a drop of saline)	Loss of sensation, paresthesia, or pain Deviation of jaw Lack of blink reflex
VI. Abducens	Lateral eye movement	M	(Test with CN III and IV)	
VII. Facial	Facial expression Salivary and lacrimal glands Taste	B	Have the patient wrinkle the forehead, grimace, raise eyebrows, smile, and frown Taste: sweet, sour, and bitter substances to anterior tongue	Asymmetry of face Deviation of mouth Weakness of forehead Inability to close eyes Loss of taste Excessive tearing
VIII. Acoustic	Hearing Equilibrium	S	Rinne and Weber's tests Whisper Ticking watch Equilibrium	Unilateral deafness Tinnitus Lateralization Vertigo, dizziness, or ataxia
IX. Glossopharyngeal	Taste on posterior tongue Gag or swallow	B	Taste: sweet, sour, and bitter substances to posterior tongue Gag and swallow	Loss of taste Loss of gag or swallow Dysphagia

*B, Both sensory and motor; *M*, motor; *S*, sensory.

Table I–4	Cranial Nerve Examination—cont'd				
CRANIAL NERVE	**FUNCTION**	**TYPE***	**TESTS**	**ABNORMAL FINDINGS**	
X. Vagus	Gag or swallow	B	Inspect soft palate Uvula in midline Stimulate pharyngeal wall Voice quality	Loss of voice or hoarseness Deviation of uvula Coughing and choking	
XI. Accessory	Fluid movement of head and neck in flexion, extension, and rotation	M	Palpate sternocleidomastoid and trapezius muscles Have the patient turn his or her head against resistance Have the patient shrug his or her shoulders against resistance	Paralysis or weakness Atrophy Spasticity	
XII. Hypoglossal	Tongue movement	M	Have the patient move his or her tongue side to side Observe for symmetry and rhythmicity	Spastic paralysis Deviation from midline Dysarthria Spastic speech	

*B, Both sensory and motor; *M*, motor; *S*, sensory.

- Coordination
  - □ Can patient perform rapid alternating movements?
  - □ Finger-to-nose: ask the patient to touch his or her nose and the examiner's finger alternately with rapid repetition
  - □ Heel-to-shin: have the patient place his or her heel on the opposite knee and slide the heel down the shin to the foot and back up the shin
  - □ Balance: have the patient stand unsupported (evaluates truncal balance)
  - □ Romberg's test evaluates the patient's ability to stand unsupported with eyes closed; a positive test means the patient is unable to perform

Inability to perform any of the tests*

Tremors

- Gait
  - □ Ask the patient to walk forward, sideways, and backward
  - □ Observe for tandem gait (ability to walk a straight line)

Foot drop

Spasticity or bradykinesia

---

*Italicized conditions are not to be missed.

- Sensory: peripheral
  □ Compare right to left sides with the patient's eyes covered or closed
  □ Definitions

  Hyperesthesia: excessively sensitive to touch

  Paresthesia: sensations without the examiner's stimulation

  □ Evaluate the patient's ability to discern the following:

  Vibration: use a tuning fork on a bony prominence

  Light touch: use a wisp of cotton

  Two-point discrimination: touch the patient in various places using sharp and dull objects and note any differences

  Temperature: blow gently on patient's skin (medial wrist is best) with lips apart (warm) and lips pursed (cool); may also use very warm and cold water in test tubes

  *Inability to discern any of these sensory tests**

- Reflexes
  □ Assess for symmetry
  □ Check for DTRs

	REFLEX	LEVEL	NORMAL RESPONSE
	Biceps, A	C5–C6	Elbow flexion
	Triceps, B	C7	Elbow extension
	Brachioradialis, C	C6–C7	Wrist flexion
	Patellar, D	L3–L4	Knee extension
	Achilles, E	S1	Foot extension

Scoring: 0 absent; 1+ weak; 2+ normal; 3+ exaggerated; 4+ clonus.

□ In patients with altered LOC or possible CVA or paralysis, the following reflexes may also be checked:

Abdominal: stimulate above and below the umbilicus; normally, the umbilicus moves toward the side stimulated

Bulbocavernous or cremasteric: stimulate the foreskin or glans; normally, the muscle at the base of the penis contracts

Plantar: stimulate the sole of the foot from the heel to the big toe with a blunt object; normally, the toes flex; a positive (abnormal) Babinski's sign occurs when the big toe moves up and the toes fan out

---

*Italicized conditions are not to be missed.

Pathologic Reflex Findings (Adult)

REFLEX	HOW TO TEST	PATHOLOGIC FINDING
Glabella	Tap forehead	Spasmodic closing of eyes
Snout	Tap above or below mouth at midline	Pursed lips (similar to rooting reflex)
Sucking	Touch lips with blunt object	Similar to sucking reflex of infant
Grasp	Stimulate palm of hand	Hand "grasps" object
Babinski's	Stroke sole of foot with blunt object	Great toe goes upward and toes fan out

History & Physical Exam

Chief Complaint:

PMH: immunizations current   chicken pox   rheumatic fever   TB   CA   DM   HTN   MI
     CVA   renal disease   jaundice   thyroid problems

Surgeries/hospitalizations:

Injuries: fractures   burns

FH: DM _____   CA _____   CV _____
    renal disease _____   Asthma _____

Allergies:

Social: occupation _____   S   M   W   D
    living arrangements _____   caffeine _____
    tobacco _____   ETOH _____   drugs _____

Current meds:

ROS: <u>General</u>
  ☐ weakness
  ☐ fatigue
  ☐ chg in weight
  ☐ fever
  ☐ night sweats

<u>Hematopoietic</u>
  ☐ abnormal bleeding
  ☐ excessive bruising

<u>Integumentary</u>
  ☐ pruritis
  ☐ hair loss
  ☐ skin lesions or
    discolorations
  ☐ nail changes

Continued

HEENT

☐ glasses/contacts
☐ last eye exam
☐ vision changes/loss
☐ blurred/double vision
☐ cataract/glaucoma

☐ hearing changes
☐ tinnitus
☐ ear drainage
☐ nasal drainage
☐ epistaxis

☐ mouth lesions
☐ voice changes
☐ dental problems
☐ dysphagia
☐ sore throat

Respiratory

☐ SOB
☐ painful breathing
☐ wheezing
☐ sputum production
☐ bloody sputum
☐ recurrent infection
☐ O_2 use
☐ # pillows used
☐ positive TB test

Cardiovascular

☐ chest pain
☐ SOB when lying flat
☐ palpitations
☐ edema
☐ murmur
☐ varicose veins
☐ claudication
☐ DVT

Gastrointestinal

☐ food intolerances
☐ loss of appetite
☐ abdominal pain/ulcer
☐ heartburn/nausea
☐ blood in vomit
☐ fecal incontinence
☐ changes in stool
   color, consistency or
   frequency

Genitourinary

☐ dysuria
☐ excess urination
☐ pain in flank
☐ pain in groin
☐ hematuria
☐ hx of stones
☐ incontinence
☐ hx of STD

Female reproductive

☐ LMP _____
☐ G   P   M   A
☐ possible PG
☐ vag. discharge/itch
☐ labial lesions
☐ dysmenorrhea
☐ menopausal symptoms
☐ PMS symptoms
☐ contraception/HRT

Male reproductive

☐ penis/testicle pain
☐ penile discharge
☐ impotence
☐ dimin. urine stream
☐ hesitancy
☐ last PSA _____

Musculoskeletal

☐ joint pain/stiffness
☐ tendon, ligament or
   muscle strain or tear
☐ bone aches/pains
☐ fractures
☐ myalgias

Neuro-psych

☐ blackouts/seizures
☐ loss of memory
☐ loss of coordination
☐ paralysis
☐ weakness/numbness
☐ tremors
☐ anxiety/irritability
☐ depression/apathy
☐ hallucinations
☐ sleep disturbances
☐ suicidal/homicidal thoughts

Endocrine

☐ excess thirst/hunger
☐ cold/heat intolerance
☐ excess sweating

Exam

General: This _____ year old (race) (sex) is alert, cooperative, and a good historian. (S)he is in no acute distress. Vital signs: BP   P   R   T

Ht.   Wt.

HEENT
- [ ] normocephalic
- [ ] PERRLA
- [ ] sclera/conjunctiva
- [ ] nystagmus
- [ ] hearing
- [ ] otoscope exam
- [ ] nasal mucosa
- [ ] teeth/dentures
- [ ] oral mucosa/pharynx

Neck
- [ ] supple
- [ ] thyroid

Chest
- [ ] symmetrical
- [ ] barrel chest
- [ ] SOB
- [ ] retraction/ accessory muscle
- [ ] breath sounds
- [ ] breast exam

Cardiovascular
- [ ] PMI
- [ ] HRRR or HIRR
- [ ] murmur
- [ ] S_3 or S_4
- [ ] JVD/carotid bruits
- [ ] abd/femoral bruits
- [ ] peripheral pulses
- [ ] edema
- [ ] varicosities

Abdomen
- [ ] size/shape
- [ ] tender/pain
- [ ] rebound signs
- [ ] CVAT
- [ ] bowel sounds
- [ ] liver/spleen
- [ ] masses/scars
- [ ] rectal exam (also hemoccult)

Male genitalia
- [ ] circumcised
- [ ] discharge
- [ ] testicular mass
- [ ] hydro-/varicocele
- [ ] hernia

Female genitalia
- [ ] external genitalia
- [ ] BUS
- [ ] vagina (including discharge)
- [ ] CMT
- [ ] bimanual exam

Skin/lymph
- [ ] texture/turgor
- [ ] pigmentation
- [ ] petechia/purpura
- [ ] lesions
- [ ] hair
- [ ] nails
- [ ] lymph glands

Neurological
- [ ] LOC
- [ ] coordination/gait
- [ ] cranial nerves
- [ ] Babinski
- [ ] motor/sensory deficits

Musculoskeletal
- [ ] kyphosis/scoliosis
- [ ] paravertebral spasm
- [ ] joint ROM
- [ ] joint deformities

Lab/X-ray and other test results:

Assessments

Plan

Focused Examinations

RESPIRATORY

History-of-present-illness emphasis
- SOB, dyspnea, orthopnea, and nocturnal dyspnea
- Wheezing
- Cough, sputum, and hemoptysis
- Sore throat
- Earache

Past medical history
- Asthma (include ED visits and hospitalizations)
- Bronchitis
- Pneumonia or TB
- Frequent strep throat or ear infections
- Chest trauma or spontaneous pneumothorax
- Occupational exposure and tobacco use
- Last influenza or pneumonia vaccine, TB test

Family history
- Asthma
- Chronic airway disease

Referral guidelines
- Patients in acute distress
- Suspected epiglottitis (see p. 438)
- Peritonsillar abscess

Include cardiovascular and abdominal examinations with respiratory complaints

CARDIOVASCULAR

History-of-present-illness emphasis
- Cardiac (e.g., chest pain, palpitations, dysrhythmias, tachycardia, cyanosis, cough, exertional dyspnea, orthopnea, nocturnal dyspnea, edema, dizziness, syncope, diaphoresis)
- Vascular (e.g., phlebitis, intermittent claudication, skin color changes, cold or painful extremities)

Past medical history
- Rheumatic fever
- Murmurs
- Mitral valve prolapse (MVP)
- Ischemic heart disease or dysrhythmia (e.g., atrial fibrillation)
- CHF
- CVA
- HTN
- DM
- Gallbladder disease
- Peptic ulcer

- DVT
- Marfan syndrome (see p. 193)

Family history
- Sudden death of family member before age 55
- ASHD
- CAD
- HTN
- Raynaud's disease or other peripheral vascular disease
- DM

Referral guidelines
- Chest pain of cardiac origin (e.g., suspected MI or new angina)
- Suspected aortic dissection
- Pulmonary embolism
- New or refractory CHF
- Acute arterial insufficiency
- Suspected DVT
- Childhood murmurs and new onset adult murmurs

Include respiratory and abdominal examination with cardiovascular complaints

ABDOMINAL

History-of-present-illness emphasis
- Onset, causes, and characteristics (e.g., N/V, diarrhea, constipation, flatulence, belching, and heartburn)
- See p. 217 for pain sites
- Review of 24-hour dietary intake and presence of similar symptoms in the patient's family

Past medical history
- Usual elimination patterns
- Ulcer
- Irritable bowel syndrome
- Gallbladder disease
- Abdominal operations
- Women: LMP, type of contraception used
- Recent travel

Family history of GI tract disorders

Referral guidelines
- Patients with an initial diagnosis of hepatic cirrhosis or Cushing's disease
- Symptoms suggestive of an acute abdomen or aortic aneurysm
- Any abdominal bruit
- Rectal mass or lymphadenopathy

Include respiratory and cardiovascular examinations with abdominal complaints; also pelvic examination if indicated (e.g., lower abdominal pain in woman of child-bearing age)

ROUTINE WELL-WOMAN EXAMINATION

History-of-present-illness emphasis
- Menstrual history (age at menarche, LMP, age at menopause)
- Sexual history (age at first intercourse, number of sexual partners, STDs)
- Obstetric history (number of pregnancies, live births, abortions/miscarriages)
- Use of contraception

Past medical history
- Gallbladder disease
- Heart disease
- Varicose veins
- History of abnormal Pap smears, date of last Pap smear
- Menopausal symptoms, dyspareunia, vaginal discharge, lesions, incontinence
- Last mammography
- Nutritional history

Family history
- Breast or reproductive tract cancer
- Heart disease
- HTN
- DM
- Osteoporosis
- Thyroid problems

Sports Physical Examination

HISTORY

Type of sport to be played: consideration of contact vs. noncontact sports

Emphasis on cardiovascular, respiratory, and musculoskeletal systems

Family history: emphasis on cardiovascular disorder or sudden death in family

Past medical history
- Cardiovascular disorder
  - Murmur
  - HTN
  - Persistent cough or SOB or chest tightness
  - Dizziness, palpitations or faintness with exercise
  - Marfan syndrome (see p. 193)
  - Rheumatic fever
- Asthma (allergic or exercise induced)
- Neurologic disorder
  - Head injury (concussion) or neck injury
  - Syncope or convulsions
  - Frequent headaches
- Musculoskeletal disorder (e.g., fracture, joint dislocation, or injury)

- Eyes, ears, nose, and throat (EENT)
  - □ Impaired vision, temporary loss of vision, history of detached retina
  - □ Use of contact lenses or glasses
  - □ Perforated eardrum, use of hearing aid(s)
  - □ Orthodontia
- Metabolic disorder
  - □ DM (especially insulin dependent)
  - □ Tendency to bleed or bruise easily, anemia
  - □ Mononucleosis
  - □ Weight problems or eating disorders
- Allergies
  - □ Hay fever
  - □ Bee sting reactions
  - □ Medication reactions
- Previous surgery (e.g., orthopedic, absence of kidney or testicle)
- Habits (e.g., tobacco, caffeine, alcohol, drug, and herbal use)
- Medications (e.g., prescription, emergency, or prn use)

PHYSICAL EXAMINATION

Vital signs: BP and pulse while the patient is resting, immediately after the patient has exercised for 3 minutes, and 3 minutes after the patient has completed exercise

Weight and height

Visual acuity (Snellen's chart)

Level of conditioning

General appearance, nutritional status

*Acute systemic infection**

Vision and hearing impairment

Teeth and mouth impairment

Cardiovascular

- Heart sounds (see Figure 1–5)

Murmur (see p. 161 and Table 6–1)

Bruits

- Peripheral pulses (see Figure 1–6)

Dysrhythmias

Abdomen

Enlarged spleen or liver

---

*Italicized conditions are not to be missed.

Musculoskeletal (back and extremities)
- ROM
- Flexibility ("duck walk" four steps)
- Strength

*Congenital anomalies**

Limitation of or pain with movement

Neuromuscular
- Test DTRs (see p. 20).
- Assess cranial nerves (see Table 1–4)
- Test coordination (see p. 19)

Genitourinary (GU) tract (male athletes): use examination to reinforce normality
- Check for inguinal hernia

Inguinal hernia

- Testicular examination

Undescended testicle

Right testis lower than left (consider situs inversus or renal cell cancer; obtain renal sonogram)

Epispadias (refer to urologist)

Varicocele (refer to urologist)

SCREENING TESTS (MAY NOT BE REQUIRED)

Urine dipstick for sugar and albumin

Hct or Hgb (female athletes)

Consider ECG with a history of palpitations or dysrhythmia

Obtain echocardiogram with new or changed murmur or findings suggestive of Marfan syndrome (see p. 193).

REFERRAL GUIDELINES

History of syncope, SOB, or palpitations

FH of sudden death before age 55 years

Physical findings of
- BP higher than 140/90 mm Hg
- Cardiac murmur, bruits, or findings suggestive of idiopathic hypertrophic subaortic stenosis (IHSS)

Contraindications for participation until physician consultation/referral
- History of detached retina
- Enlarged spleen or liver associated with systemic disease
- Absent kidney or testicle

---

*Italicized conditions are not to be missed.

- Posttraumatic convulsive disorders
- Multiple concussions (more than three per season or head injuries that demonstrate residual symptoms, neurologic changes, or evidence of altered activity on EEG)
- Inadequately controlled diabetes
- Acute systemic infection
- History of or active cardiovascular disorders
- Pregnancy

Employment Physical Examination

HISTORY

Complete review with emphasis on vision, hearing, and musculoskeletal system disorders

Previous work history; previous injury

Permanent partial disabilities or limitations

Habits (type and amount of tobacco, alcohol, and street drug use)

Allergies

Current medications

Type of work being hired to do

Immunization status

PHYSICAL EXAMINATION

Vital signs: BP; pulse while the patient is resting, immediately after the patient has exercised for 2 minutes, and 2 minutes after the patient has completed exercise

Weight and height

General appearance
- Age appropriateness
- Nutritional status
- Developmental state

Speech and cognition

Vision and hearing

*Significant vision or hearing loss**

Head, neck, and lymph nodes

Cardiovascular
- Normal heart sounds (see Figure 1–5)

Murmur (see p. 161 and Table 6–1)

Bruits
- Peripheral vascular pulses (see Figure 1–6)

---

*Italicized conditions are not to be missed.

Musculoskeletal (back and extremities)
- ROM, flexibility, strength

Limitation of or pain with movement*

- Assess lifting technique

Neuromuscular
- Test DTRs (see p. 20)
- Assess cranial nerves (see Table 1–4)
- Test coordination (see p. 19)
- Perform Phalen's and reverse Phalen's maneuvers and Tinel's test

Carpal tunnel syndrome

GU tract: assess for inguinal hernia in males

Inguinal hernia

Rectal examination if indicated; stool for guaiac

Rectal mass

Malignancy

Examination specific to essential functions of the job (EFJ): focus examination on job description (have copy of job description on hand during examination)

Inability to perform EFJ

DIAGNOSTIC TESTING (AS INDICATED)
CBC

UA

Blood chemistry

PFT

Drug screening

TB skin testing

Hepatitis panel (A, B, and C)

PREVENTION (AS INDICATED)
Hepatitis A and B vaccines

Health Appraisal and Risk Factors
See Table 1–5

Anticipatory Guidance and Counseling
See Table 1–6

---

*Italicized conditions are not to be missed.

Table 1–5 Health Appraisal and Risk Factors for Patients Aged 19 Years and Older

	19–29 yr	30–39 yr	40–49 yr	50–59 yr	>60 yr
History					
Reason for visit	Each visit	Each visit	Each visit	Each visit	Each visit
Status: medical, surgical, family	q1–3y	q1–3y	q2y	q2y	q2y
Dietary intake	q1–3y	q1–3y	q2y	q2y	q2y
Physical activity	q1–3y	q1–3y	q2y	q2y	q2y
Tobacco/alcohol/ drug use	q1–3y	q1–3y	q2y	q2y	q2y
Sexual practices	As indicated	As indicated	As indicated	As indicated	As indicated
Change in life arrangements	q3y	q3y	q2y	Yearly	Yearly
Complete physical examination	Once				
Weight	Periodically				
Height	Once			As indicated, with postural changes	
BP	q2y	q2y	q2y	q2y	q2y
Tonometry by ophthalmologist			q2–4y	q2–4y	q2y
Dental examination	Yearly	Yearly	Yearly	Yearly	Yearly
Screening					
Stool for occult blood				Yearly	Yearly
Digital rectal examination			q1–2y	Yearly	Yearly
Pap smear	q1–3y	q1–3y	q1–2y	q1–3y	q1–3y
Pelvic examination	q1–3y	q1–3y	q1–2y	Yearly	Yearly
Breast, skin, testes examination	q1–3y	q1–3y	q1–2y	Yearly	Yearly
Mammography		Once	Yearly	Yearly	Yearly
Serum cholesterol		q5y	q5y	q5y	As indicated
PSA				Yearly	Yearly
Sigmoidoscopy				q5y	q5y
Immunizations					
Tetanus and diphtheria	q10y	q10y	q10y	q10y	q10y
Pneumovax					Once, >65 yr
Influenza	As desired	As desired	As desired	Yearly	Yearly, >65 yr

Continued

Table 1-5 Health Appraisal and Risk Factors for Patients Aged 19 Years and Older—cont'd

	19–29 yr	30–39 yr	40–49 yr	50–59 yr	>60 yr
High-risk screening/ testing STDs TB skin test ECG Fasting blood glucose Hearing Thyroid function tests			Periodically, as indicated		
Leading causes of death	Ages 19–39 yr Motor vehicle accidents Heart disease Homicide AIDS Breast and uterine cancer Cerebrovascular disease		Ages 40–64 yr Heart disease Breast, lung, colorectal cancer Cerebrovascular disease COPD Ovarian cancer		Age 65 yr and older Heart disease Cerebrovascular disease Pneumonia and influenza COPD Colorectal, lung cancer
Counseling	With each visit, as indicated (see Table 1–6)				

Table 1–6 Anticipatory Guidance/Counseling for Patients Aged 19 Years and Older

TOPIC	19–39 yr	40–64 yr	>65 yr
Nutrition and exercise	Fat (especially saturated fat) and cholesterol Fiber Sodium (see Appendix B) Iron and calcium (for women) (see Appendix B) Selection of exercise program	Fat (especially saturated fat) and cholesterol Fiber Sodium (see Appendix B) Calcium (for women) (see Appendix B)	Fat (especially saturated fat) and cholesterol Fiber Sodium (see Appendix B) Calcium (for women) (see Appendix B)
Substance use	Tobacco*: cessation/primary prevention Alcohol, drugs Limiting alcohol consumption Driving, other activities while under the influence Treatment for abuse Sharing, using unsterilized needles and syringes	Tobacco*: cessation Alcohol, drugs Limiting alcohol consumption Driving, other activities while under the influence Treatment for abuse Sharing, using unsterilized needles and syringes	Tobacco*: cessation Alcohol, drugs Limiting alcohol consumption Driving, other activities while under the influence Treatment for abuse Sharing, using unsterilized needles and syringes
Sexual practices	STDs: partner selection, condom use Unplanned pregnancy, contraception	STDs: partner selection, condom use Unplanned pregnancy, contraception	

*Includes cigarettes and smokeless tobacco.

Continued

Table 1-6 Anticipatory Guidance/Counseling for Patients Aged 19 Years and Older—cont'd

TOPIC	19–39 yr	40–64 yr	>65 yr
Injury prevention	Safety belts	Safety belts	Prevention of falls
	Safety helmets	Safety helmets	Safety belts
	Violent behavior (especially for young men)	Smoke detector	Smoke detector
	Firearms	Smoking near bedding or upholstery	Smoking near bedding or upholstery
	Smoke detector		Hot water heater temperature
	Smoking near bedding or upholstery		
Other	Prevention of childhood injuries (with children in home)	Prevention of childhood injuries (with children in home)	Prevention of childhood injuries (with children in home)
	Falls in elderly persons (with elderly in home)	Falls in elderly persons (with elderly in home)	Regular toothbrushing, flossing, dental visits
	Regular toothbrushing, flossing, dental visits	Regular toothbrushing, flossing, dental visits	Glaucoma testing by eye specialist
	Skin protection from ultraviolet light	Skin protection from ultraviolet light	Discuss HRT with women
		Discuss ASA therapy	Discuss ASA therapy
		Discuss HRT with women	Skin protection from ultraviolet light

NOTES

NOTES

2

Pediatric Assessment

The goals of pediatric assessment are to record and monitor overall growth and development from birth through late adolescence, identify problems with psychosocial maturity and problem solving, identify any genetic anomalies, and seek appropriate referral when necessary. Assessment varies with each visit depending on what stage of growth and development the infant/child is in. Focus should be on normal milestones plus any deviations or problems that the parent/caregiver has identified.

Pediatric assessment can be as difficult as geriatric assessment at times. The infant/toddler cannot tell you specifically what the problem is in words, and many times the caregiver cannot either. Your eyes and ears are sometimes the best tools for assessment. As the child matures the problems are easier to focus on; however, many times, outward behaviors indicate clues to the practitioner of the particular difficulty. Your assessment should always consist of normal patterns of development, and when illness is considered, identify deviations from normal patterns as the cause of illness.

Your approach to the pediatric assessment depends on the goal of the encounter: is this a well-child checkup or illness, and how severe is the illness at this time? During the encounters, the caregiver is the usual informant, and many times the informant has hidden agendas that reveal the real problem. Always try to establish rapport with both the caregiver and the child. Pediatric assessment relies a lot on trust between the caregiver, the pediatric patient, and the practitioner.

There are many tools developed for assessment of normal growth and development, behavioral characteristics, and cognitive and social development. Some examples are given in this chapter. Remember there are normal variations in all growth and development (Tables 2–1 and 2–2).

HEALTH HISTORY
Practice Pearls
- Document the patient's name, age, birth date, sex, and ethnic background
- Be aware of current living arrangements/situation (e.g., lives with parent[s] or foster care)
- Observe caregiver and patient's relationship
- A quiet room with some minor distractions (e.g., coloring books, reading books, handheld toys/games) is helpful
- Always allow the toddler/child some personal space during the interview; this will facilitate trust with the examiner

| Table 2–1 | Tanner's Sexual Maturity Rating |

Pubic Hair
1. Sparse, slightly darker hairs along labia and at base of penis
2. Hair darker, coarser, curlier; spreading over entire pubis
3. Hair thick and dark like adult; covers pubis but not on thighs
4. Adult type and quantity; also on medial thighs

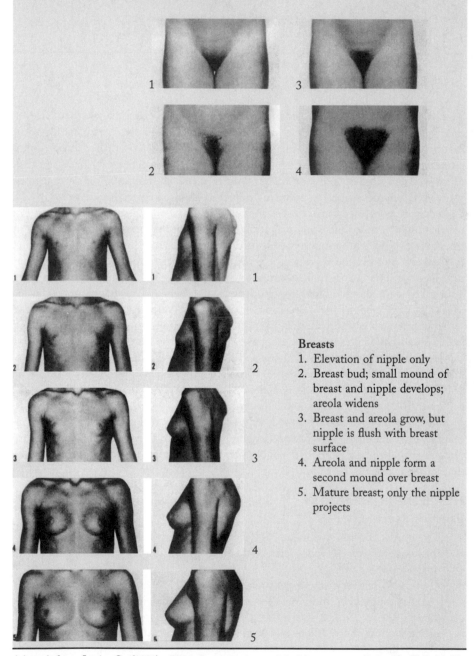

Breasts
1. Elevation of nipple only
2. Breast bud; small mound of breast and nipple develops; areola widens
3. Breast and areola grow, but nipple is flush with breast surface
4. Areola and nipple form a second mound over breast
5. Mature breast; only the nipple projects

Adapted from Jarvis, C. (2002). *Physical examination and health assessment* (3rd ed.). Philadelphia: W.B. Saunders.

Table 2–1   Tanner's Sexual Maturity Rating—cont'd

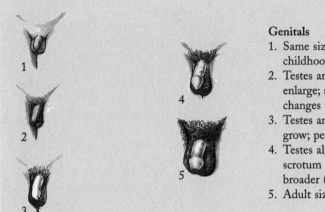

Genitals
1. Same size and proportion as early childhood
2. Testes and scrotum begin to enlarge; scrotum reddens and changes texture
3. Testes and scrotum continue to grow; penis longer
4. Testes almost fully grown; scrotum darker; penis larger and broader (glans develops)
5. Adult size and shape

Adapted from Tanner, J. M. (1962) *Growth at adolescence*. Oxford, England: Blackwell Publishing Ltd.

Table 2–2   Stages of Growth and Development

AGE	NORMAL GROWTH RATE	SPECIAL CONSIDERATIONS
Birth–12 mo	9–11 in. (22–27 cm)/yr Birth weight doubles by 6 mo; triples by 12 mo; quadruples by 24 mo Average weight gain is 4.4–6 lb (2–2.75 kg)/yr until puberty	Rapid, highly variable rate of growth, "catch-up" and "catch-down" growth Refer if the height or weight falls more than two standard deviations on growth chart Nutritional factors Psychosocial adjustment (e.g., inorganic failure to thrive) Infants should be weighed and measured at least twice a year and more often if a growth problem is suspected
12–36 mo	3–5 in. (7.5–13 cm)/yr 2 yr–adolescence ~5-lb (2.3-kg) weight gain per year	Growth rate declines from neonatal period Between 18 and 24 mo the growth "channel" (percentile on the growth chart) is established Patterns and velocity established by 36 mo Weight and measurements at least once a year

Continued

Table 2–2 Stages of Growth and Development—cont'd

AGE	NORMAL GROWTH RATE	SPECIAL CONSIDERATIONS
3 yr–puberty	2–2.5 in (5–6.5 cm)/yr	Linear growth stabilizes Changes in growth velocity signal potential growth or health disorder Weight and measurements at least once a year
Adolescence	Growth rate is rapid and highly variable Onset of pubertal growth spurt: average age in girls is 10 yr; average age in boys is 12.5 yr ~10-lb (4.5-kg) weight gain per year	Refer precocious puberty (before 9 yr) Menarche occurs ~2 yr after breast buds appear Girl must weigh 88–90 lb (29.5–40.5 kg) before menarche will occur Once puberty begins, growth plates begin to close Refer if puberty is delayed beyond 13 yr for girls or 15 yr for boys

- Allow the infant/toddler/child to sit with the caregiver during the interview and as much as possible during the initial exam
- Initially, when you first touch the child, always touch nonthreatening body parts first, such as head/hair, legs, feet
- Always assume a very calm and matter-of-fact attitude; kids know when you are uncomfortable or nervous
- Try to compliment the toddler/child/adolescent on something, whether it is clothing, hair, or toy
- Use puppets or stuffed animals to distract toddlers/children while examining them and allow them to hold objects during exam if needed

COMPLETE HEALTH HISTORY*

Chief complaint
- Try to elicit the child's and caregiver's perspectives of the problem
- Caregiver may have other reasons for seeking health care

History of present illness
- Prodromal symptoms
- Associated symptoms
- Situational factors
- Developmental factors
- Change in appetite, sleep patterns, activity

*Only additions/differences to a normal health history are listed here.

- If the child is in preschool or school, ask if there have been missed days at school and if there are other students in same class with similar problems

Past medical history
- Prenatal history (especially mother's use of drugs, tobacco, or alcohol)
- Birth and neonatal history, including any difficulty with delivery; Apgar score (if known); preterm birth; intensive care stay and why; any hearing screening performed at birth; first hepatitis B immunization
- Any delays in growth and development, social, personal, language milestones since birth
- At what age was the toddler/child toilet trained; if toilet trained, does the toddler/child have accidents and when
- Nutritional status (bottle/breast-fed, number of feedings per day and amount, does infant seem satisfied after eating); type of foods offered; amount of whole milk, if provided; weight gain
- Pica habits
- Sleep habits
- Type of discipline and any problems identified at home, at school, in social settings
- School progress
- Immunization history and any problems with immunizations; obtain written immunization record
- Illnesses, hospitalizations, and surgeries
- Allergies to food, medication, or seasonal pollens

Personal and social history
- Home environment (exposure to smoke, alcohol, drugs, or unsafe practices)
- Use of any medications—over-the-counter, prescribed, or illicit; does child like to take medications, and is this a risk at home; vitamins/fluoride intake
- Leisure activities and amount of time spent watching television or playing computer or video games
- Habits such as nail biting, temper tantrums, hair pulling/twisting

Family history and dynamics
- Composition of family
- Congenital abnormalities in family
- Interaction between patient and caregiver, patient interaction with siblings and playmates, patient interaction with authority figures
- Parental satisfaction with patient's behavior
- Is child in daycare or school

Review of systems
- Try to obtain the caregiver's and the patient's perspectives of each component of the review of systems; do they perceive any problems and what are they
- Dentition and progression with dentition (Figure 2–1)
- Sexual maturity (see Tanner's staging, Table 2–1)
- Attention span and perceived hyperactivity

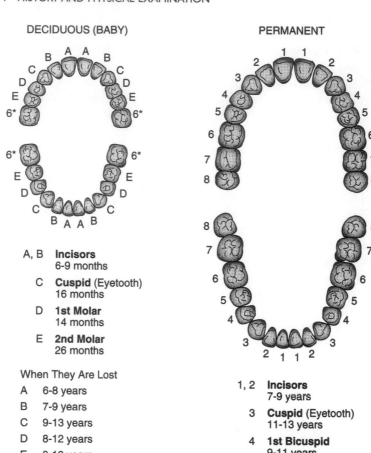

DECIDUOUS (BABY)   PERMANENT

A, B   **Incisors**
       6-9 months

C   **Cuspid** (Eyetooth)
       16 months

D   **1st Molar**
       14 months

E   **2nd Molar**
       26 months

When They Are Lost

A   6-8 years
B   7-9 years
C   9-13 years
D   8-12 years
E   8-12 years

Expected number of teeth up to 24 months = age of child in months −4 (e.g., 18 month-old should have 14 teeth)

* The 6th year Molar is a PERMANENT TOOTH.
  It is not shed, nor does it replace a baby tooth.
  It is there for a lifetime!

1, 2   **Incisors**
       7-9 years

3   **Cuspid** (Eyetooth)
       11-13 years

4   **1st Bicuspid**
       9-11 years

5   **2nd Bicuspid**
       10-12 years

6   **6th Year Molar***
       1st permanent tooth

7   **2nd Molar**
       12-14 years

8   **3rd Molar** (Wisdom)
       16-20 years

FIGURE 2–I Dental chart.

COMPREHENSIVE PEDIATRIC ASSESSMENT

The overall physical examination for pediatrics is the same as that for adults, but there are some variations specific to pediatrics that are focused on in the following list. The practitioner may have to change the order of the exam and may not be able to perform the entire exam in one visit, but the end product should be similar to that of an adult encounter. Note that any discrepancies between history and physical findings may alert the examiner to the possibility of neglect/abuse and should be further investigated.

Practice Pearls
- During the "warming up" period and interview, assess the child's behavioral patterns and interaction with the caregiver and surroundings
- Assess overall health status, general symmetry of movement, speech patterns, and nutritional status
- Note child's attention to sounds and sights and overall curiosity to environment
- Observe the child for unusual characteristics that might indicate genetic abnormalities
- Examine affected areas last and focus on the normal healthy body parts
- Perform traumatic procedures last (EENT, genitalia)
- Plot height, weight, and head circumference (when appropriate) on standardized chart for each visit or more often if abnormality is noted; measure head circumference above eyebrows, above pinnae, and over occipital prominence; use same chart with each encounter so you can see progress or delay; discuss chart with caregiver at each visit
- Always obtain vital signs, TPR (BP >3 years), with each visit; monitor for deviation from normal; these can be plotted on standardized charts

Vital Signs: Approximate Normal Findings

AGE	RR	HR	BP
0–2 mo	30–50	80–170	70/50
2–6 mo	20–30	80–150	91/50–53
6–11 mo	20–30	80–150	90/47 + age in mo
1–5 yr	20–30	70–120	90 + age in yr/56
6–18 yr	10–30	60–110	83 + (2 × age in yr)/52 + age in yr

BP, Blood pressure; *HR,* heart rate; *RR,* respiratory rate.

PHYSICAL EXAMINATION

	CLINICAL OBSERVATIONS	NOT TO BE MISSED
Integumentary System	Variations in color	Cyanosis
		Jaundice
	Characteristic rashes of possible	Viral rash
	communicable diseases	Impetigo
	Ecchymosis, petechiae	Abuse
	Lesions suggesting abuse	
	Birthmarks, color changes with	Café au lait spots
	position	Mongolian spots
		Port-wine stains, stork
		bite marks
	Skin turgor and eczemic changes	Milia, dermatitis
		Dehydration
	Palmar creases and hair whorls	Congenital deformity
HEENT	Observe overall symmetry of head	Birth trauma to head
(Nares and throat	and placement of facial parts	Low-set ears, which
covered under	especially ears	can be connected
respiratory		with renal disease
section)	Palpate fontanelles (posterior closes	Craniofacial
	by 8 wk, anterior closes by 18 mo)	malformations
		Dehydration or
		increased ICP
	Dentition and general appearance of	Dental malocclusions
	teeth (see Fig. 2–1)	Gingival disease
	Note abnormal appearance of pupils,	Nystagmus, infection,
	presence of red reflex, tearing,	strabismus, loss of
	redness of sclera, strabismus	red reflex,
		retinoblastoma,
		cataracts
	Perform cover-uncover test, test	Blindness
	EOMs, funduscopic exam	
	when indicated	
	Palpate lymph nodes (small,	Hodgkin's disease
	nontender and mobile are normal	
	and called "shotty")	
	Assess vision or ability to see and	
	grasp objects without difficulty;	
	visual acuity at birth: 20/200;	
	visual acuity at 6 mo: 20/100;	
	visual acuity at 1 yr: 20/50;	
	visual acuity at 18 mo: 20/20	

	CLINICAL OBSERVATIONS	NOT TO BE MISSED
HEENT—cont'd	Testing charts are available to use for young patients such as Allen picture cards, "E" chart, Sheridan-Gardiner geometric designs, and Snellen charts	
	Hearing should be assessed at birth either with auditory brain stem testing or with startle reflex response	Deafness Laryngeal disease, hoarseness, poor phonation, inability to verbalize by 18 mo
	Refer school-age child without physical reason for failure to hear any frequency >25 dB on audiometer	
	Language skills correspond to hearing abilities: infants localize sounds by 6–8 mo; know several words by 12 mo; can articulate short sentences by 2 yr	
	Speech sound development: 3 yr (p, m, h, n) 4 yr (k, g, d, f, y) 5–6 yr (t, ng, r, l) 7–8 yr (s, ch, sh, z, j, v, zh)	
Respiratory System	Infants are obligatory nasal breathers until about age 6 mo; nares may swell because of allergies in the home or enlarged adenoids; ask about snoring and unilateral nasal discharge	Nasal obstructions or foreign objects
	Nasal sounds can be heard throughout the lung fields in infants, but usually better in the upper lobes because of the size of the infant and the proximity of the bronchial tree	
	Children have smaller airways and poor cartilage development until adolescence	
	Sinus cavities are present at birth but are very small and function poorly; child may have unusual symptoms if sinus infection is present	Sinusitis

Continued

	CLINICAL OBSERVATIONS	NOT TO BE MISSED
Respiratory System —cont'd	Epiglottis is longer and flatter, more prone to viral infections	Epiglottitis, pharyngitis
	Alveoli increase tenfold by 3 yr of age	Bronchiolitis, pneumonia, asthma
	Lungs are not mature until about 8 yr	Pneumothorax that usually occurs in the right apex
	Question caregiver about history of skin allergies, atopy, hay fever	
	Observe for specific S/S of inherited respiratory diseases such as asthma or cystic fibrosis	Cystic fibrosis Pulmonary fibrosis
	Was an apnea monitor ever used and why	
	Was infant hypoxic at birth and how long was oxygen used	Vision disturbances Cataracts Blindness
Cardiac System	Assess for congenital heart defects	Congenital heart defects (ASD, VSD, etc.)
	Differentiate between innocent (functional) heart murmurs and pathologic murmur; *any undiagnosed murmur should be evaluated by echocardiogram and possibly referred to cardiologist* (see Table 6–1)	Pathologic murmurs
	S_3 is normal in some children	
	PMI is best observed in children <7 yr at fourth intercostal space; in children >7 yr best observed at fifth intercostal space; if PMI is felt lower, may indicate cardiac enlargement; if bounding may indicate anemia, fever, or fear	CHF Anemia Fever Cardiomegaly
	Sternal nodules may signal vitamin D deficiency (rickets)	Rickets
	Observe child's activity level and response to exercise; observe for any posturing after exercise and the color of the skin at rest and with activity	
	Peripheral pulses should be palpable and equal on both sides of the body (see Fig. 1–6)	Coarctation of the aorta (delayed or absent femoral pulses)

	CLINICAL OBSERVATIONS	NOT TO BE MISSED
Abdominal System	Assess for peristaltic waves, hernias, abnormal masses, organomegaly	Pyloric stenosis Incarcerated hernia Wilms' tumor Dysplastic kidney Neuroblastoma
	Abdomen is usually prominent in infants and children while standing and is flat when lying down	
	In infants and children, liver may be felt 1–3 cm below rib edges, but in older children liver should not be felt below rib edges	
	Observe umbilicus for drainage, inversion, eversion, hernia	Umbilical hernia Infection or fissure in umbilicus
Genitourinary System	Take a "matter-of-fact" approach to exam	Extreme uncomfortableness with exam may alert examiner to possibility of abuse
	Examine a boy with him in a "tailor-sit" position to avoid testicular retraction (cremasteric reflex); observe for placement of testicles, urethral position and penis size and shape, circumcision	Undescended testicles Hypospadias Testicular torsion or any severe scrotal pain should be referred immediately to either ED or urologist
	Examine a girl while she is in the "hands and knees" position for imperforate hymen or adhesions of labia (see Table 15–4 for treatment)	Hematuria UTI (refer boys for first-time UTI; girls for second-time UTI) Nephrotic syndrome
	Assess rectal sphincter tone; note any masses, fissures, or bleeding	
	Assess sexual maturity using Tanner's staging (see Table 2–1)	XY genetic abnormality

Continued

	CLINICAL OBSERVATIONS	NOT TO BE MISSED
Musculoskeletal System	Note any opisthotonoid curvatures and asymmetric body movements Perform Barlow-Ortolani test to detect hip dislocation, observe buttock creases for asymmetry	Delayed growth and development Congenital musculoskeletal abnormality Congenital hip dysplasia Cerebral palsy
	Observe shape, contour, tone and strength of muscles; there should be equal movements bilaterally Test joint flexibility and ROM Assess spine for scoliosis (see p. 426) Child may appear to be "flat footed" until about age 3 yr, when the fat pad starts to resolve	
	Observe child while walking and running for coordination and how the feet move; observe for foot flapping and toe walking Genu varum (bowed leg) is normal until about 18 mo of age Genu valgum (knock-kneed) appearance is common between 2 and 4 yr Ascertain from caregiver any gradual degeneration of previously mastered mobility skills	Shortening of the Achilles tendon Clubfoot
	Evaluate any hip or knee pain that causes limited or painful ROM and/or limping	Legg-Calvé-Perthes disease Osteomyelitis Osgood-Schlatter disease
Neurologic System	Assessment begins when the child enters the room with observations related to mobility, facial expressions, and overall symmetry of limbs and any gait disturbances, balance, coordination, and neuromuscular development	

	CLINICAL OBSERVATIONS	NOT TO BE MISSED
Neurologic System —cont'd	Monitor HC at each visit until age 2 yr, unless abnormal	Hydrocephaly, macrocephaly, microcephaly
	Assess cranial nerve function	
	Developmental assessment tools include Denver Developmental Screening Tool, Denver Articulation Screening Exam, Dubowitz scale and various other scales for determining cognition and response to stimuli	Benign intracranial hypertension Increased intracranial pressure due to trauma or increased fluid around brain Seizure disorders
	Observe infant developmental reflexes for presence or absence:	

REFLEX	DISAPPEARS BY
Sucking	Toddler age
Palmar grasp	3 mo
Rooting	4 mo (except during sleep)
Tonic neck	6 mo
Moro	6 mo
Plantar grasp	8–10 mo
Stepping	Varies
Babinski's	12–18 mo

	Assess cerebellar function by watching infant or child at play; watching a toddler/child walk or run determines the toddler's/child's cerebellar function, motor strength, peripheral nerve function and identifies any abnormalities of tone	
	Observe for cutaneous abnormalities, dimples, vascular malformations, and tufts of hair over the lower back	Neural tube abnormality
	Assess limb length for asymmetry	

Feeding schedule (Table 2–3)

Table 2–3 Feeding Schedule: Birth to 18 Months

AGE (MO)	FEEDINGS PER DAY	OUNCES (ml) PER FEEDING	CEREAL	VEGETABLES	FRUITS
Birth–1	6–8	2–4 (60–120)			
2–3	4–5	5–7 (150–210)			
4–5	4–5	5–7 (150–210)	Rice (if breast-feeding, cereal with iron)		
5–6	4–5	5–7 (150–210)	Rice	Any type (strained)	
6–7	3–4	8 (240)	Rice	Any type cooked or canned	Any type cooked or canned, including juice
7–8	3–4	8 (240)	Rice	Vary types	Vary types
8–10	3–4	8 (240)	Whole grains	Vary types	Vary types
10–12	3	8 (240) Intake from formula should be <28–32 oz (840–960 ml) qd	Any type cereal	Vary types, usually table food	Vary types, usually table food; good snack food
12–18	3	8 (240) Intake from milk should not exceed that of food: 24–30 oz (720–900 ml) qd	Any type cereal; usually want commercial brands	Vary; can try some raw	Vary; can try some raw fruits

MEATS	WHOLE MILK	ATTEMPTS TO FEED SELF	TABLE FOOD	INTRODUCE CUP
			Mashed or soft	Start sippy cup
			Mashed or soft Teething biscuits	Continue cup
Mashed, processed			Mashed or soft	Continue cup
Mashed; start soft finger foods	Introduce cheeses and egg products	Initial attempts at feeding self	Usually eating same foods as family and with family	Gaining proficiency with cup; decreasing need for bottle
Chopped but soft; do not use small pieces that can cause choking	Slowly begin whole milk, good snack food	Continues to improve; begins to be more aggressive	Usually eating same foods as family and with family	Gaining proficiency with cup; may only want bottle at bedtime
Chopped but soft; beware of choking potential	Switch from formula to whole milk; do not worry about fat content; do not let milk be the sole food	Wants to feed self	Usually eating same foods	Has gained more proficiency; may not want bottle now

Practice Pearls

- Introduce new foods one at a time; wait 1 week before introducing another food; if an allergic reaction occurs, it is then easier to identify which food caused it
- Beware of too many orange-colored foods in the initial feeding period because this can discolor the skin orange; this does not affect the color of the sclera, however
- Start with vegetables instead of fruits; fruits are sweeter than vegetables, and the infant may refuse the vegetables; start with vegetables that have less acid content
- Fruit juices should be mixed with water (half and half) for the first few months after they are introduced
- Fluoride usually is started after the infant is at least 6 months of age and continued until school age; many rural communities do not supplement water supply with fluoride
- Do not give infants younger than 12 months honey or corn syrup because infants do not possess the enzyme to breakdown *Clostridium botulinum*
- Encourage parents to use the food pyramid to achieve a balanced diet; always supervise infants and small children while they are eating to prevent choking
- Avoid extreme dietary practices; avoid the more allergenic foods, such as citrus, egg whites, chocolate, wheat, nuts, fish, and berries until the child is older than 12 months
- Suspect anemia if the diet of a toddler (primarily between 18 and 24 months) is largely whole milk with scant solid food; obtain CBC by 2-year checkup; babies are born with 6 to 9 months of iron reserves, but low birth weight or prematurity may speed up loss of iron reserves; all infant diets should contain iron-fortified foods and formulas by 6 months of age
- Let the babies put their fingers in their mouth while eating; this helps the baby learn to swallow foods by the same sucking methods they use with the breast or bottle
- Infants receiving formula do not need extra meat or protein; if baby is eating a variety of foods, change to whole milk at 12 months; do not switch from formula to whole milk if child is not eating a good variety of table foods
- Colic can be very difficult to treat and very hard on parents
  - □ Carefully palpate all extremities and abdomen, check anal ring for fissures or stenosis
  - □ Treatment options start with education of parents about normal crying
  - □ Switch to lactose-free formula, low sugar, and low iron
  - □ Avoid fruit juices until 6 months of age
  - □ Start soothing measures such as rocking, gentle vibration, car rides, pacifiers, swaddling in warm blanket

▫ Simethicone (Mylicon) drops 40 mg/0.6 ml for colic:
  Younger than 2 years: give 0.3 ml qid (after meals and at bedtime)

  Older than 2 years: give 0.6 ml qid (after meals and at bedtime)

Constipation in infants is usually due to lack of water in diet; have parents increase water intake with formula or with breast-feeding
- As child gets older and can chew, try sugar-free Gummy Bears (sorbitol is laxative); parents choose amounts
- Psyllium (Metamucil) or methylcellulose (Citrucel) can be mixed with fruit juice; may freeze on a wooden stick; give one frozen fruit bar a day
- Mix 2 tbsp applesauce + 1 tbsp chopped prunes + 1 tbsp psyllium (Metamucil), season with cinnamon, brown sugar, and nutmeg to taste; give 1 to 2 tbsp qd
- Docusate (Colace) liquid 10 mg/ml or syrup 20 mg/5 ml
  - ▫ 0 to 3 years: 10 to 40 mg qd
  - ▫ 3 to 6 years: 20 to 60 mg qd
  - ▫ 6 to 12 years: 40 to 120 mg qd

Breast-feeding guidelines
- Nurse when baby shows signs of hunger: crying, "hunger" sound to cry, increased alertness, increased activity, mouthing or rooting
- Nurse approximately 8 to 12 times in a 24-hour period; nursing time approximately 10 to 15 minutes with each breast or until baby is satisfied
- Breast-feeding can be sole diet until infant is 6 months old; then gradually add solid foods
- Babies usually do not need water or formula during the first 6 months of life if sole intake is breast milk
- A total of 12 months of breast-feeding is recommended

Failure to thrive (FTT)
- Infants and children who fail to gain weight, fall below the fifth percentile on the growth charts, or drop more than 2 standard deviations on the growth curve without obvious organic etiology are defined as having a nonorganic failure to thrive
- History should include any symptoms that might suggest organic illness; psychosocial evaluation and how this might affect the infant's/child's behavior; detailed feeding and dietary history, including amounts of formula/breast feedings and did infant/child appear satisfied
- Family history is necessary to determine if other family members have had FTT; include parents' height, weight, and any chronic illnesses present
- Involve family services or home visits to observe infant/child in home setting and the interaction between caregivers and infants/children
- Perform complete physical exam with attention to developmental milestones; abuse/neglect issues; chronic illness or genetic abnormalities
- Nutritional recovery includes intake of calories (should start with 150 kcal/kg/day and may need to be even higher); feeding should be on ad lib basis depending on the infant's/child's demands; during the recovery period intake may exceed 150% of daily requirements; during recovery period many infants/

children will develop fidgetiness or mild hyperactivity, sweatiness, hepatomegaly, widening of the sutures (growth of brain exceeds growth of skull if suture lines are still open)
- Follow-up should continue until growth and development have begun to normalize; involvement of the family, extended family, community, and governmental support programs will aid in accomplishing recovery
- One fourth to one half of children with FTT remain small and some have cognitive and behavioral problems
- Treatment should begin as soon as the problem is identified

Health Maintenance Guidelines

See Tables 2–4, 2–5, and 2–6

Alerts for Child Abuse and Neglect

- Many factors contribute to the issue of child abuse, which can be physical or emotional in nature
- Abuse is usually committed by family, caretakers, or other persons in the family setting
- Recognizing the factors that contribute to child abuse is of the utmost importance for the practitioner because this may be the child's first entry into the health care system
- Family characteristics contributing to abuse may include the following:
  □ Family patterns of violence
  □ Poverty or very low socioeconomic status
  □ Lack of parenting skills
  □ Lack of extended family support
  □ Single-parent status (with or without financial support from other parent)
  □ Poor coping skills
  □ Drug or alcohol abuse or overuse
- Community characteristics contributing to child abuse may include the following:
  □ Unwanted birth
  □ Hyperactive or demanding
  □ Mentally or physically disabled
- Types of abuse are varied from minor to major, with some leading to death:
  □ Neglect of basic needs or education, or abandonment by caregiver
  □ Emotional abuse involves detachment from child's needs; unrealistic expectations and angry outbursts over insignificant actions/issues
  □ Physical abuse of child results in obvious injuries such as lacerations, bruises, burns, fractures to bones; may result in death from shaking, suffocation, poisoning, or beating; if there are repeated visits to health care facility with questionable causes for injury or condition, suspect Munchausen syndrome by proxy

Table 2-4 Health Appraisal and Risk Factors and Anticipatory Guidance/Counseling: Newborn (NB)–18 Years

	NB–2wk	2mo	4mo	6mo	12mo	15mo	24mo	3–4yr	5–6yr	7–10yr	11–14yr	16yr	18yr
History	X	X	X	X	X	X	X	X	X	X	X	X	X
Height and weight	X	X	X	X	X	X	X	X	X	X	X	X	X
Head circumference	X	X	X	X	X	X	X						
Blood pressure												Every 2yr	
Vision screening	Based on history and observation							X	X	As needed, using age-appropriate materials			
Hearing screening	Based on history and observation							X	As needed, using pure-tone audiometry		X	X	X
Developmental/behavioral screening	X	X	X	X	X	X	X	X	X	X	X	X	X
Immunizations						See Table 2–5							
TB test					X		X		X—		As indicated		
Hematocrit/hemoglobin				X	X		X		X				
Urinalysis				X	X		X—	X—		X			
Lead screening*					X		X	X—					
Cholesterol								As indicated, if parent has value >240 mg/dl or family history of early CAD					
Dental referral								X	As determined by dentist				
Anticipatory guidance/counseling	With each visit, as indicated (see Table 2–6 for specifics)												

Leading causes of death

Birth–1yr	2–6yr	7–12yr	13–18yr
Perinatal conditions	Injuries (non-MVC)	MVC	MVC
Congenital anomalies	MVC	Injuries (non-MVC)	Homicide
Heart disease	Congenital anomalies	Congenital anomalies	Suicide
Injuries (non-MVC)	Homicide	Leukemia	Injuries (non-MVC)
Pneumonia/influenza	Heart disease	Homicide	Heart disease
		Heart disease	

*Assess risk using a lead questionnaire; if any answer is "yes," consider high risk and test more often.
CAD, Coronary artery disease; *MVC*, motor-vehicle-crashes; *TB*, tuberculosis; *X*, with each visit; *X—*, once in time space.

2

| Table 2-5 | Immunization Guidelines* |
| | |

AGE	IMMUNIZATIONS	COMMENTS
Birth	Hepatitis B vaccine	
1 mo	Hepatitis B vaccine	
2 mo†	DTaP, Hib (or HbCV), OPV/IPV	DTP and HbCV are available as a combined vaccine (tetramune)
4 mo†	DtaP, Hib (or HbCV), OPV/IPV	
6 mo†	DtaP, Hib (or HbCV), hepatitis B vaccine	Influenza vaccine yearly, starting at 6 mo
12 mo	Consider Varivax	Give if no history of chickenpox Varivax is a single injection given between 12 mo and 13 yr; after child is 13 yr old, give 2 injections 8 wk apart
15 mo	MMR, HbCV	If prior TB skin test is positive, MMR may increase TB symptoms, so wait until treatment is established
15–18 mo	DTP/DTaP, OPV/IPV	
4–6 yr	DTP/DTaP, OPV/IPV, MMR	Second MMR can also be given at 11–12 yr or before college admission depending on child's age; check with state health department for recommendations
11–12 yr	Hepatitis B vaccine series	Give if child not previously immunized
14–16 yr	Td	Repeat q10y throughout life

*If the child does not start the series at the recommended age, charts are available outlining sequencing and spacing.
†Pediarix is a DTaP, IPV, Hib, and hepatitis B vaccine and can be given at 2, 4, and 6 mo (instead of as indicated on this chart).
DTaP, Diphtheria-tetanus-acellular pertussis; *DTP,* diphtheria-tetanus-pertussis; *HbCV, Haemophilus influenzae* b conjugate vaccine; *Hib, Haemophilus influenzae* type B; *IPV,* inactivated poliomyelitis vaccine; *MMR,* measles-mumps-rubella; *OPV,* oral polio vaccine; *TB,* tuberculosis; *Td,* tetanus-diphtheria toxoid.

- □ Sexual assault may go undetected for long periods of time because of child's embarrassment over situation or lack of experience to know that the actions of the abuser are wrong
- History of present illness may alert the practitioner if:
  - □ The history is inconsistent with the illness or injury
  - □ Stories of illness or injury keep changing over time
  - □ Inappropriate emotional concern shown by caregiver
  - □ Delay in seeking medical care
- Most common signs of abuse are soft tissue injuries such as burns, bruising, or lacerations in identifiable shapes or patterns or bites with imprint of teeth
- Skeletal fractures in rib area, multiple fractures in various stages of healing, or femur fractures in nonambulating child should raise suspicions of abuse

Table 2-6 Anticipatory Guidance and Counseling: Newborn–18yr

TOPIC	BIRTH–18 mo	2–6yr	7–12yr	13–18yr
Nutrition and exercise	Breast-feeding Baby bottle tooth decay Nutrient intake (see Table 2-3)	Sweets and between meal snacks Iron-enriched foods (see Appendix B) Physical activity	Fat (especially saturated fat) and cholesterol Sweets and between meal snacks Selection of exercise and physical activity	Fat (especially saturated fat) and cholesterol Calcium (girls) Selection of exercise program
Injury prevention	Child safety seats Smoke detectors Hot water heater temperature Stairway gates, window guards, pool fence Storage of drugs and toxic chemicals Syrup of ipecac, poison control number	Safety belts Smoke detectors Hot water heater temperature Window guards, pool fence Bicycle safety helmets Storage of drugs, toxic chemicals, matches, firearms Syrup of ipecac, poison control number	Safety belts Smoke detectors Storage of firearms, drugs, toxic chemicals, matches Bicycle safety helmets	Safety belts Safety helmets Violent behavior (especially for boys) Firearms (especially for boys) Smoke detectors
Other	Effects of passive smoking	Skin protection from ultraviolet light Effects of passive smoking Toothbrushing and dental visit	Skin protection from ultraviolet light Regular toothbrushing	Regular toothbrushing and flossing, dental visits Skin protection from ultraviolet light
Substance use			Tobacco,* drugs: primary prevention	Tobacco*: cessation, primary prevention Alcohol, drugs: Cessation, primary prevention Driving, other activities while under the influence Treatment for abuse Sharing, using unsterilized needles and syringes
Sexual practices				Sexual development and behavior STDs: partner selection, condoms Unplanned pregnancy, contraception Pap smears

*Includes cigarettes and smokeless tobacco.
STDs, Sexually transmitted diseases.

- Urinary complaints and vaginal or rectal pain with or without itching in a young child may be a sign of sexual abuse; if this is suspected the child should be examined by a certified examiner to ensure adequate documentation
- If the practitioner is concerned for the welfare of the child, the authorities should be notified, and the child can be sent to the hospital for his/her protection

NOTES

NOTES

3

Geriatric Assessment

The goal of geriatric assessment is maintaining and enhancing the daily functioning of the elderly patient. If the nurse practitioner performed only a physical examination, the most critical and revealing parts of the assessment would be missed. With a comprehensive assessment the nurse practitioner reviews as many parameters of health as possible, including nutrition, gait and balance, toileting, ability to perform ADLs, and visual and auditory, social, and psychologic assessment, in addition to the physical examination and laboratory assessment.

Comprehensive assessment is important in caring for elderly patients. The normal changes of aging are often complicated by many different chronic and acute illnesses. The clinical presentation of a health problem may be confusing in an older patient because the symptoms often appear in an atypical fashion and may mimic many different illnesses.

Because there is limited time in the primary care setting, the assessment tools presented in this chapter can be conducted within a few minutes and have been documented in terms of their validity and reliability. By using the objective assessment tools, the nurse practitioner can identify functional status decline, which so often is slowly progressive. With early identification of the problem, early nursing intervention may ameliorate the condition or slow the progress.

Health History

Practice Pearls

- Use the patient's last name when addressing him or her
- Sit level with the patient during the interview
- Make sure that the patient is comfortable with starting the interview
- Make sure room is well lit; do not stand in front of strong light or window
- Get rid of as much background noise as possible
- Note reliability of the health history information

COMPLETE HEALTH HISTORY*

Chief complaint
- Complaints may be multiple
- Help patient identify which complaint is personally of greatest concern

---

*Only additions to a normal health history are listed here.

Patient profile
- Marital status and relationship with spouse
- Children (e.g., relationship and frequency of contact with them, their telephone numbers)
- Living arrangements
- Support systems (e.g., family, friends, community services)
- Recent losses, including pets
- Education, occupation, and retirement
- Adequacy of finances and health insurance
- Transportation, especially to health care facilities
- Typical day's activities

Present illness

Self-rated health (elderly patients often see themselves as healthier than practitioners do)

Past medical history
- Ask patient specifically about reported illnesses; do not accept a diagnosis
- Ask about past blood transfusions
- Medication history is extremely important (including pain medications, laxatives, OTC sleep aids, and cold or allergy medicines); it is often advantageous to have patients bring all of their current medications and prescriptions in their bottles to the visit

Health prevention practices (see Tables 1–5 and 1–6)

Nutrition
- Determine if diet is adequate and if patient is at risk for malnutrition
- Conditions associated with malnutrition include chronic alcoholism, chronic myocardial or pulmonary diseases, cognitive disorders, malabsorption syndromes, and polypharmacy

Sleep patterns
- What time does patient go to bed and get up?
- How often does he or she wake at night and for how long?
- Is the sleep restful?

Safety (see pp. 73–79)

Comprehensive Geriatric Assessment

Note: If there are discrepancies between the history answers and physical findings, consider hidden problems such as falls or abuse.

Additional Questions to Ask
- What changes have you noted in your skin's condition over the last few years?

Integumentary System

PHYSIOLOGIC CHANGES	CLINICAL CORRELATION	NOT-TO-BE-MISSED POINTS
Loss of elasticity	Wrinkles	Abnormal skin lesions (e.g., actinic keratosis, skin cancers)
Loss of elastin, collagen, subcutaneous fat	Paper-thin skin prone to breakdown and injury	Dehydration Hypothermia
Decreased sweat and oil glands	Dry skin and pruritus Difficulty in regulating body temperature, especially with changes in environmental temperatures	Pruritus secondary to renal or hepatic disease, hyperthyroidism, DM, drug allergy, iron deficiency anemia, parasitic infections Heat stroke
Increased vascular fragility	Senile purpura	Bruising or purpura secondary to falls or abuse
Slower epidermal growth rate	Slower wound healing	
Hair turns gray or white and feels thin and fine	Potential effect on self-esteem	
Hair distribution changes	"Male pattern" baldness Decreased axillary and public hair Women may develop bristly facial hair	Localized hair loss due to PVD Diffuse alopecia due to hypothyroidism, iron deficiency, hypoproteinemia
Nails grow more slowly and develop longitudinal ridges	Nails prone to splitting	

- Has there been any delayed wound healing?
- Have you had any skin itching or pain?
- Do you have a history of DM or PVD?

Practice Pearls

- Pulling a patient up in bed can damage the skin
- Elderly patients are at higher risk of ulcer formation because of decreased turgor and subcutaneous fat
- With skin changes, remember to ask about history of allergies or atopy, work history, and environmental exposure (including sun)
- The incidence of herpes zoster peaks in people 50 to 70 years old, and postherpetic neuralgia is near 40% in people over the age of 60 years

Sensory System

PHYSIOLOGIC CHANGES	CLINICAL CORRELATION	NOT-TO-BE-MISSED POINTS
Eye skin loses elasticity	Wrinkling and drooping May have ectropion or entropion	
Distorted depth perception	Incorrect assessment of height of curbs and steps	Falls due to other conditions (e.g., stroke or arrhythmia)
Changes in retina, choroid, and skin	Decreased visual acuity Visual fields narrow Slower light-to-dark adaptation (patient needs more light to see)	Macular degeneration DM
Increased intraocular pressures	Increased incidence of glaucoma	Glaucoma
Lens turns yellow and loses elasticity	Decreased visual acuity Color vision may be impaired (blue, green, violet)	Cataract
Decreased tear production	Dry or burning eyes	
Cilia in ear canal become coarse and stiff	May cause cerumen build-up	Impaired hearing due to cerumen impaction
Gradual sensorineural hearing loss, starting in the 50s	Harder to hear consonants and to localize sound Difficulty hearing whispered words or in a noisy background	Social isolation due to hearing loss Hearing loss due to Paget's disease, ototoxic medications, or vascular or mass lesions
Decreased number of olfactory nerve fibers	May have decreased sense of smell	Potential hazard if patient cannot detect harmful odors
Altered taste sensation		Zinc deficiency Medications that may affect taste DM neuropathy
Reduced tactile sensation	Decreased ability to sense pressure, pain, and temperature	Vascular diseases DM Neurologic disorder

Additional Questions to Ask

- Do you have any difficulty climbing steps or driving?
- When were you last tested for glaucoma? If you have glaucoma, how do you manage the eye drops?
- Do you have any problem with night vision?
- Do your eyes feel dry or burning? How do you manage this?

- Have you noticed a change in your hearing or taste?
- Have you noticed any burns, bruises, or cuts that you were not aware of?

Practice Pearls

- The degree of pain in elderly patients may not accurately reflect the seriousness of the underlying condition
- Blue or yellow nightlights are safer than white ones (less glare)

Respiratory System

PHYSIOLOGIC CHANGES	CLINICAL CORRELATION	NOT-TO-BE-MISSED POINTS
Rib cage less mobile	Commonly results in an increased AP diameter May obscure heart and lung sounds	Thorax changes due to COPD Decreased breath sounds due to effusion, atelectasis, pneumonia, COPD
Decreased lung tissue elasticity	Decreased vital capacity Increased residual volume	SOB or rales due to CHF or pneumonia Deconditioning
Cilia atrophy	Change in mucociliary movement	Pulmonary infection

Additional Questions to Ask

- Do you have any shortness of breath or fatigue with your normal activities?
- What is your usual level of physical activity?
- For those patients with COPD: How are you getting along each day? Has your weight changed?

Practice Pearls

- Elderly patients may not have respiratory signs and symptoms until late in the course of a disease (e.g., patients with pneumonia may have a decreased level of responsiveness, poor appetite, or evidence of falls)
- Using a stethoscope with a pediatric diaphragm may be helpful in patients with prominent ribs
- The most common respiratory complaint is dyspnea; the cause may be cardiac, respiratory, metabolic, mechanical, or hematologic
- Rales (or crackles) are the most common physical finding; the cause may be age-related fibrotic changes, infection, or cardiac or pulmonary disorders

Cardiovascular System

PHYSIOLOGIC CHANGES	CLINICAL CORRELATION	NOT-TO-BE-MISSED POINTS
"Physiologic changes" are so interrelated with lifestyle changes that it is difficult to determine which are truly physiologic changes.		
Atherosclerosis and arteriosclerosis	Increased incidence of HTN and CAD	HTN secondary to anemia or hyperthyroidism
	Pedal pulses may be difficult to palpate	Changes indicating PVD Aneurysms
Decreased compliance of left ventricle	S_4 may be audible	
Decreased sensitivity of baroreceptors	Valsalva maneuver may cause sudden drop in BP	Falls secondary to postural hypotension Volume depletion
ECG changes may include: Decreased precordial QRS voltage ST and T wave changes Prolonged PR and QT intervals (QRS remains normal) Ectopic (extra) heartbeats		ECG changes secondary to ischemia, injury or infarction (see p. 176)
Heart valves thicken	Increased incidence of murmurs, especially aortic stenosis and mitral regurgitation	Pathologic murmur (see Table 6–1)
Decreased number of pacemaker cells	Slower or irregular heartrate	Atrial fibrillation

Additional Questions to Ask

- Do you get dyspneic with activity? Is it increasing?
- Do you ever experience edema?
- Have you ever experienced dizziness or syncope?
- If you have CHF, how often do you use OTC antiinflammatory medicines such as ibuprofen (Motrin)?

Practice Pearls

- Systolic murmurs are common in the elderly and frequently indicate aortic stenosis
- Although an S_4 can be normal, an S_3 warrants looking for other signs of CHF
- Check BP while patient is lying, sitting, and standing to evaluate for orthostatic hypotension; wait 2 minutes between position changes to allow time for

baroreceptors to compensate; evaluate further if systolic BP drops 20 mm Hg (10 mm Hg in symptomatic patient)
- Chest pain is not always present with severe disease or even with an MI
- Edema may be caused by CHF, protein malnutrition, PVD, venous varicosities, or lymphatic obstruction

Gastrointestinal System

PHYSIOLOGIC CHANGES	CLINICAL CORRELATION	NOT-TO-BE-MISSED POINTS
Dental enamel thins and gums begin to recede	Tooth and gum decay Tooth loss may lead to malocclusion	Insufficient nutrition Periodontal disease Poorly fitting dentures
Decreased saliva production	Dry mouth Increased susceptibility to injury and infection	Dry mouth due to medications or systemic disease
Delayed esophageal emptying	Occasional discomfort if food stays in esophagus longer	Gastroesophageal reflux disease or hiatal hernia Barrett's esophagus Medication reaction or side effect Dysphagia due to esophageal stricture or tumor or CNS dysfunction
Decreased gastric acid secretion	May delay absorption of certain vitamins and minerals (e.g., iron, calcium, vitamin B_{12}) and medications	Pernicious anemia Gastric cancer
Decrease in liver size with concomitant decrease in production of albumin	May have significant effect on drug metabolism	Drug toxicity due to fewer albumin-binding sites results in more "free" drug (e.g., digoxin, warfarin)
Decreased muscle tone and atrophy of mucosa	May contribute to constipation, esophageal spasm, diverticulosis	Bowel changes due to tumors, dehydration, loss of defecation reflex

Additional Questions to Ask
- Have you lost any teeth?
- Can you chew all types of food? Do you have trouble with any foods?
- Are you able to care for your teeth or dentures?
- How do you obtain groceries and prepare your meals?
- Do you eat alone or share meals with others?
- What did you eat yesterday for meals and snacks?
- How often do your bowels move? Do you take anything for constipation?

Practice Pearls

- Abdominal pain in the elderly can be a vague symptom of a serious or life-threatening disease—do not take this lightly
- With abdominal pain, obtain an ECG to rule out an MI
- Abdominal pain associated with confusion and shoulder pain may be found with lower lobe pneumonia
- Because of diminished muscle mass, an elderly patient may not have a rigid abdomen with peritoneal irritation
- Elderly people are prone to an atonic bowel, which often leads to laxative abuse
- Elderly patients can also have anorexia or bulimia; for a poor appetite, try mirtazapine (Remeron) 7.5 to 15 mg a day or cyproheptadine hydrochloride (Periactin) 4 mg 2 to 3 times a day or doxepin hydrochloride (Sinequan) 25 to 50 mg a day

Musculoskeletal System

PHYSIOLOGIC CHANGES	CLINICAL CORRELATION	NOT-TO-BE-MISSED POINTS
Loss of muscle mass and muscle strength		Accelerated changes due to immobility Increased falls
Tendons shrink	Decreased ROM	Decreased ROM due to fractures, osteoporosis, inflammation, or contractures
Deterioration of joint cartilage	May lead to pain and limited movement	Pain due to fracture Bursitis "Frozen" joint
Decreased bone mass and osteoblastic activity	Osteoporosis Postural changes (e.g., kyphosis) Decrease in height	Fracture Gait and posture changes

Additional Questions to Ask

- Have you noticed any weakness in the past year?
- Have you noticed an increase in falls or stumbling?
- Do you use anything to help you get around (e.g., cane)?
- How often and for how long do you exercise? What type of activity?

Practice Pearls

- Inspect muscles for atrophy and bones for any deformities; muscle tone is evaluated by passive movement (increased tone: marked resistance or spasms; decreased tone: no or minimal resistance)
- ESR and alkaline phosphatase levels rise in the elderly

- Pain and stiffness are the most common musculoskeletal complaints in elderly people
- A change in gait may result from deconditioning or from a musculoskeletal or neurologic cause
- Muscle *weakness* is not a normal aging process; look for a cause (e.g., DM or thiamine deficiency due to alcohol abuse or hypokalemia); evaluate by having patient stand from sitting in a chair; if patient must use his or her arms, there is muscle weakness; falls may be an early sign of underlying illness

Neurologic System

PHYSIOLOGIC CHANGES	CLINICAL CORRELATION	NOT-TO-BE-MISSED POINTS
Loss of neurons and nerve fibers	Decreased Achilles tendon reflex	
Slower impulse conduction between neurons	Decreased reaction time and vibratory sensation	Falls or injuries (e.g., burns) Changes due to PVD, CNS disease, or neuropathies
	Decreased pain sensation	
Atrophy of brain	Loss of follow-through or memory loss	Subdural hematoma
Modest decline in short-term memory	Benign loss, usually involving more trivial events	Dementia Delirium Depression Medication related
Changes in sleep-wake cycle	More or less time sleeping May have nightmares	Sleep changes due to dementia, depression, medications

Additional Questions to Ask
- Have you noticed any dizziness? If so, does it seem associated with changes in position?
- Have you noticed any change in memory or mental functioning?
- Have you noticed any muscle weakness or tremors?
- Have you had any sudden vision change or brief blindness?

Practice Pearls
- Because there are few significant neurologic changes associated with aging, most neurologic decline is evidence of a disease process
- Mental (cognitive) status can be evaluated during the history and examination (Table 3–1); also, consider a brief screening tool for depression (see Table 3–2)
- Sensory testing is crucial in elderly patients. Test distal arms and legs bilaterally for both light touch and pain
- A gait evaluation is essential in most elderly patients (see Table 3–5)

- To increase memory potential, encourage patient to "use the brain" (e.g., crossword puzzles, games, or reading); Ginkgo biloba 90 to 120 mg bid or vitamin E 400 IU bid may help
- The most common peripheral neuropathies are caused by type 2 DM, alcohol abuse (thiamine deficiency), and vitamin B_{12} deficiency
- Tremors should be evaluated
- Dizziness may be caused by problems with the eyes or ears or with the cardiovascular, musculoskeletal, or neurologic systems

Genitourinary

PHYSIOLOGIC CHANGES	CLINICAL CORRELATION	NOT-TO-BE-MISSED POINTS
Males		
Decreased testosterone level	Slower and less intense sexual response	Impotence
Decrease in size and firmness of testicles	Less rugae in scrotal skin, and contents hang lower	
Decrease in scrotal muscle tone		
Prostatic hypertrophy	Urinary frequency	Prostate cancer UTI due to difficulty emptying the bladder
Females		
Decreased estrogen level	Vaginal dryness and fragility Narrowing of the vagina UTI symptoms without infection Cessation of menses	UTI Incontinence Palpable ovaries Postmenopausal bleeding
Decreased elasticity of pelvic ligaments		Cystocele (see p. 289) Uterine prolapse
Atrophy of breast tissue	Breasts become more pendulous	Breast cancer
Both Sexes		
Loss of glomeruli and reduced renal mass	Decreased kidney function; may need to modify medication doses	Creatinine clearance less than 90 ml/hr (see p. 297)
Reduced bladder muscle tone	Decreased bladder capacity may lead to increased nocturia or urge to urinate only when bladder is full	Nocturia due to BPH, renal insufficiency, CHF, or DM

Table 3-1 Short Portable Mental Status Questionnaire (SPMSQ)

1. What is the date today (month/day/year)?
2. What day of the week is it?
3. What is the name of this place?
4. What is your telephone number? (If no telephone, what is your street address?)
5. How old are you?
6. When were you born (month/day/year)?
7. Who is the current president of the United States?
8. Who was the president just before him?
9. What was your mother's maiden name?
10. Subtract 3 from 20 and keep subtracting 3 from each new number all the way down.

Scoring: 0–2 errors = intact
        3–4 errors = mild intellectual impairment
        5–7 errors = moderate intellectual impairment
        8–10 errors = severe intellectual impairment

Allow one more error if subject had no grade school education.
Allow one fewer error if subject has education beyond high school.

Reprinted with the permission of Blackwell Publishing Ltd., A short portable mental status questionnaire for the assessment of organic brain deficit in elderly patients, by E. Pfeiffer, *Journal of the American Geriatrics Society.* 1975, 23(10), 433–441.

- For insomnia, try mirtazapine (Remeron) 7.5 mg or trazodone (Desyrel) 25 mg at hs

Additional Questions to Ask

Males
- Do you have difficulty urinating: hesitancy, weaker force of stream, or dribbling?
- How many times at night do you get up to urinate?

Females
- Have you noticed any bleeding since menopause?
- Do you have any vaginal itching, burning, or dryness or pain with intercourse?
- Do you feel any pressure in the genital area or loss of urine when coughing, laughing, or sneezing?

Practice Pearls

- With nocturia, ask when diuretics are taken and what the fluid intake is before bedtime
- With impotence, look for a cause; it may be psychologic, physiologic, or pharmacologic
- With decreased renal function and use of ACE inhibitors, do not use NSAIDs

Endocrine/Immune Systems

PHYSIOLOGIC CHANGES	CLINICAL CORRELATION	NOT-TO-BE-MISSED POINTS
Decreased hormone secretion and diminished tissue sensitivity to hormones	Stresses, such as surgery or trauma, may increase mortality	
Fibrosis of thyroid gland	Hypothyroidism signs and symptoms	Myxedema
Decreased basal metabolic rate	Increased incidence of obesity and altered carbohydrate tolerance	DM
Defects in temperature regulation	Reduced sweating / Fever not always present with infection	Infection
Decreased number of T cells and T cell function	Delayed hypersensitivity reactions	Reactivation of latent infectious diseases
	Increased incidence of infections	Autoimmune disorders
	Increased prevalence of autoimmune disorders	
Increased IgA and decreased IgG levels	Increased prevalence of infection	
Decreased activity in the renin-angiotensin-aldosterone system		Hyperkalemia

Practice Pearls

- Atypical presenting symptoms of DM in elderly persons include altered mentation, behavior changes, sleep disturbances, incontinence, weight loss, anorexia, and falls
- Earlier warning signs of DM include shin spots and recurrent skin infections
- Any changes in eye appearance or heart rate warrant evaluation for a thyroid problem
- The usual symptoms of infection (e.g., fever, chills, leukocytosis, and tachycardia) may be blunted or absent in the elderly
- The most common atypical signs and symptoms of infection include failure to thrive and changes in mental status, activity, appetite, or weight
- Pneumonia and influenza are the most common causes of death
- Overlooked sites of infection include the lining of the heart, the teeth, feet, and GI tract
- Encourage a yearly influenza vaccine; the pneumococcal vaccine (23-valent) should be given once to patients older than 50 years and repeated once after 5 years in immunocompromised patients

Assessing Cognitive and Emotional Status

Can create anxiety for the patient
- Develop rapport with the patient before beginning an assessment
- Provide a quiet, private environment
- Ensure the patient has the necessary aids (e.g., glasses or a hearing aid)
- Interspersing the assessment questions throughout the interview or examination can reduce stress

Assessment tools
- Short Portable Mental Status Questionnaire (SPMSQ) (see Table 3–1)
  - Test detects intellectual impairment in the elderly
  - Score can be adjusted to reflect education
- Mini-Mental State Examination (MMSE)
  - It is the most commonly used test of cognitive status
  - This standardized set of 10 questions specifically tests attention, memory, language, and spatial ability

Assessing Depression

Provide privacy and build rapport before conducting an assessment
Geriatric Depression Scale (GDS) (Table 3–2)

Table 3–2 Yesavage Geriatric Depression Scale (GDS): Short Form	
1. Are you basically satisfied with your life?	Yes/NO
2. Have you dropped many of your activities and interests?	YES/No
3. Do you feel that your life is empty?	YES/No
4. Do you often get bored?	YES/No
5. Are you in good spirits most of the time?	Yes/NO
6. Are you afraid that something bad is going to happen to you?	YES/No
7. Do you feel happy most of the time?	Yes/NO
8. Do you often feel helpless?	YES/No
9. Do you prefer to stay at home rather than going out and doing new things?	YES/No
10. Do you feel you have more problems with memory than most?	YES/No
11. Do you think it is wonderful to be alive now?	Yes/NO
12. Do you feel pretty worthless the way you are now?	YES/No
13. Do you feel full of energy?	Yes/NO
14. Do you feel that your situation is hopeless?	YES/No
15. Do you think that most people are better off than you are?	YES/No

Score 1 for answer in capitals.
   0–5: not depressed
   6–15: depressed

- Completed by the patient directly or by interviewing the patient
- Short form with 15 questions; can be completed in 5 to 7 minutes

Functional Assessment

Functional ability must be the focus when providing care to the elderly

Physical examination and identification of disease(s) do not sufficiently define the functional ability of the patient

Using structured assessment tools identifies problems and monitors patients over time

Assessment tools
- Index of Independence in Activities of Daily Living (Table 3–3)
  - Valid measure of ADLs
  - Completed by interviewer in approximately 3 to 4 minutes
  - Helps to identify the ADLs with which the patient needs assistance (e.g., through rehabilitative therapy, adaptive devices, or personal care assistance)
- Instrumental Activities of Daily Living Scale (Table 3–4)
  - Assesses more complex activities (e.g., shopping, laundry, food preparation, and managing finances)
  - There are 9 possible points for men and 17 possible points for women; the score difference reflects the difficulty in measuring the competence of tasks that are influenced by early life experiences (e.g., women are more likely to have more experience with housekeeping tasks)

Table 3–3 Activities of Daily Living Index Evaluation Form

Name _____ Date _____

For each area of functioning listed below, check the description that applies. (The word "assistance" means supervision, direction, or personal assistance.)

Bathing: Sponge bath, tub bath, or shower.

❏ Receives no assistance (gets into and out of tub by self if tub is the usual means of bathing).	❏ Receives assistance in bathing only one part of the body (such as the back or a leg).	○ Receives assistance in bathing more than one part of the body (or not bathed).

Dressing: Gets clothes from closets and drawers, including underclothes and outer garments, and uses fasteners, including suspenders if worn.

❏ Gets clothes and gets completely dressed without assistance.	❏ Gets clothes and gets dressed without assistance except for tying shoes.	○ Receives assistance in getting clothes or in getting dressed or stays partly or completely undressed.

From Katz, S., Ford, A., Moskowitz, R., et al. (1963). Studies of illness in the aged: The index of ADL—a Standardized Measure of Biological and Psychosocial Function. *JAMA 185*, 914–919. Copyright 1963 American Medical Association.

Table 3–3 Activities of Daily Living Index Evaluation Form—cont'd

Toileting: Goes to the room termed "toilet" for bowel movement/urination, cleans self afterward, and arranges clothes.

☐ Goes to the toilet room, cleans self, and arranges clothes without assistance. (May use object for support such as cane, walker, or wheelchair and may manage night bedpan or commode, emptying it in morning.)	○ Receives assistance in going to toilet room or in cleaning self or arranging clothes after elimination or in use of night bedpan or commode.	○ Does not go to toilet room for the elimination process.

Transfer

☐ Moves into and out of bed as well as into and out of chair without assistance. (May use objects such as cane or walker for support.)	○ Moves into or out of bed or chair with assistance.	○ Does not get out of bed.

Continence

☐ Controls urination and bowel movement completely by self.	○ Has occasional accidents.	○ Supervision helps keep control of urination or bowel movement, catheter is used, or is incontinent.

Feeding

☐ Feeds self without assistance.	☐ Feeds self except for assistance in cutting meat and buttering bread.	○ Receives assistance in feeding or is fed partly or completely through tubes or by IV fluids.

Index ☐ Indicates Independence   ○ Indicates Dependence

A: Independent in all six functions.

B: Independent in all but one of these functions.

C: Independent in all but bathing and one additional function.

D: Independent in all but bathing, dressing, and one additional function.

E: Independent in all but bathing, dressing, toileting and at least one additional function.

F: Independent in all but bathing, dressing, toileting, transferring, and one additional function.

G: Dependent in all six functions.

Other: Dependent in at least two functions but not classifiable as C, D, E, or F.

Table 3–4 Instrumental Activities of Daily Living Scale

	SCORING	
	MEN	WOMEN
A. Ability to use telephone		
1. Operates telephone on own initiative, looks up and dials numbers, etc.	1	1
2. Dials a few well-known numbers.	1	1
3. Answers telephone but does not dial.	1	1
4. Does not use telephone at all.	0	0
B. Shopping		
1. Takes care of all shopping needs.	1	1
2. Shops independently for small purchases.	0	0
3. Needs to be accompanied on any shopping trip.	0	0
4. Completely unable to shop.	0	0
C. Food preparation		
1. Plans, prepares, and serves adequate meals independently.		1
2. Prepares adequate meals if supplied with ingredients.		0
3. Heats and serves prepared meals or prepares meal but does not maintain adequate diet.		0
4. Needs to have meals prepared and served.		0
D. Housekeeping		
1. Maintains house alone or with occasional assistance (e.g., "heavy work—domestic help").		1
2. Performs light daily tasks such as dishwashing, bedmaking.		1
3. Performs light daily tasks but cannot maintain acceptable level of cleanliness.		1
4. Needs help with all home maintenance.		1
5. Does not participate in any housekeeping tasks.		0
E. Laundry		
1. Does personal laundry completely.		1
2. Launders small items, rinses socks, stockings, etc.		1
3. All laundry must be done by others.		0
F. Mode of transportation		
1. Travels independently on public transportation or drives own car.	1	1
2. Arranges own travel via taxi but does not otherwise use public transportation.	1	1
3. Travels on public transportation when assisted or accompanied by another.	0	1
4. Travel limited to taxi or automobile with assistance of another.	0	0
5. Does not travel at all.	0	0

From Lawton, M. P., & Brody, E. (1969). Assessment of older people: Self-maintaining and instrumental activities of daily living. *Gerontologist, 9,* 179.

Table 3–4 Instrumental Activities of Daily Living Scale—cont'd

	SCORING	
	MEN	WOMEN
G. Responsibility for medications		
1. Is responsible for taking medication in correct dosage at correct time.	1	1
2. Takes responsibility if medication is prepared in advance in separate dosages.	0	0
3. Is not capable of dispensing own medication.	0	
H. Ability to handle finances		
1. Manages financial matters independently (budget, writes checks, pays bills, goes to bank), collects and keeps track of income.	1	1
2. Manages day-to-day purchases but needs help with banking, major purchases, etc.	1	1
3. Incapable of handling money.	0	0

- Complete by interviewing the patient, family, or friends
- It is used to provide insight into areas with which an elderly patient needs assistance to continue to live in the community

Falls

Assessment
- Must include the evaluation for balance and gait problems
- Performed as part of an annual examination, as well as when there appears to be a change in the patient's health status
- May be critical to include a home visit to assess both the patient and the environment for prevention and safety

Assessment tools
- Tinetti Balance and Gait Evaluation (Table 3–5)
  - Assesses for musculoskeletal and neurologic disorders
  - Requires no equipment
  - Administered in the clinical setting by observing actual function
  - Activity-based test that asks the patient to perform tasks, such as sitting and rising from a chair, turning, and bending
- Timed "Up and Go" Test
  - It is a reliable, valid, and practical test of balance and gait speed
  - To perform, time the patient as he or she rises from a standard arm chair, walks 3 meters (10 feet), turns 180 degrees, returns to the chair, and sits down again
  - The score is the number of seconds taken to complete the test; a freely mobile person can complete it in less than 10 seconds
  - The score(s) can be monitored to note clinical changes over time

Table 3–5 Tinetti Balance and Gait Evaluation*

BALANCE

Instructions: Seat the subject in a hard armless chair. Test the following maneuvers. Select one number that best describes the subject's performance in each test and add up the scores at the end.

1. **Sitting balance**
   Leans or slides in chair: 0
   Steady, safe: 1
2. **Arising**
   Unstable without help: 0
   Able but uses arms to help: 1
   Able without use of arms: 2
3. **Attempt to arise**
   Unable without help: 0
   Able but requires more than one
      attempt: 1
   Able to arise with one attempt: 2
4. **Immediate standing balance (first
   5 seconds)**
   Unsteady (staggers, moves feet, marked
      trunk sway): 0
   Steady but uses walker or cane or grabs
      other objectsfor support: 1
   Steady without walker, cane, or other
      support: 2

5. **Standing balance**
   Unsteady: 0
   Steady but wide stance (medial heels
      more than 4 inches apart) or uses
      cane, walker, or other support: 1
   Narrow stance without support: 2
6. **Nudging (With subject's feet as close
   together as possible, push lightly on
   the sternum with palm of hand three
   times.)**
   Begins to fall: 0
   Staggers and grabs but catches self: 1
   Steady: 2
7. **Eyes closed (at same position as in
   No. 6)**
   Unsteady: 0
   Steady: 1
8. **Turning 360 degrees**
   Discontinuous steps: 0
   Continuous steps: 1
   Unsteady (grabs and staggers): 0
   Steady: 1
9. **Sitting down**
   Unsafe (misjudges distance, falls into
      chair): 0
   Uses arms or lacks smooth motion: 1
   Safe, smooth motion: 2

Reprinted with permission of Blackwell Publishing Ltd., Performance-oriented assessment of mobility problems in elderly patients, by ME Tinetti, *Journal of the American Geriatrics Society,* 1986, *34*(2), 119–126.
*Requires 5 to 15 minutes and an armless, unupholstered chair; walking space, such as a large room or hallway; and the patient's usual ambulatory aids. The maximum achievable score is 28 (balance, 16; gait, 12), and the lowest score is zero. Like other assessment tests this one can be administered occasionally to detect possible deterioration in a patient's condition.

Table 3–5 Tinetti Balance and Gait Evaluation—cont'd

GAIT

Instructions: The subject stands with the examiner and then walks down hallway or across room, first at the usual pace and then back at a rapid but safe pace, using a cane or a walker if accustomed to one.

10. **Initiation of gait (immediately after being told to go)**
    Any hesitancy or several attempts to start: 0
    No hesitancy: 1
11. **Step length and height**
    Right swing foot
       Fails to pass left stance foot with step: 0
       Passes left stance foot: 1
       Fails to clear floor completely with step: 0
       Completely clears floor: 1
    Left swing foot
       Fails to pass right stance foot with step: 0
       Passes right stance foot: 1
       Fails to clear floor completely with step: 0
       Completely clears floor: 1
12. **Step symmetry**
    Right and left step length unequal: 0
    Right and left step equal: 1

13. **Step continuity**
    Stopping or discontinuity between steps: 0
    Steps appear continuous: 1
14. **Path (Observe excursion of either left or right foot over about 10 feet of the course.)**
    Marked deviation: 0
    Mild to moderate deviation or uses walking aid: 1
    Walks straight without aid: 2
15. **Trunk**
    Marked sway or uses walking aid: 0
    No sway but flexion of knees or back or spreads arms out while walking: 1
    No sway, flexion, use of arms, or use of walking aid: 2
16. **Walking stance**
    Heels apart: 0
    Heels almost touch when walking: 1

Balance Score: _____/16
  Gait Score: _____/12
  Total Score: _____/28

NOTES

Unit II

Common Conditions

4

Skin Disorders

Disorders Causing Inflammation

CONDITION	DESCRIPTION	TREATMENT
Atopic dermatitis 691.8	Cases usually stem from familial disposition of eczema Lesions are diffuse erythematous papules to scaly plaques Lesions seem to be result of itch-scratch cycle May produce exudation with wet crusts and fissures; this increases risk of infections Patient usually has abnormally dry skin that itches more at night Distribution of lesions is common to face, antecubital and popliteal spaces, wrists, lateral legs; distribution of lesions is symmetric Patient may have acute exacerbations, with periods of remission Increased prevalence of atopic dermatitis flare-ups with known food allergies, smoke exposure, and perfumes and cosmetics	*General treatment* Increase ambient moisture Increase oral hydration Wear all-cotton clothing Decrease number of baths per week; use only tepid water and mild soap (Dial, Dove, Aveeno) Apply sunscreen to all exposed areas anytime person is outside Moisturizers should be used 3–4 times a day routinely Apply moisturizers onto skin immediately after bathing (Eucerin, Aquaphor, mineral or baby oil); can use after steroid application Vitamin E 400–800 IU daily Always be aware of flare ups or infections and start treatment quickly to keep symptoms under control *Drug therapy* First-line therapy: topical steroids (Table 4–1) High potency steroids should be used for short-term therapy for <7 days, then decrease to low-potency steroids until lesions are resolving, and then stop treatment (if possible) Mid-potency steroids can be used to control flare-ups for short term, then resume the use of low-potency topical steroids

Continued

83

Disorders Causing Inflammation—cont'd

CONDITION	DESCRIPTION	TREATMENT
		Second-line therapy: topical immunomodulators can be used for short-term, moderate-to-severe symptoms: Tacrolimus (Protopic) 0.03% for children older than 2yr; 0.1% for children older than 15yr; apply to lesions bid Pimecrolimus (Elidel) 0.1% for persons older than 2yr; apply bid to lesions; can be used in sensitive areas where steroids may cause harm Oral steroids, in "burst" therapy, or immunosuppressants can be used short term for severe, refractory cases; must monitor closely for side effects Oral antihistamines for sedative effect: Diphenhydramine (Benadryl) 12.5–50mg q6h po Hydroxyzine (Atarax) 10–100mg q6–8h po Cyproheptadine (Periactin) 2mg/5ml syrup or 4mg tab tid Drugs under investigation (not FDA approved): montelukast (Singulair) and zafirlukast (Accolate)
Contact dermatitis 692.9	Inflammation of epidermis and dermis caused by irritative agents or allergens Characteristics are itching, burning, redness, swelling with well-demarcated areas where irritant/allergen has touched skin; scaly, vesicular, or papular lesions appear in scattered, linear, or clustered groupings Lesions are pruritic with occasional lymphadenopathy Uncontrolled scratching can cause skin infections and scars Latex dermatitis affects health care providers and lay people	Remove irritant and cleanse skin thoroughly with soap and water Control itching with antihistamine (e.g., diphenhydramine, hydroxyzine, cyproheptadine) (see above for dosing) Topical treatment for relief of itching: Aluminum acetate (Domeboro) Oatmeal baths Calamine lotion/spray Vinegar in water 50:50 solution Aveeno baths Topical steroids, mid-potency applied 2–3 times a day (see Table 4–1) With more severe reactions may

Disorders Causing Inflammation—cont'd

CONDITION	DESCRIPTION	TREATMENT
	Latex is found in home products and medical facilities and there are some foods that cross-react with latex IgE (Table 4–2)	need to use oral prednisone in "burst" therapy, especially if reaction is involving face
Xerosis (dry skin) 706.8	Moderate-to-severe itching with dry, scaly skin that appears on extremities and "high use" skin areas (outer thighs, buttocks, mid-back, and extremities); usually spares face and scalp Occurs predominantly in winter Pruritus with no obvious rash	Increase ambient moisture with humidifier Bathing with tepid water and mild soap, oatmeal, vinegar, or Aveeno to relieve itch Lubricants (e.g., Vaseline, mineral oil, baby oil, or Crisco) 3–4 times daily and after bathing Ammonium lactate topical (Lac-Hydrin) bid and rub in thoroughly Lactic acid creams (Eucerin Plus, Lacticare 5%); apply 3–4 times a day Low- to mid-potency topical steroids (see Table 4–1)
Urticaria (hives) 708.9	Transient eruptions of papular lesions anywhere on body; can be any size; may last minutes to days; usually pruritic Urticaria may be associated with ingestion of drugs, foods, fish, berries and occasionally with infection, trauma, stress, temperature changes	Avoid trigger if known Short-term relief with epinephrine 0.1–0.3 cc SQ and may repeat in 15–30 min H_1 blockers: hydroxyzine 10 mg, diphenhydramine 12.5–50 mg po or IM q4–6h, or nonsedating antihistamine fexofenadine (Allegra), cetirizine (Zyrtec), desloratadine (Clarinex); use daily for 2 weeks H_2 blocker may decrease reaction on daily basis (cimetidine) May need to start oral steroids in short-course "burst" therapy or dose pack Chronic urticaria may need daily antihistamines or H_2 blockers If chronic urticarial itching not relieved at night with antihistamine, switch to tricyclic antidepressant such as doxepin (Sinequan) 10–50 mg at hs Refer to dermatologist if no improvement in symptoms

Continued

Disorders Causing Inflammation—cont'd

CONDITION	DESCRIPTION	TREATMENT
Diaper dermatitis Diaper Dermatitis 691.0 Candida infection 112.3	Infection occurs in "diaper" area Usual cause is irritation from urine/stool in close contact with skin for long periods of time or highly acidic urine/stool; causes skin breakdown and colonization with normal skin flora causing infection; *Candida* is the most common agent Lesions are bright red in diaper area with papular and sometimes pustular lesions; satellite lesions are common; lesions may spare inguinal folds	Frequent diaper changes Discourage use of diaper wipes; cleanse with baby lotion and cotton cloth or place baby in tepid bath after stooling Encourage frequent air drying during day (leave diapers off) or use blow-dryer on low temperature at arm's length from baby after each diaper change Encourage use of protective ointment after each diaper change Encourage using super-absorbent diapers and avoid rubber pants Discourage use of highly acidic foods/juices when dermatitis is present Use topical antifungals if *Candida* infection is suspected (nystatin cream, clotrimazole, miconazole); apply 2–3 times a day to diaper area; still use protective cream over this Baby may need combination steroid and antifungal (Mycolog II cream) preparation bid to diaper area
Seborrheic dermatitis 690.10	Characterized by mild-to-severe red, dry, flaky, patchy lesions on face, scalp, and ears Patches are poorly defined and appear greasy Lesions typically appear on nasolabial folds, ears, eyebrows, or hairline; can occur in groin, axilla, and mid-chest areas Mild itch to burning sensation Appears where sebaceous glands are most active Usually chronic condition, bothersome appearance	Gentle cleansing with soft brush (can use soft toothbrush) to remove patches/plaques Selenium sulfide shampoo, ketoconazole shampoo to cleanse areas daily Low- or mid-potency steroids can be used to control flare-ups; caution patient not to use steroids >5 days on face
Hyperhidrosis 780.8	Excessive sweating, which can be local or generalized Can disrupt lifestyle and cause embarrassment in social settings	Start treatment with antiperspirant (not deodorant) to block sweat gland production Aluminum chloride, aluminum chlorhydrate, and buffered

Disorders Causing Inflammation—cont'd

CONDITION	DESCRIPTION	TREATMENT
		aluminum sulfate to reduce excessive sweating from glands
		Apply aluminum chloride 20% (Drysol) for 7–10 nights initially, then 1–2 times a week; wash off every morning
		Aluminum chloride 6.25% (Xerac AC) at night
		Glycopyrrolate (Robinul) 1–2 mg 1–3 times a day; systemic treatment can be used, but the side effects can be problematic
		Sweating associated with a social phobia and/or public speaking may be relieved with propranolol 10–20 mg before speaking or social activity
Psoriasis Psoriasis **696.1** Pustules **686.9**	Familial tendency, usually starts in childhood Lesions are sharply demarcated red papules and plaques with powdery white scale Lesions vary in size and distribution Pitting and dystrophy of nails Lesions may itch Distribution over extensor aspect of elbows and knees, presacral area, and scalp are most common, but lesions can occur anywhere Pustules most common on palms and soles	Mid- or high-potency steroids up to 7 days on skin for acute exacerbations; use low-potency steroid in intertriginous areas Scalp lesions often require tar shampoo and steroids under an occlusive shower cap Low-potency steroids for maintenance Calcipotriene topical 0.005% (Dovonex) applied bid; avoid face, mucous membranes, and eyes; wash hands after application Tazarotene topical 0.05%, 0.1% (Tazorac) applied qhs; if childbearing age, obtain pregnancy test before starting treatment Discourage scratching and rubbing of lesions Discourage oral steroids Small, mild hyperkeratotic lesions respond to low-potency topical steroids (hydrocortisone 1%) with tar preparations (e.g., phototar or anthralin) 1–2 times a day PUVA (psoralen ultraviolet A-range) treatment may relieve symptoms; can also try tanning bed phototherapy

Topical Steroids

Topical steroids are antiinflammatory agents that control inflammation and pruritic conditions of the skin. Remember to consider the potency, the location, and the desired duration of action when prescribing a topical steroid preparation.

Practice Pearls

- Do not use "very high" potency steroids on the face or groin area or with occlusive dressings
- Do not use topical steroids for diaper rash; children have a relatively greater body surface area; therefore absorption will be greater
- Twice-a-day application is the most useful and economical; more frequent applications do not speed improvement because topical steroids have a repository effect; start with twice-a-day applications and decrease as improvement occurs
- Topical steroids, especially in higher concentrations and in children, can affect the HPA axis; beware of the dosage and slowly withdraw the drug if it has been used for a long time
- Adverse reactions such as thinning of skin, striae, rebound flare of lesions, and HPA axis depression can occur
- For an infant younger than 6 months, nothing stronger than 1% OTC hydrocortisone should be used
- For a child older than 6 months but younger than 12 years, medium potency steroids can be used for short periods of time (e.g., 7 to 10 days)
- When a high or a very high potency steroid is ordered, indicate on the prescription "not for use on the face"

VEHICLES FOR ADMINISTRATION

Topical steroids come in various vehicles designed to maximize the effects of the steroids (see Table 4–1):

Ointments	They are more occlusive; use for dry, scaly lesions; more potent than creams or lotions in the same group; may cause maceration and folliculitis
Creams	Less occlusive; more drying; used for oozing lesions and in intertriginous areas; increases anesthetic action
Gels, lotions, aerosols	Gels have some occlusive properties; used on hairy areas; urea increases hydration of the skin, facilitates cortisone penetration, and may be cooling to the skin

Table 4-1 Selected Topical Steroid Potencies

POTENCY	PRODUCT	VEHICLE	SIZES
Very high potency	Betamethasone dipropionate (Diprolene) 0.05%	Ointment	15 and 45 g
	Clobetasol propionate (Temovate) 0.05%	Cream, ointment	15, 30, 45, and 60 g
	Diflorasone diacetate (Psorcon) 0.05%	Ointment	15, 30, and 60 g
High potency	Desoximetasone (Topicort) 0.25%	Cream, ointment	15 and 60 g
	Fluocinonide (Lidex) 0.05%	Gel, ointment, cream	15, 30, 60, and 120 g
	Halcinonide (Halog) 0.1%	Cream	15, 30, 60, and 240 g
	Triamcinolone acetonide (Aristocort) 0.1%	Ointment	15 and 60 g
	Fluticasone propionate (Cutivate) 0.005%	Ointment	15, 30, and 60 g
	Diflorasone diacetate (Florone) 0.05%	Cream	15, 30, and 60 g
Medium potency	Triamcinolone acetonide (Kenalog) 0.1%	Cream	15, 60, and 80 g
	Fluocinolone acetonide (Synalar) 0.025%	Ointment	15, 30, and 60 g
	Mometasone furoate (Elocon) 0.1%	Cream	15 and 45 g
	Flurandrenolide (Cordran) 0.05%	Cream	15, 30, and 60 g
	Hydrocortisone valerate (Westcort) 0.2%	Cream	15, 45, and 60 g
	Hydrocortisone butyrate (Locoid) 0.1%	Cream	15 and 45 g
Low potency	Alclometasone dipropionate (Aclovate) 0.05%	Cream, ointment	15, 45, and 60 g
	Fluocinolone acetonide (Synalar) 0.01%	Cream, solution	15, 30, and 60 g; 20 and 60 ml
	Desonide (DesOwen) 0.05%	Cream, lotion	15, 60, and 90 g; 60 and 120 ml
	Prednicarbate (Dermatop) 0.1%	Cream	15 and 60 g
	Hydrocortisone (Hytone) 2.5%	Cream, ointment	15, 30, and 60 g
	Hydrocortisone (OTC brands) 1%	Cream, ointment	15 and 45 g

Table 4–2 Common Products Containing Latex	
Products containing latex in home	Adhesives, balloons, baby bottle nipples, carpet backing, clothing, elastic, condoms, diaphragm, gloves, pacifiers, rubber toys, shower curtains, window insulation
Products containing latex in medical office	Ambu bags, gloves, blood pressure cuffs, IV tubing, catheter tubing/tip, rubber pillows, cervical dilators, rubber stoppers, dental dams, elastic bandages, elastic support hose, stethoscope tubing, electrode pads, surgical implants, endotracheal tubes, tourniquets
Foods that may cross-react with latex	**Common foods:** avocado, banana, chestnut, cantaloupe, kiwi, potato, tomato **Reported foods:** apple, mango, peach, spinach, celery, melon, pear, turnip, cherry, papaya, pineapple, wheat

OCCLUSIVE DRESSINGS

Occlusive dressings can be used in areas where the increased uptake of topical steroids is required. Occlusive dressings should not be used for more than 12 hours a day because of the enhanced penetration and concomitant systemic effects. The following are instructions to patients regarding occlusive dressings:

- Soak the area in warm water or wash well with warm water
- While the skin is still slightly wet, rub the topical steroid into the affected area (increased moisture increases penetration)
- Cover the area with a plastic wrap, such as Saran Wrap, and seal the edges with tape or a cloth bandage; ensure a good seal between the steroid and the skin; gloves may be worn on the hands; sandwich bags for the feet and shower caps for the scalp may also be used
- Leave the dressing in place overnight or approximately 6 hours; do not use an occlusive dressing with "very high" potency steroids
- Patient should report signs of infection such as pain, increased warmth, exudate, and worsening redness to the practitioner; discontinue occlusive dressing immediately

DISPENSING AMOUNTS

Dispensing amounts of topical steroids vary according to the number of applications and the square meters of body surface to be covered. The following are some general guidelines for application twice a day for 10 days for a normal-size adult:

AREA	AMOUNT (g)
Face, head	30
Anterior chest or back	120
One arm	60
Forearm	30
One leg	120
One hand or foot	30
Anogenital area	30
Entire body	400–850

Some conditions may require oral steroid therapy. Listed below are options for equivalent doses (Table 4–3).

Table 4–3 Oral Steroid Equivalency

NAME	5 mg	10 mg	15 mg	20 mg	25 mg	30 mg	35 mg	40 mg
Prednisone 5 mg/ 5 ml (Liquid Pred syrup)	1 tsp	2 tsp	3 tsp	4 tsp	5 tsp	6 tsp	7 tsp	8 tsp
Prednisone 5 mg tablets	1 tab	2 tab	3 tab	4 tab	5 tab	6 tab	7 tab	8 tab
Prednisolone 15 mg/ 5 ml (Prelone syrup)	$\frac{1}{3}$ tsp	$\frac{2}{3}$ tsp	1 tsp	1.3 tsp	1.6 tsp	2 tsp	2.3 tsp	2.6 tsp
Prednisolone 5 mg tablets	1 tab	2 tab	3 tab	4 tab	5 tab	6 tab	7 tab	8 tab
Dexamethasone 0.5 mg/5 ml (Decadron elixir)	1.5 tsp	3 tsp	4.5 tsp	6 tsp	7.5 tsp	9 tsp	10.5 tsp	12 tsp
Dexamethasone 0.75 mg tablets (Decadron)	1 tab	2 tab	3 tab	4 tab	5 tab	6 tab	7 tab	8 tab
Prednisolone sodium phosphate 5 mg/5 ml (Pediapred)	1 tsp	2 tsp	3 tsp	4 tsp	5 tsp	6 tsp	7 tsp	8 tsp
Methylprednisolone 4 mg tablets (Medrol)	1 tab	2 tab	3 tab	4 tab	5 tab	6 tab	7 tab	8 tab
Triamcinolone 4 mg tablets (Aristocort)	1 tab	2 tab	3 tab	4 tab	5 tab	6 tab	7 tab	8 tab

Disorders Caused by Infection

CONDITION	DESCRIPTION	TREATMENT
Impetigo 684.	Group A streptococcus infection of the skin usually appears in children Highly contagious Initially lesion is vesicular later becoming encrusted with thick, honey-colored crust Usually seen in exposed areas	Cleanse area daily with soap and water; scrub crust off gently *Antibiotic therapy* Mupirocin topical ointment tid for 5–10 days Dicloxacillin 250–500 mg po q4–6h for 5–10 days Cephalexin 125–250 mg po tid for 7–10 days Monitor all exposed persons and treat if indicated Topical antibiotics can be used if there are few lesions and none on face
Scarlet fever 034.1	Outbreak caused from exposure to streptococcal pyrogenic exotoxin Associated with streptococcal pharyngitis Rash usually appears on second day of illness Diffuse red, raised, *rough* rash with blanching on pressure Seen on chest and trunk; spares face, palms, and soles	Treat underlying infection *Antibiotic therapy 7–10 days* Penicillin VK for 10 days; adults 500 mg po tid; children 25–50 mg/kg tid Azithromycin for 5 days; adults 500 mg qd; children 12 mg/kg qd, not to exceed 500 mg qd Cephalexin for 10 days; adults 250–500 mg tid; children 25–100 mg/kg qid Rash should disappear within 48 hr
Cellulitis Cellulitis 682.9 Streptococcus 041.00 Staphylococcus 041.11	Infected skin wounds are usually caused by *Streptococcus* or *Staphylococcus* infections Erythema usually follows lymphatic channel and gives the appearance of "streaking" on the skin	Use warm, moist soaks to area minimum of qid Keep extremity elevated Inquire about last tetanus immunization (see Table 4–6) *Antibiotic therapy for 7–10 days* Dicloxacillin: adult 250–500 mg po q6h; children 25–50 mg/kg q6h Amoxicillin/clavulanate (Augmentin): adult 875 mg q12h; children 20–40 mg/kg q12h Erythromycin: adult 250–500 mg qid; children 25–50 mg/kg qid

Disorders Caused by Infection—cont'd

CONDITION	DESCRIPTION	TREATMENT
Folliculitis 704.8	Superficial inflammation of hair follicles, usually *Staphylococcus aureus* Heals without scarring Scattered discrete pustules are seen at base of hair follicles Hot tub folliculitis occurs after sitting in hot tub; usually seen on buttocks, thighs, and lower trunk *Pseudomonas aeruginosa* is common pathogen with hot tub folliculitis	*Topical antibiotic therapy until healed* Mupirocin ointment (Bactroban) bid Clindamycin bid until healed Erythromycin solution bid If *S. aureus* is suspected, may need oral antibiotic Treat hot tub folliculitis with gentamicin topical and acetic acid 0.25% solution tid-qid May need oral therapy with ciprofloxacin 500 mg po bid Hot, moist packs minimum of qid
Furuncle and carbuncle Furuncle 680.9 Carbuncle 680.9	Furuncle is an acute, red, hot, very tender nodule that evolves from folliculitis Carbuncle is conglomerate of multiple coalescing furuncles May have fever and malaise Due to the increase in methicillin resistant *staphylococcus aureus* (MRSA) infections, treat as MRSA until wound culture confirmation; ask about other exposure at home, school, or recent hospitalizations	Incision and drainage of abscess *Antibiotic therapy (non-MRSA) for 10 days* Dicloxacillin 250–500 mg q6h Amoxicillin/clavulanate (Augmentin) 875 mg q12h Erythromycin 250 mg tid *Antibiotic therapy (MRSA) for 10–14 days* Bactrim DS bid; clindamycin 150–300 mg q6h; doxycycline 100 mg bid If furuncle recurs or fails to resolve, can add rifampin 300 mg bid for 5 days; may need eradication protocol* for recurrent infections Screen family members for carrier status (consider nasal, axillary, groin)

*Eradication protocol (may vary): Bactroban intranasal and under fingernails bid for 5 days with Hibiclens showers daily for 3 days, then 3 times a week for 3 weeks.

Acne

Acne (Pustular) (Vulgaris)	706.1	Acne (Mechanica)	706.1	Flushing (Transient)	782.62	
Acne (Mild)	706.1	Acne (Excoriée)	706.1	Telangiectasis	448.9	
Acne (Grade II)	706.1	Acne (Cosmetica)	706.1	Rhinophyma (usually in men)		695.3
Acne (Grade III)	706.1	Rosacea	695.3			

Condition
- Disorder involving chronic inflammation of the pilosebaceous follicles, probably involving an increase in androgenic hormones; usually occurs in adolescents and has a familial tendency; may disrupt lifestyles due to appearance of skin

- Therapies for acne are time-consuming and involve commitment of the person for a daily regimen of care; resolution is very slow, and continual reinforcement is needed
- Sunscreens greater than 30 SPF and moisturizers are required daily
- Tea tree oil may reduce number of papules and comedones
- Topical gels seem to work better on females; topical solutions (roll-ons) are better tolerated by males; if skin is dry, use creams; if skin is oily, use gels
- Keratolytics decrease follicular plugging but cause erythema to skin; encourage use of moisturizers over keratolytics at night
- Discourage picking at papules or squeezing bumps
- Makeup brands that do not irritate acne are Almay, Neutrogena, Clinique, or any that are accurately labeled as hypoallergenic

Grades of acne and treatment
- Grade 1: mild acne, few comedones, few papules, and no acute erythema
  □ Wash skin once or twice daily using hands to avoid trauma, not a cloth or buff puff; do not rub skin
  □ Avoid harsh soaps; use OTC acne wash such as Neutrogena acne wash, Whitedove, or Cetaphil; pat skin dry; do not rub skin
  □ Start with benzoyl peroxide 2.5% or higher with current regimen initially for 4 weeks; if no improvement, begin keratolytic
  □ Apply keratolytic; start with low dose and gradually increase as needed
  □ Apply moisturizer over keratolytic to prevent erythema and drying to skin

Keratolytics	Moisturizers
Benzoyl peroxide 4%–5%	Cetaphil lotion
Retin-A (tretinoin)	Purpose
Differin (adaptaline)	Neutrogena
Azelex (azelaic acid)	Clinique
Tazorac (tazarotene)	
Desquam-X5	
Epiduo (adapalene + benzoyl peroxide)	

Topical Antibiotics

DRUG	SOLUTION	LOTION	GEL	CREAM	PADS
Akne-Mycin				X	
A/T/S	X				X
Erycette					X
Eryderm	X				
T-Stat	X				X
Cleocin T	X	X	X		
Topicycline (tetracycline)	X				
Sulfacetamide/sulfur		X			
Benzoyl peroxide/clindamycin (BenzaClin)			X		
Benzoyl peroxide/erythromycin (Benzamycin)		X	X	X	

- □ Apply topical antibiotic cream, gel, or solution in morning and keratolytic at night; always use moisturizer over keratolytic at night and moisturizer in combination with sunscreen in daytime
- □ Continue same treatment for 4 weeks before changing medications
- Grade II: moderate amount of comedones with increasing papular and pustular lesions and mild to moderate erythema
  - □ Treatment is same as with grade I, but add an oral antibiotic twice daily until lesions start to resolve; then patient may need daily dosing until condition is resolved

Oral Antibiotic Drugs (acute or exacerbation)	Precautions
Tetracycline 250–500 mg bid (on empty stomach)	sun sensitivity
Minocycline 50–100 mg bid	sun sensitivity
Doxycycline 100 mg bid	sun sensitivity
Erythromycin 333 mg or 500 mg bid	gastritis
Ampicillin 250–500 mg bid	diarrhea
Trimethoprim/sulfamethoxazole 160 mg/800 mg bid	sun sensitivity

- □ Maintenance antibiotics are same as those listed except dosing is daily; a patient could take antibiotics for years
- □ If androgen excess is the predominant cause of acne, the patient can try oral contraceptives or spironolactone
- Grade III: severe pustular, nodular and cystic lesions, and erythema; dermatologist referral for isotretinoin (Accutane) and other therapies if needed

Variants of acne
- *Acne mechanica* is acne resulting from pressure, friction, or rubbing (acne beneath hatband)
- *Acne excoriée* (excoriated acne) is a form of acne that is seen with self-inflicted scratching; mostly seen in young women; considered a psychologic or emotional problem and will require in-depth counseling by specialist
- *Acne cosmetica* is caused by certain oil-based cosmetics that will cause comedones; acne is usually resolved when cosmetics are not used
- Acne can also be caused by the overuse of topical steroids, and when the steroid is stopped, acne will be resolved; lesions are in the same stage of development with rapid onset and may only appear in certain areas
- Always obtain a detailed history of the patient's symptoms, including all OTC and prescription drugs used and the use of "friends'" cures for acne

Rosacea

Condition
- *Rosacea* is a cutaneous vascular disorder that arises later in life, usually between the ages of 30 and 50 years, and is most common in fair-skinned people; women are affected 3 times more often than men, but men have more severe symptoms, including rhinophyma

- Distribution of lesions occurs on the center of the face (cheeks, chin, nose, or forehead) with inflammatory papules and pustules on an erythematous base; patients often have telangiectases; many have flushing and blushing reactions to emotional or environmental triggers before actual lesions occur
- Triggers for flush/blush reaction
  □ Alcohol ingestion
  □ Irritating cosmetics
  □ Excessive washing of face
  □ Emotional stress
  □ Spicy foods, smoking, caffeine, or sun exposure

Signs and symptoms
- Flushing (transient)
- Nontransient erythema or persistent redness of the face
- Papules and pustules in clusters
- Telangiectasia
- Burning or stinging, which can occur with the use of sunscreens or moisturizers
- Plaques and dryness with itchy, scaly skin (resembles xerosis)
- Edema after prolonged flushing
- Rhinophyma (usually in men)
- Symptoms occur bilaterally, without comedones; there is very little to no scarring
- Watery, bloodshot eyes; dryness with photophobia

Treatment
- Topical treatment
  □ Use metronidazole 1% cream once daily or metronidazole 0.75% twice daily; initially may need to add an oral antibiotic (tetracycline) until remission; metronidazole therapy may take several weeks to take effect
  □ Second-line topical antibiotics include clindamycin 1% lotion, erythromycin 2% solution, or sulfacetamide/sulfur 10% lotion (Sulfacet-R)
- Systemic therapy is used to treat hard-to-control rosacea with or without ocular or skin manifestations
  □ Tetracycline 250–500 mg bid
  □ Doxycycline 100 mg bid
  □ Minocycline 50–100 mg bid
- As symptoms improve, decrease oral antibiotics and return to topical antibiotics
- Avoid using steroids on the face
- Refer to dermatologist if symptoms worsen or persist

Pediculosis Capitis (Head Lice)

Capitis (Head Lice)	132.0

- Head lice is a common infestation by a small parasite called *Pediculus humanus capitis*
- It is found worldwide and is most common in small children ages 3 to 12 years

Text continued on p. 101

Disorders Caused by Viral Infections

CONDITION	DESCRIPTION	TREATMENT
Molluscum contagiosum 078.0	Smooth, flesh- to pink-colored, raised, umbilicated papule; caused by pox virus; may have redness or scaling around lesions Found anywhere on body: face is common area in children; genitals and anal area are common in adults Lesions are considered contagious Even with treatment lesions may recur	Nick lesions with scalpel and extrude white material Curette excision of lesion Liquid nitrogen application lightly to lesion Imiquimod (Aldara) applied to lesion 3 times a wk with or without occlusion Tretinoin (Retin-A) applied twice daily until lesions resolve
Verruca vulgaris (warts) Verruca Vulgaris (warts) 078.10 Human Papillomavirus 079.4	Caused by human papillomavirus Lesions are discrete, raised, pink-to- flesh colored, irregularly shaped and scaly appearing, with roughened, villous texture May be singular or grouped lesions May be found anywhere on body Does not itch, but may be painful if in high stress area such as sole of foot Lesions may spontaneously resolve without any treatment	Treatment is destructive Flat warts may respond to tretinoin acid cream 0.05% (Retin-A) qd with or without occlusion; can use benzoyl peroxide 5% or salicylic acid cream 5% with Retin-A until healed Plantar warts may respond to occlusive salicylic acid 40%; plaster kept in place for 2–3 days then pare down wart and use liquid nitrogen Hand warts may respond to: Cryotherapy every week for 3 wk Salicylic acid plasters or imiquimod (Aldara) 5% cream 3 times a week up to 16 wk; use small amount and rub into wart well; if wart is keratinized, soak first before applying For children >10 yr, try cimetidine 30 mg/kg/day or 300 mg tid until wart is resolved; if using liquid cimetidine and taste is a problem, mix with butterscotch or marshmallow topping

Continued

Disorders Caused by Viral Infections—cont'd

CONDITION	DESCRIPTION	TREATMENT
		Duct tape can also be tried over wart; apply tape and leave on for several days, then remove tape and pare down wart and reapply tape; may take several months but this procedure is relatively painless
		Cryotherapy can be used for all warts and may require several treatments before resolution
		Remember: whenever using liquid nitrogen, let the lesion thaw between treatments; watch for ring around lesion to ensure an adequate freeze
		Do not leave liquid nitrogen on skin for >15 sec at a time; if using this on children, have them count or recite letters to distract them or sing songs during treatment
Erythema infectiosum (fifth disease) 057.0	Viral rash starts on the cheeks as a red, macular blush that looks like a "slapped cheek" Eruption then moves to extensor surfaces of extremities and then develops into a lacy, reticulated pattern on upper legs or arms May last up to 1 mo, and exacerbations occur with sun or temperature changes No other symptoms noted	No treatment indicated Rash will resolve Caution with pregnancy; may cause fetal harm, consult with obstetrician
Roseola 057.8	Before rash, child will have 3–4 days of high fever without other symptoms As fever decreases, rash appears as rose-pink maculopapular rash that will fade with pressure Appears first on trunk and may spread to face, neck, and extremities Child does not appear ill Symptoms last about 7 days	No treatment Increase fluids to prevent dehydration Use antipyretics routinely while fever is present

Disorders Caused by Viral Infections—cont'd

CONDITION	DESCRIPTION	TREATMENT
Hand-foot-and-mouth disease 074.3	Abrupt onset of scattered papular and vesicular lesions found on palms, between fingers and on soles of feet; has oral lesions on soft/hard palate, buccal mucosa, and tongue Fever, malaise, joint aches, and cervical adenopathy	No treatment indicated, self-limited illness May have occasional itching Use antipyretics for fever Increase fluid intake May try diphenhydramine (Benadryl) liquid as a mouthwash to decrease pain or sucralfate (Carafate) suspension 1 g/10 ml ½ to 1 tsp 3–4 times a day as swish and rinse; this will coat and soothe mucosa in mouth
Herpes simplex (fever blisters) 054.9	Lesions appear as grouped vesicles, followed by erosions and ulcerations May appear on lips, oral mucosa, epidermal areas, and genitalia Outbreak may be preceded by fever, malaise, H/A, and adenopathy Lesions are very painful Outbreak may start as "tingling" sensation; this is contagious period Recurrent episodes are common, especially after stress, fevers, and sun exposure	Keep lesions moist at all times with OTC products such as Carmex or lip balm Lysine, orally or as topical ointment, may shorten illness or lessen intensity of symptoms Abreva sold OTC; apply 5 times a day at first sign of illness; apply with fingercot or rubber glove; use until healed *Initial episodes* Apply penciclovir (Denavir) cream every 2 hours while awake for 4 days; use rubber glove or fingercot to apply Valacyclovir (Valtrex) oral 2 g bid for 1 day; start with first sign of tingling, burning, or itching Acyclovir (Zovirax) oral: 200 mg 5 times a day for 5 days *Recurrent episodes* Acyclovir (Zovirax) oral: 400 mg tid for 5 days Valacyclovir (Valtrex) oral: 2 g bid for 2 days Famciclovir (Famvir) oral: 500 mg tid for 5 days (unlabeled use)

Continued

Disorders Caused by Viral Infections—cont'd

CONDITION	DESCRIPTION	TREATMENT
Herpes zoster (shingles) Herpes zoster (shingles) 053.9 Postherpetic Neuralgia (PHN) 053.19	Discrete, vesiculopustular grouped lesions; follows dermatomal line Lesions do not cross the midline. Very painful, occasional itching that may precede actual eruption *Initiate treatment as soon as possible* Postherpetic neuralgia (PHN) occurs after initial episode of zoster; this is a residual burning pain that occurs at site of lesions after rash is gone; may disrupt life activities; initiate medical therapy immediately	Topical calamine lotion or Domeboro solution can be used to start drying lesions and will help decrease itch *Systemic antiviral medication* Acyclovir (Zovirax): 800 mg 5 times a day for 7 days Famciclovir (Famvir): 500 mg q8h for 7 days Valacyclovir (Valtrex): 1 g tid for 7 days *PHN treatment* Amitriptyline (Elavil): 10–25 mg at hs Nortriptyline (Pamelor): 10–25 mg at hs (better tolerated than Elavil); monitor side effects (the higher the dose, the more side effects) Gabapentin (Neurontin): start 300 mg on day 1, and then take 300 mg bid for 2 days, then tid Lidocaine transdermal (Lidoderm) 5% patches: apply for up to 12 hr a day in 24-hr period; may be cut to size; no more than three patches at a time; never reuse a patch; contraindicated with Class 1 antiarrhythmics Benzoyl peroxide 10%: apply liberally as needed (not to orbital area); shower daily to prevent build-up Capsaicin (Zostrix) cream: apply to skin 3–4 times a day; it may take 2–6 wk to see improvement; wash hands well after rubbing on or use gloves

Disorders Caused by Viral Infections—cont'd

CONDITION	DESCRIPTION	TREATMENT
		Lidocaine/prilocaine topical (EMLA) cream: apply over painful area and cover; may leave it on up to 24 hr, then wash area
		Consider Zostavax for adults >50 yr; may receive even if outbreak has occurred; should wait until lesions are resolved prior to immunization
Varicella (chickenpox) Varicella (chickenpox) 052.9 Pruritus 698.9	Multistaged papular, vesicular, pustular lesions on red base that crust Lesions begin on trunk and are scattered Pruritus is common Usually seen in young children	Adults, elderly, or immunocompromised persons need to be treated to prevent complications Treat adults and children older than 2 yr with acyclovir 20 mg/kg qid for 5 days (do not exceed 800 mg/dose)

- Area most commonly affected is the scalp, but the louse can inhabit the eyelashes, eyebrows, and beard
- Nit infestation is most commonly found behind the ears, nape of neck, and crown of head; nits are usually located near the hair shaft and are usually a dark color; as the eggs hatch the casing turns white and is easier to see
- Adult louse is small, grayish in color and very agile; it is approximately 3 mm long with 6 legs
- Transmission occurs when hats, combs, hairbrushes, and caps are shared; lice are spread through direct contact
- In many areas of the United States, head lice are becoming resistant to standard medications used for treatment
- Treatments for head lice should always involve removing the nits; this can be time-consuming, and many parents will not take the time to remove all nits; shaving the head is an easy treatment for boys, but not for many girls; instruct the parent to get a bright light and several hair clips and section off the hair for easier identification of nits; the nit combs are not very good because they miss nits or cannot pull the egg off the hair shaft
- Some hair rinses will facilitate nit removal by loosening the eggs attachment; try a vinegar and water rinse
- All head lice preparations are applied at bedtime after washing the hair, and a shower cap can be worn to increase the effectiveness of the product; avoid getting product in eyes or mouth; rinse it out in the morning

- Topical head lice preparations:
  - Permethrin 1% cream rinse
  - Lindane 1% shampoo or lotion
  - Pyrethrin 0.3%/piperonyl butoxide 3% to 4% liquid, gel, or shampoo
  - Malathion 0.5% lotion
  - Elimite 5% cream
- Oral head lice medications for resistant head lice
  - Bactrim 5 mg/kg bid × 10 days; works best if used with Nix shampoo
  - Ivermectin 200 mcg/kg initially and repeated in 7 days (not for children)
- Tea tree oil can be used daily and may eliminate live head lice; eggs still have to be removed manually
- Environmental cleaning must be started with other treatments; wash all clothing worn in the last 3 days in hot water and dry for 20 minutes on hot cycle; for nonwashable items, store in closed plastic bag for 2 weeks

Sarcoptes scabiei (Scabies)

Sarcoptes scabiei (Scabies)	133.0
Vesicles	709.8

- Scabies is a skin infestation caused by a mite, which is spread by close contact
- Nocturnal itching is the presenting symptom
- Primary lesions are papules with burrows, but they can have vesicular lesions without burrows
- In adults, scalp, face, and upper back are spared; in infants these areas are not spared, and lesions may be found on palms and soles
- Burrows are common between fingers and flexor areas of wrist, penis, vulva, nipples, axilla, and buttocks
- Vesicles can be found on sides of fingers
- To test for scabies, place one drop of mineral oil on slide, touch blade to oil, and then touch skin after scraping four to five vesicular lesions or burrows (scrape almost to point of bleeding); place all samples on slide and cover; it is difficult to collect a live mite
- Treatments for scabies:
  - Permethrin 5% cream (Elimite): apply to skin from the neck down, leave on for 8 to 12 hours, and then wash off; may repeat once in 7 days
  - Crotamiton (Eurax) 10% cream/lotion: apply from neck down, leave on for 24 hours, and then wash off; repeat in 24 hours and leave on for 48 hours
  - Lindane 1% cream: apply to skin from the neck down, leave on for 6 hours, and then wash off; the patient may repeat treatment in 1 week
  - Benzyl benzoate 10% to 25% lotion: apply to whole body and wash off in 24 hours
  - Ivermectin 200 mcg/kg orally once, repeat in 2 weeks
- Treat all close contacts; wash all linens and clothes in hot water and dry on hot cycle in dryer; if an item is not able to be machine washed or dried, place it in a tightly closed plastic bag for 2 weeks

- The patient may need antihistamines for itching, which may continue because of increased sensitivity to dead mites and mite by-products
- If itching continues for more than 7 days, consider re-treatment

Disorders Caused by Fungal Infection

CONDITION	DESCRIPTION	TREATMENT
Tinea Tinea 110.9 Tinea Pedis (feet) 110.4 Tinea Manum (hand) 110.2 Tinea Corporis (body) 110.5 Tinea Capitis (head) 110.0 Tinea Cruris (groin) 110.1	Superficial infection caused by dermatophytes Well-demarcated plaques with or without pustules or papules; usually have scaling at edges with central clearing Feet may appear macerated, especially between toes Scalp lesions can be large with exudate that mats hair Predisposes person to bacterial infections or dyshidrotic eczema Scrape leading edge of lesion with scalpel and place scraping on slide; add one drop of KOH and then heat slide; examine under microscope for hyphae and spores Mildly pruritic *Monitoring for systemic therapy: do baseline testing every 4 wk* Griseofulvin AST/ALT, CBC, Cre Nizoral and Lamisil AST/ALT	Tinea capitis usually requires systemic antifungal and antibiotics: Micronized griseofulvin: 15 mg/kg a day for 4–6 wk Terbinafine (Lamisil): 1 mg/kg a day for 2–6 wk Ketoconazole (Nizoral): Take 200–400 mg po qd for 4 wk; for children >2 yr: 3.3–6.6 mg/kg qd ×4 wk (maximum dose: 400 mg/dose) Topical medications for other forms of tinea are usually effective: Butenafine topical (Mentax): apply to affected areas and surrounding skin once a day for 4 wk Terbinafine (Lamisil AT): apply bid for 1–4 wk Ketoconazole 2% (Nizoral) cream or shampoo: apply 1–2 times daily for 2–6 wk Person needs to wear white socks and shoes with ventilation
Onychomycosis 110.1	Fungal infection of the nail bed or nail plate Causes unsightly, discolored, thickened, and dystrophic nails More common in toenails than fingernails Fingernails are easier to treat Thickened nails cause pain when shoe doesn't fit well	Keep nails trimmed and filed Tell person to soak feet in warm water with a small amount of cooking oil in pan; this will soften nails and speed clipping *Topical therapy* Ciclopirox 8% solution nail lacquer (Penlac): apply daily

Continued

Disorders Caused by Fungal Infection—cont'd

CONDITION	DESCRIPTION	TREATMENT

	and can lead to injury and infection under the nail plate
	Testing is difficult; scrape under nail or clip nail and send to laboratory for analysis
	Thickened nails can also lead to decreased circulation and exacerbate venous stasis
	Many insurance companies will not pay for treatment; infection must be life-threatening or surgery inevitable before coverage is approved
	When using systemic treatments, practitioner must monitor liver enzymes closely (AST/ALT) every 8 wk
		Have person fill pan with warm water and add 2–3 capfuls of bleach to water; soak feet in this solution for 10–15 min twice daily for 2 wk (wash feet after each treatment); toenails will turn white; new nails should regrow in 2–3 mo
		Another remedy that has become popular is applying Metholatum to toenails every night until fungus is resolved; may take months to see results
		Systemic treatment
		  Terbinafine (Lamisil): 250 mg/day for 6–12 wk
		  Itraconazole (Sporanox): 200 mg qd for 12 wk
		Surgical treatment
		  Used as last resort; not proven to cure

Disorders of Pigmentation

CONDITION	DESCRIPTION	TREATMENT

Melasma
 	
Melasma   709.09
Macular
Hyperpigmentation
709.00
	Facial bronzing (macular hyperpigmentation)
	Distributed over cheeks, forehead, nose, chin, jaw angle, and above upper lip
	Seen most often in dark-complected women who have sun exposure
	Can be seen with pregnancy, initiation of OCs, sun exposure, and some antiepilepsy drugs
	May spontaneously resolve when stimulus is removed
	Is considered a chronic disease
		Sun protection and sunscreens containing zinc oxide or titanium are most beneficial and *must* be used for any sun exposure
		Treatment
		  Hydroquinone (Melanex) 3%–4% cream: apply bid (apply small amount to arm to test for hypersensitivity first)
		  Tretinoin (Retin-A) 0.05%: apply bid
		  Azelaic acid (Azelex) 20%: apply bid
		  Fluocinolone acetonide (Synalar) 0.01% (low potency): apply bid

Disorders of Pigmentation—cont'd

CONDITION	DESCRIPTION	TREATMENT
		Any of the listed products can be compounded together and applied bid in conjunction with sunscreen Tri-Luma: used nightly for short-term moderate to severe melasma up to 8 wk
Tinea versicolor <u>111.0</u>	Chronic, asymptomatic, superficial fungal infection Found mainly on the trunk, upper arms, abdomen, thighs, neck, and groin Macular lesions appear brownish to off-white with well-defined borders and occasionally a fine scale that is easily wiped off Use skin scraping and microscopic evaluation with KOH; if positive, will see "spaghetti and meatballs" hyphae Very difficult to eradicate; causes no long-term problems	*Topical treatment* Selenium sulfide 2.5%: apply and leave on for 10 min daily for 7–10 days; then use monthly to prevent recurrence Ketoconazole 2% cream: apply 1–2 times a day for 6 wk Miconazole cream (Monistat): apply 1–2 times daily until resolved *Systemic treatment* Ketaconazole: 200-mg tablet daily for 10 days; for prevention or recurrent symptoms, try 400 mg once a month
Lichen sclerosus <u>701.01</u>	Hypopigmentation disorder resulting in loss of color, tissue thinning, and scarring in the vulvar area Dry, papery thin skin starting above the clitoral arch and going down labia majora; does not involve vaginal tissue Pruritus is severe Can result in stenosis and fusion of vaginal introitus Common in older women, but can occur in children Biopsy is indicated because 5% can progress to squamous cell carcinoma	Avoid harsh soaps Wear ventilated cotton clothes and avoid panty liners Use Cetaphil as cleanser and moisturizer Use mild vaginal lubricants daily and with intercourse For severe pruritus, try Domeboro solution in cool water as a sitz bath High-potency steroids are useful (clobetasol or halobetasol 0.05%); start with bid treatment then decrease to daily or PRN Other hormone creams may relieve some symptoms Refer to dermatologist or gynecologist for persistent problems

Sunburn Precautions

Skin sensitivity varies from person to person and requires different sunscreen protection. After the skin type is determined (Table 4–4), the optimal product can be selected. SPF indicates the resistance a product affords based on exposure time to nonprotected skin; for example, an SPF of 30 gives 30 times the user's natural protection from the sun. As a general rule, broad-spectrum sunscreens with SPF >15 are effective for blocking ultraviolet A and B rays when applied appropriately.

Practice Pearls

- For maximum protection, reapply sunscreen every hour as long as the person is in the sun; all products have specific durations, but applying lotion every hour will greatly minimize the chance of sunburn
- Apply sunscreen at least 30 minutes before exposure to allow absorption into skin
- Discontinue if signs of a rash or itching occur
- Discontinue if the individual is allergic to "caines," sulfa, thiazides, or PABA (para-aminobenzoic acid)
- If there is eczema or inflamed skin, do not use an alcohol-based product
- PABA can permanently stain clothing yellow
- Do not use sunscreens on infants younger than 6 months; there is a potential for skin reaction or sensitivity and a greater risk that the alcohol content in the sunscreen will have systemic effects on this age group
- Limit sun exposure between 10 am and 2 pm

Screening Skin Lesions

- Screen all patients for precancerous and cancerous skin lesions annually
- Inspect the skin in well-lit surroundings, paying particular attention to the posterior thorax, AP cervical areas, "bra" and "panty" lines, and posterior lower legs
- If a suspicious lesion is found, determine the length of time the lesion has been present and ask if there have been any changes in the lesion; use the ABCDE mnemonic for evaluating the skin lesion:

  A Asymmetry such as lumpy, bump-on-bump appearance

  B Border irregularity such as scalloped, cauliflower, or spreading pattern

  C Color variation such as two or more colors present in the lesion (e.g., red, white, blue, brown, or black)

Table 4–4 Skin Sensitivity Type

SKIN TYPE	PATIENT HISTORY	SPF
1	Always burns easily, rarely tans	30
2	Always burns easily, tans minimally	12–20
3	Burns moderately, tans gradually	8–12
4	Burns minimally, always tans well	4–8
5	Rarely burns, tans deeply	2–4
6	Never burns, deeply pigmented	2–4

D Diameter more than 0.6 cm (approximate size of a pencil eraser); growth
either vertical (indicated by puckering of surrounding skin–poor prognosis)
or horizontal (slightly improved prognosis)

E Elevation; any change in elevation in any lesion that was previously flat

• If malignant melanoma is suspected, *refer* the patient to a surgeon immediately
• Perform a biopsy on any red, scaly lesion that persists

Skin Lesions

LESION	DESCRIPTION	TREATMENT
Skin tag 701.9	Flesh-colored papilloma on stalk; occurs anywhere on body, but mostly in intertriginous areas Varying sizes; small at base <1 mm up to 10 mm Papillomas are always soft and pliable Causes cosmetic disfigurement and discomfort at site because of friction; nonmalignant	Remove by snipping off, cryotherapy, or punch biopsy (can send to pathology lab, if needed) If many lesions noted in local area, use EMLA cream 30 min before appointment to decrease pain with removal
Epidermoid cyst (sebaceous) 706.2	Dermal nodule with keratin-filled pore Can become inflamed with persistent irritation Cyst contents are usually cream colored with cottage cheese–appearing material with foul odor Can be small (0.5 cm) to large (5 cm); usually a solitary nodule.	Incision and removal of sac lining or surgical excision of entire lesion
Actinic keratosis 702.0	Lesions are symmetric and have scaling appearance Found on sun-exposed skin Usually have been present for a long time as a chronic scale that can be removed but will always come back	Cryotherapy Curette excision Refer to dermatologist if large area of skin is involved
Keratoacanthoma 238.2	Found on extremities and face Lesions are symmetric and elevated, with a central plug and crust; borders are smooth, well demarcated; nodule is firm and not painful	Cryotherapy to lesion; if unresolved, perform surgical excision and send for pathology

Continued

Skin Lesions—cont'd

LESION	DESCRIPTION	TREATMENT
	Size can be up to 2 cm (some larger) Found primarily on sun-exposed areas Can be rapid-growing lesion May mimic basal or squamous cell carcinoma	
Basal cell carcinoma (BCC) 173.9	Found on sun-exposed skin Usually develops in middle-age, fair-skinned persons with significant outdoor exposure Lesions are asymmetric and raised, with dilated blood vessels around the rim; borders are smooth, but irregular Color variation from tan to blue-black	Remove lesion with surgical excision, cryotherapy, or punch biopsy If lesion is >10 cm, in area of high recurrence (nasolabial fold, nose) or is recurrent after removal, *refer* to dermatologist
Squamous cell carcinoma (SCC) 172.9	Found mainly on sun-exposed areas Lesions are slightly raised with scaling, having irregularly shaped borders that are sharply demarcated; may be ulcerated with crust in center on firm, moveable base Diameter varies	Surgical excision for larger lesions and send to pathologist Smaller lesions can be removed with cryotherapy or 5-FU treatment
Melanoma 172.9	Malignant lesion with poor prognosis Found anywhere on body, especially in areas where visibility is poor (on posterior back and posterior legs) Lesions are asymmetric (one half unlike other half) with irregular notched borders Color is variegated with blues, reds, blacks, and pinks with haphazard pattern Diameter is 8–12 mm (larger than end of pencil eraser) but can be larger; vertical growth appears elevated with dimpling of surrounding skin	If melanoma is suspected, refer immediately to surgeon or dermatologist for excision and biopsy

4

Wound Care

BURN CARE (Table 4–5)

- Burns should be kept clean and covered with silver sulfadiazine (Silvadene) cream; dressings should be changed daily and monitored closely
- Tar burns can cause deep tissue injury because of constant burning until removed; use mayonnaise or mineral oil to remove tar
- Refer burns that involve the palms, fingers, feet, and genital area; are greater than second degree; involve the fascia and tendons, ligaments, or muscle; or are electrical burns

MINOR ABRASIONS, SCRATCHES, SUPERFICIAL LACERATIONS

- Thoroughly clean area with soap and water
- Keep covered with a clean, dry bandage while working; may remove at night
- May need to use a butterfly dressing for a small, superficial laceration to hold edges together
- May use Dermabond (an adhesive similar to Super Glue) with a simple, clean laceration that is easily approximated
- Ask about tetanus prophylaxis (Table 4–6)

HUMAN BITES

- Clean thoroughly with soap and water, followed by irrigation with normal saline
- Ask about tetanus prophylaxis (see Table 4–6)
- Antibiotics often used are cephalexin (Keflex) qid and amoxicillin-clavulanate (Augmentin) bid-tid
- Use hot moist soaks or hot packs minimum of qid
- Monitor for cellulitis; recheck in office at least once if the bite is large or patient delayed seeking care
- Do not suture human or animal bites

PUNCH BIOPSY

- Can easily remove small skin lesions and imbedded ticks and can facilitate obtaining a sample for pathologic examination
- After anesthetizing and prepping the skin, stretch skin around the lesion 90 degrees to the proposed direction of the linear closure
- Lightly depress the instrument over the lesion while turning it; remove the instrument and release skin tension
- Remove the cored-out lesion from the punch; the resulting incision should be an ellipse that can be easily sutured

LACERATIONS AND SUTURING (Table 4–7)

- Before using a local anesthetic on the wound, drizzle a small amount into the laceration to decrease pain with infiltration
- EMLA cream can be applied 30 minutes to 1 hour before infiltration to decrease pain

Table 4–5 Burn Care

BURN CLASSIFICATION	APPEARANCE	PAIN SENSATION	WOUND PROGNOSIS	TREATMENT
First degree 949.1	Erythematous No blisters Dry	Painful Hyperesthetic	Heals in 3–7 days No scarring	Clean with mild soap and water May try aloe either as gel or spray for pain relief Apply scant amount of silver sulfadiazine cream 1% bid
Second degree 949.2				
Superficial	Blisters with reddened moist base	Painful Hyperesthetic	Heals <21 days May have pigment changes	Clean daily with mild soap and water using sterile technique Change dressing daily Use scant amount of silver sulfadiazine cream 1% bid If burn is extensive, refer to emergency department or burn unit
Deep dermal	Usually blisters with blanched moist base	Painful Hyperesthetic Numb in places	Heals in >21 days May have severe hypertrophic scarring	Refer to emergency department or burn unit
Third degree 949.3				
Full-thickness skin	Leathery Pearly white or charred dry	Not painful Numb	Eschar sloughs in 2–3 wk Grafting necessary	Refer to emergency department or burn unit

Table 4–6 Postexposure Tetanus Prophylaxis for Persons Who Previously Had Received Tetanus Toxoid Doses

	SIGNIFICANT WOUNDS		MINOR WOUNDS*	
	VACCINE†	TETANUS IMMUNE GLOBULIN	VACCINE†	TETANUS IMMUNE GLOBULIN
Unsure of tetanus status or <3 doses	Yes	Yes (do not mix vaccines and do not give in the same extremity)	Yes	No
Has had at least 3 doses	Yes, if last dose was >5 yr ago	No	Yes, if last dose was >10 yr ago	No

*Including contaminated wounds, those related to necrotizing infections, or those from crush injury, burns, frostbite, bullets, or shrapnel.
†Patients ≥7 years old receive adult dT vaccine; patients <7 years old receive pediatric dT vaccine.
Note: Tdap (Adacel ages 11–64 yr; Boostrix 65 yr or older) to boost tetanus, diphtheria, and pertussis immunity can be given anywhere in the series one time, then return to every-10-yr schedule.

- Anesthetize wound using the smallest needle possible (e.g., 27 gauge); inject *slowly* into wound edges, not into the intact skin; inject each side of laceration with as few punctures as possible
- Methods of primary closure for wounds that occur within 8 hours of injury (except face and scalp) include sutures, Steri-strips, staples, and Dermabond
- Secondary closure/healing involves allowing the wound to close on its own; the wound must be cleansed *very well* and debrided if necessary; assess wounds more frequently during healing process
- Before suturing lacerations that involve extremities, assess the distal digits' neurovascular status such as sensation, strength, and movement
- Wound care rechecks should be done in 24 hours if contaminated wound, in 5 to 7 days, or before removing sutures
- Instruct person to keep wound dry and clean; if dressing accidentally gets wet, change dressing immediately
- Have person (or caregiver) gently clean the edges of the wound daily with a cotton swab saturated with peroxide to remove crusts (this will decrease scarring by facilitating the healing of wound's edges)
- Caution person to return immediately if signs of infection occur
  - Redness
  - Increasing pain
  - Swelling
  - Fever
  - Red streaks progressing up an extremity
- Suture points to consider when repairing wounds:
  - Assess the degree of wound tension by observing the wound edges; if edges are close, there is minimal tension and good cosmetic closure should result

□ If the edges are greater than 5 mm apart, there is increased tension and wound should be repaired in layers for best results

□ When removing a lesion, make the incision parallel to skin tension lines; this will decrease the scarring (gently pull intact skin in different directions and see which way the natural line of the skin moves)

□ To check wound thickness, use stick end of applicator and set into injury; if it will not drop through the skin, this is considered *partial thickness*

□ Digital blocks work well for providing anesthesia in finger and toe lacerations

□ *Never* use anesthetic with epinephrine in or on fingers, toes, ears, nose, or penis

• After wound is anesthetized, clean vigorously and irrigate profusely (the cleaner the wound, the less likely infection will occur)

□ Do not suture highly contaminated wounds, human or animal bites, wounds older than 24 hours, or puncture wounds

• Use broad-spectrum antibiotics for lacerations with

□ Traumatic injury with contamination

□ Untidy wound with inadequate debridement

□ Joint wounds

□ Wounds older than 6 to 12 hours

□ Animal and human bites

□ Compromised host

• Ask about tetanus prophylaxis (see Table 4–6)

• It takes approximately 12 to 18 months for a scar to fully develop in strength, color, and size

Table 4–7 Suture Points

LOCATION	SUGGESTED SUTURE SIZE		SUTURE REMOVAL	
	SKIN	DEEP ABSORBENT	ADULT	CHILD
Scalp	4–0, 5–0	4–0	6–7 days	5–6 days
Face or forehead	6–0	5–0	4–5 days	3–4 days
Eyebrow	5–0, 6–0	5–0	4–5 days	3–4 days
Lip, nose, or ear	6–0	5–0 (n/a for ear)	4–5 days	3–4 days
Trunk	4–0, 5–0	3–0	7–10 days	6–8 days
Arm or leg	4–0, 5–0	3–0	Joint spared: 7–10 days Joint (extensor surface): 8–14 days Joint (flexor surface): 8–10 days	Joint spared: 5–9 days Joint (extensor surface): 7–12 days Joint (flexor surface): 6–8 days
Hand	5–0	5–0	Dorsal 7–9 days Palm 7–12 days	Dorsal 5–7 days Palm 7–10 days
Plantar foot	3–0, 4–0	4–0	7–12 days	7–10 days

Things That Bite and Sting

This section gives a general overview of common animal, snake, and insect bite and sting injuries with common treatments to help practitioners in caring for patients with such injuries.

BITES	SIGNS AND SYMPTOMS	TREATMENT

Rattlesnake, water moccasin, copperhead
 	
 Rattlesnake 989.5
 Water Moccasin 989.5
 Copperhead 989.5
	Proteolytic venom causes hemorrhage and hemolysis
	 Pain and puncture wounds are the hallmark of snakebite
	 Onset of symptoms relates to severity of envenomation
	 Minimal envenomation:
	    Moderate pain
	    Erythema within 15 cm, without systemic symptoms
	 Moderate envenomation:
	    Severe pain
	    Erythema beyond 15 cm, edema spreading up to 40 cm
	    Petechiae
	    Fever, vomiting, and weakness
	 Severe envenomation:
	    Extreme pain
	    Edema beyond 40 cm
	    Ecchymosis
	    Vertigo and confusion
	    Convulsions, shock, and respiratory failure
		Be calm and keep the victim calm
		 Transport to emergency department
		 Remove any constricting jewelry/clothing
		 Note amount of time between bite and symptoms
		 Keep extremity affected below heart level
		 Minimal wounds are treated supportively with cleansing, Td prophylaxis, and broad-spectrum antibiotics
		 More severe envenomations will require hospitalization and possibly antivenin
		 Will need to assess CBC, U/A, chemistry profile, PT/PTT, ECG, DIC panel, and type and crossmatch for possible transfusion
		 Do not use tourniquet, ice, or alcohol

Coral snake bites 989.5	Venom causes paralysis Few local symptoms initially but within 30 min may have numbness, sore throat, ptosis, ataxia, increase salivation, dysphagia, N/V, and mydriasis If bite is severe, may see respiratory distress and failure Symptoms occur within 8–72 hr	Monitor closely Have entubation equipment available Treatment is the same as above

Continued

BITES	SIGNS AND SYMPTOMS	TREATMENT
Animal bites (domestic) 879.8	Multifaceted bacteria are embedded in wound after bite Signs of infection include Swelling at site Redness and heat to wound Pain Fever Lymphadenopathy	Cleanse area thoroughly with soap and water immediately Use clean dressing with antibiotic ointment (mupirocin) *Systemic antibiotics for 10 days:* Amoxicillin/clavulanate (Augmentin) adult: 875 mg q12h; children: 20–40 mg/kg q12h Clindamycin (Cleocin) 150–300 mg qid Dicloxacillin 250–500 mg q6h Td prophylaxis as indicated Follow state laws for reporting animal bites
Feral or wild animal bites 879.8	**Principle carriers of rabies:** Bats Fox Raccoon Skunks Coyote Cats/dogs **Rarely carry rabies:** Squirrels Mice Rats Rabbits Symptoms of rabies may not appear for up to 10 days Bat bites may go undetected because of size of bite area and painless act of biting Initial symptoms include H/A Jaw pain Photophobia Dizziness Numbness Fever, N/V As disease progresses, symptoms include changes in mentation and gait disturbances Final stage of disease is cardiovascular collapse	Any exposure to bats requires prophylaxis with RIG (rabies immune globulin) followed by 5 days of rabies vaccine Keep all wounds chean Use antibiotic creams Td prophylaxis as indicated

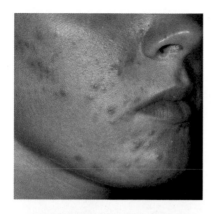

COLOR PLATE 1. Papular and pustular acne (mild). Several papules are localized on the cheeks. (From Habif, T. P. [1996]. *Clinical dermatology: A color guide to diagnosis and therapy* [3rd ed.]. St. Louis: Mosby.)

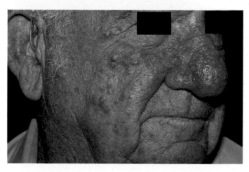

COLOR PLATE 2. The classic appearance of rosacea. Multiple papules and a few pustules are scattered on the nose and cheeks. The nose shows almost confluent erythema. (From White, G. M., & Cox, N. H. [2002]. *Diseases of the skin: A color atlas and text.* St. Louis: Mosby.)

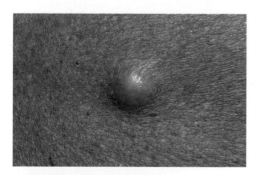

COLOR PLATE 3. Epidermal inclusion cyst. (From White, G. M., & Cox, N. H. [2002]. *Diseases of the skin: A color atlas and text.* St. Louis: Mosby.)

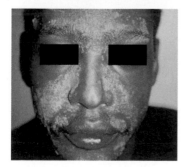

COLOR PLATE 4. Seborrheic dermatitis. (Courtesy William D. James, MD. From Habif, T. P. [1996]. *Clinical dermatology: A color guide to diagnosis and therapy* [3rd ed.]. St. Louis: Mosby.)

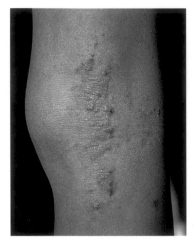

COLOR PLATE 5. Flexural atopic dermatitis with lichenification. (From White, G. M., & Cox, N. H. [2002]. *Diseases of the skin: A color atlas and text.* St. Louis: Mosby.)

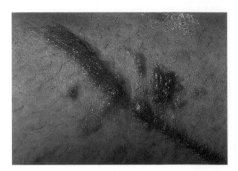

COLOR PLATE 6. Allergic contact dermatitis to *Rhus.* The classic appearance of allergic contact dermatitis is illustrated in this patient who came into contact with poison oak. The lesions are linear but not following Blaschko's lines. The eruption is microvesicular and extremely pruritic. (From White, G. M., & Cox, N. H. [2002]. *Diseases of the skin: A color atlas and text.* St. Louis: Mosby.)

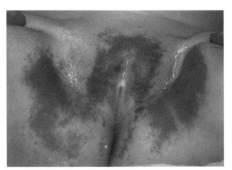

COLOR PLATE 7. Diaper dermatitis. (From White, G. M., & Cox, N. H. [2002]. *Diseases of the skin: A color atlas and text.* St. Louis: Mosby.)

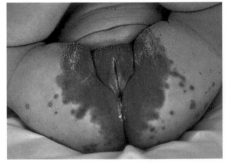

COLOR PLATE 8. Candida dermatitis. (From White, G. M., & Cox, N. H. [2002]. *Diseases of the skin: A color atlas and text.* St. Louis: Mosby.)

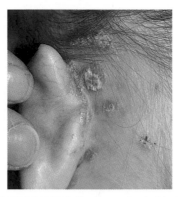

COLOR PLATE 9. Scaly papules behind the ear and on the scalp in psoriasis. (From Weston, W. L., Lane, A. T., & Morelli, J. G. [2002]. *Color textbook of pediatric dermatology* [3rd ed.]. St. Louis: Mosby.)

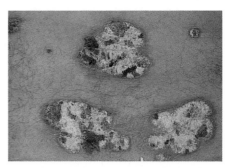

COLOR PLATE 10. Psoriasis vulgaris. (From Callen, J. P., Greer, K. E., Paller, A. S., & Swinyer, L. J. [2000]. *Color atlas of dermatology* [2nd ed.]. Philadelphia: W.B. Saunders.)

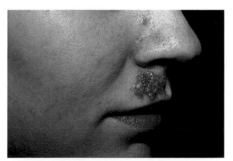

COLOR PLATE 11. Impetigo. Honey-colored moist crust just above the upper lip. (From Weston, W. L., Lane, A. T., & Morelli, J. G. [2002]. *Color textbook of pediatric dermatology* [3rd ed.]. St. Louis: Mosby.)

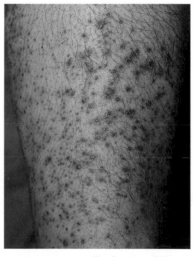

COLOR PLATE 12. Perforating folliculitis. From Callen, J. P., Greer, K. E., Paller, A. S., & Swinyer, L. J. [2000]. *Color atlas of dermatology* [2nd ed.]. Philadelphia: W.B. Saunders.)

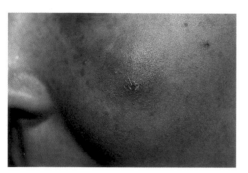

COLOR PLATE 13. Cellulitis following self-manipulation of acne pustule. (From Weston, W. L., Lane, A. T., & Morelli, J. G. [2002]. *Color textbook of pediatric dermatology* [3rd ed.]. St. Louis: Mosby.)

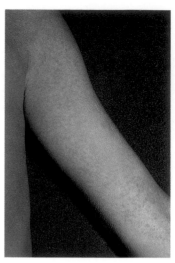

COLOR PLATE 14. Red, rough eruption of trunk and arm in streptococcal scarlet fever. (From Weston, W. L., Lane, A. T., & Morelli, J. G. [2002]. *Color textbook of pediatric dermatology* [3rd ed.]. St. Louis: Mosby.)

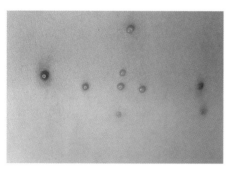

COLOR PLATE 15. Molluscum contagiosum. Small papules with a central umbilication. (From Callen, J. P., Greer, K. E., Paller, A. S., & Swinyer, L. J. [2000]. *Color atlas of dermatology* [2nd ed.]. Philadelphia: W.B. Saunders.)

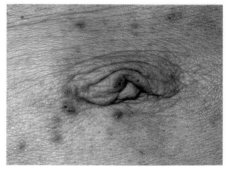

COLOR PLATE 16. Lesions about the umbilicus. The lower abdomen and umbilicus are commonly affected by nondescript, excoriated lesions in scabies. (From White, G. M., & Cox, N. H. [2002]. *Diseases of the skin: A color atlas and text.* St. Louis: Mosby.)

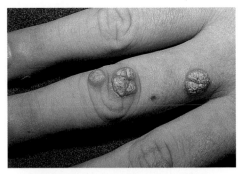

COLOR PLATE 17. Common warts on a child's fingers. (From Weston, W. L., Lane, A. T., & Morelli, J. G. [2002]. *Color textbook of pediatric dermatology* [3rd ed.]. St. Louis: Mosby.)

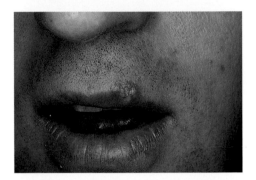

COLOR PLATE 18. Herpes simplex labialis-recurrent lesions. (From Callen, J. P., Greer, K. E., Paller, A. S., & Swinyer, L. J. [2000]. *Color atlas of dermatology* [2nd ed.]. Philadelphia: W.B. Saunders.)

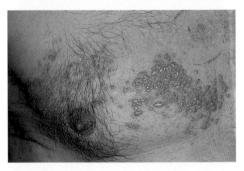

COLOR PLATE 19. Herpes zoster. (From Callen, J. P., Greer, K. E., Paller, A. S., & Swinyer, L. J. [2000]. *Color atlas of dermatology* [2nd ed.]. Philadelphia: W.B. Saunders.)

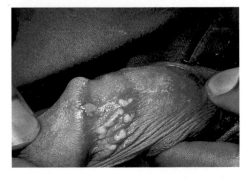

COLOR PLATE 20. Herpes genitalis, male. (Courtesy of Michael O. Murphy, MD. From White, G. M., & Cox, N. H. [2002]. *Diseases of the skin: A color atlas and text.* St. Louis: Mosby.)

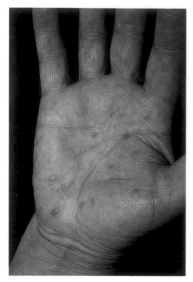

COLOR PLATE 21. Hand-foot-and-mouth disease. (From Callen, J. P., Greer, K. E., Paller, A. S., & Swinyer, L. J. [2000]. *Color atlas of dermatology* [2nd ed.]. Philadelphia: W.B. Saunders.)

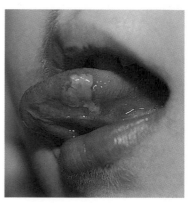

COLOR PLATE 22. Erosion of the tongue in a child with hand-foot-and-mouth syndrome. (From Weston, W. L., Lane, A. T., & Morelli, J. G. [2002]. *Color textbook of pediatric dermatology* [3rd ed.]. St. Louis: Mosby.)

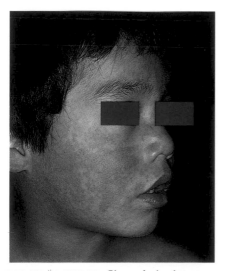

COLOR PLATE 23. Slapped-cheek appearance of a child with parvovirus B19 infection (erythema infectiosum). (From Weston, W. L., Lane, A. T., & Morelli, J. G. [2002]. *Color textbook of pediatric dermatology* [3rd ed.]. St. Louis: Mosby.)

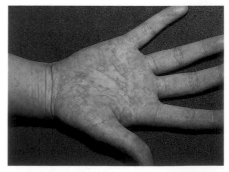

COLOR PLATE 24. Lacy pink eruption over the palms in erythema infectiosum. (From Weston, W. L., Lane, A. T., & Morelli, J. G. [2002]. *Color textbook of pediatric dermatology* [3rd ed.]. St. Louis: Mosby.)

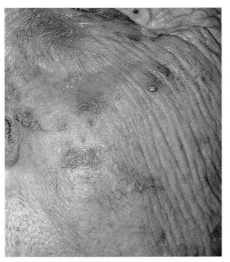

COLOR PLATE 25. Multiple actinic keratoses. (From Callen, J. P., Greer, K. E., Paller, A. S., & Swinyer, L. J. [2000]. *Color atlas of dermatology* [2nd ed.]. Philadelphia: W.B. Saunders.)

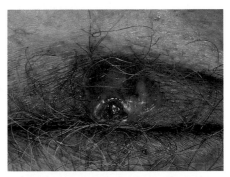

COLOR PLATE 26. Basal cell carcinoma of nodular type with ulceration affecting the vulva. (From White, G. M., & Cox, N. H. [2002]. *Diseases of the skin: A color atlas and text.* St. Louis: Mosby.)

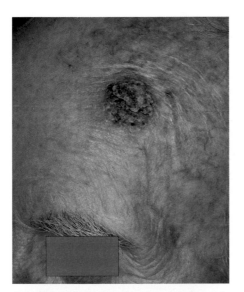

COLOR PLATE 27. Squamous cell carcinoma. Malignant degeneration occurred in an actinic keratosis that had been present for years. (From Habif, T. P. [1996]. *Clinical dermatology: A color guide to diagnosis and therapy* [3rd ed.]. St. Louis: Mosby.)

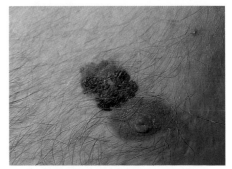

COLOR PLATE 28. Malignant melanoma on the chest of an adolescent male. (From Weston, W. L., Lane, A. T., & Morelli, J. G. [2002]. *Color textbook of pediatric dermatology* [3rd ed.]. St. Louis: Mosby.)

COLOR PLATE 29. Tinea cruris. (From Callen, J. P., Greer, K. E., Paller, A. S., & Swinyer, L. J. [2000]. *Color atlas of dermatology* [2nd ed.]. Philadelphia: W.B. Saunders.)

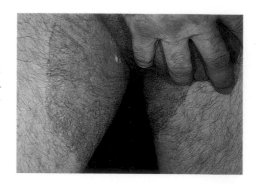

COLOR PLATE 30. Tinea pedis as a result of *Trichophyton rubrum.* (From Callen, J. P., Greer, K. E., Paller, A. S., & Swinyer, L. J. [2000]. *Color atlas of dermatology* [2nd ed.]. Philadelphia: W.B. Saunders.)

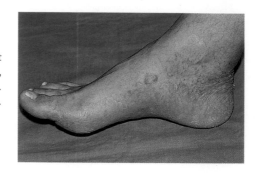

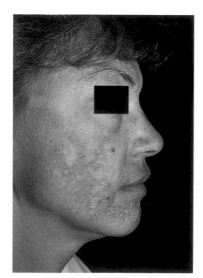

COLOR PLATE 31. Melasma. (From Callen, J. P., Greer, K. E., Paller, A. S., & Swinyer, L. J. [2000]. *Color atlas of dermatology* [2nd ed.]. Philadelphia: W.B. Saunders.)

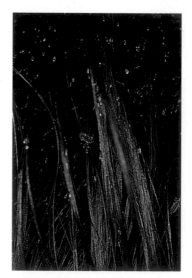

COLOR PLATE 32. Head lice. Numerous white nits attached to hairs. (From Weston, W. L, Lane, A. T., & Morelli, J. G. [2002]. *Color textbook of pediatric dermatology* [3rd ed.]. St. Louis: Mosby.)

BITES	SIGNS AND SYMPTOMS	TREATMENT
Tick bite, Lyme disease, spirochete infection with *Borrelia burgdorferi* Tick 919.4 Lyme Disease 088.81 Spirochete Infection 104.9	Bites are common April–August Incubation period is 7–10 days Tick needs to be attached for >24 hr for transmission of disease Symptoms may not appear for >30 days *Stage I symptoms:* Erythema migrans Fever Malaise Myalgia *Stage II symptoms* are the same as above with Migratory arthritis Bell's palsy Myocarditis (rare) *Stage III symptoms* same as Stage I and above with Scleroderma-like lesions on knees and elbows Severe fatigue Sleep disorders and confusion	Diagnosis is difficult because of unreliable testing Supportive care with rest, hydration, and NSAIDs for pain Early intervention with antibiotics may prevent adverse effects: *Adult dosing:* Doxycycline 100 mg bid for 10–21 days Amoxicillin 250–500 mg tid for 14–21 days Cefuroxime 500 mg bid for 20 days (Can use macrolides if allergic to these antibiotics, but they are less effective.) *Child dosing:* Amoxicillin 50 mg/kg/day po divided tid × 14 days Cefuroxime 30 mg/kg/day po divided bid × 14 days If >8 yr, doxycycline 4 mg/kg/day po divided bid × 14 days For more severe symptom management, refer to infectious disease specialist
Rocky Mountain Spotted Fever (RMSF) rickettsial disease Rocky Mountain Spotted Fever (RMSF) 082.0 Rickettsial (Tick) 082.9	Bites frequently occur April–September Transmission occurs within hours of bite Symptoms occur within 2–10 days Symptoms occur suddenly with: H/A Fever, chills Photophobia Myalgias, malaise, and N/V Maculopapular rash starts on extremities (wrists or ankles) and spreads to trunk and face Petechial rash is common on extremities Thrombocytopenia and elevated liver enzymes are common	Diagnosis relies on heightened suspicion, endemic area, and season Always ask about tick exposure in history of illness Treatment is supportive for fever control and arthralgia and to prevent dehydration *Antibiotic therapy for 7–10 days for adults:* Doxycycline 100 mg bid Tetracycline 250–500 mg qid Chloramphenicol 50–75 mg/kg qid (do not exceed 4 g/day, and monitor for side effects)

Continued

BITES	SIGNS AND SYMPTOMS	TREATMENT
Ehrlichiosis 082.4	Bites frequently occur between May and July Transmission occurs immediately after bite *Symptoms occur within 7–10 days:* H/A Malaise Myalgia Abdomen pain N/V/D Lymphadenopathy Maculopapular or petechial rash occurs on trunk and extremities (spares hands/feet)	Diagnosis based on suspicion of disease and history of tick bite before symptoms *Ehrlichia* organisms are resistant to most antibiotics Therapy is limited to Doxycycline for 14 days Adult dose: 100 mg bid Child dose: Weight >45 kg = 100 mg bid Weight <45 kg = 3 mg/kg a day bid The younger the child, the shorter the course of treatment Supportive treatment for other symptoms
Spider bites: brown recluse spider 989.5	Symptoms occur 1–24 hr after bite Spiders like dark, little used areas; not an aggressive spider; bites usually occur when spider is caught in clothing or bed linens Person complaining of "pin-pricking" sensation followed by irritation, itch, and redness After 24 hr, site of bite turns deep blue purple surrounded by white ring and large outer ring; may be raised or bullous; will experience pain at site After 48 hr, site will develop an ulceration in center that will gradually enlarge and slough May experience headache, body aches, rash, fever, and N/V Wound is usually worse if occurs in highly adipose tissue	Cleanse area thoroughly Use antibiotic ointment Apply ice packs Use NSAIDs or acetaminophen for pain There is no specific treatment for bite; not all bites progress to tissue sloughing Treat with systemic antibiotic if cellulitis or tissue breakdown occurs Refer to surgeon if lesion is enlarging and sloughing Td prophylaxis if indicated Antihistamine for any itching Dapsone has been tried to slow slough process down; no proven benefit Nitroglycerin patch has been tried to increase circulation to ulcer by applying over wound; again no proven benefit Steroid injections into site have been tried with little success

BITES	SIGNS AND SYMPTOMS	TREATMENT
Black widow spider bite 989.5	Slightly aggressive spider; lives in dark, secluded places Symptoms may not occur immediately after bite, but person will complain of severe pain, burning, redness, and swelling at site followed by more severe symptoms Headache Dizziness Rash Itching Restlessness Anxiety Sweating Eyelid edema Salivation, weakness N/V Muscle tremor, fasciculations, and leg pain	Treatment is usually supportive Significant analgesia with morphine is needed Antihistamine: Diphenhydramine 25–50 mg q6h Hydroxyzine 10–50 mg q6h Muscle relaxants: Diazepam 6–10 mg IM or po Methocarbamol 15 mg/kg IM Calcium gluconate 10% solution, 1–2 mg/kg slow IVP Antivenin is available, but side effects are significant Td prophylaxis if indicated
Mosquito-borne disease (West Nile Virus [WNV]) 066.4	Disease is spreading throughout the United States Illness can be very mild, similar to "cold" symptoms or can be very severe and lead to death Incubation period is 3–14 days Symptoms include acute febrile illness followed by Malaise Anorexia N/V Headache Eye pain Myalgia Rash Lymphadenopathy Symptoms may progress to severe neurologic disease with encephalitis, ataxia, seizures, and neuritis	Diagnosis is made with positive IgM antibody to WNV in serum or spinal fluid Treatment: IV fluids and respiratory support Antipyretics, analgesics, rest, and hydration This is a reportable illness; notify local HD Prophylaxis should be directed toward mosquito control by draining all standing water, cleaning out drains, and removing all items that might hold water If going out at night, use mosquito repellant with DEET and wear long sleeves

Continued

BITES	SIGNS AND SYMPTOMS	TREATMENT

Malaria
084.6
	Disease is a major problem for world travelers
	Symptoms usually occur 7–9 days after exposure
	Symptoms include
	  Fever
	  Shaking chills
	  Headache
	  N/V/D
	  Abdominal pain
	  Muscle aches
	  Back pain
	  Dark urine
		Diagnosis can be made from history of recent visit to endemic tropical area
		Blood smears for plasmodium species is confirmative
		Call the CDC toll-free at 1-888-232-3299 for information on prevention and treatment that can be faxed; request document #000005
		Preventive treatment depending on destination:
		  Mefloquine (Lariam) 250 mg weekly, starting 1–2 wk before travel and continuing for 4 wk after returning (do not give if person has any history of psychiatric illness)
		  Doxycycline 100 mg qd starting 1–2 days before travel and for 4 wk after returning
		  Malarone 250/100 mg po daily, starting 1–2 days before travel and for 7 days after returning
		Take all medications same time of day with food
		See prescriptive information for full prescribing details
		Use insect repellant to all exposed skin whenever outside; use mosquito netting and avoid going outside between dusk and dawn.

Stinging injuries: bee stings (Hymenoptera) 989.5	Non-Africanized bees sting only once and never in swarms Africanized bees can sting multiple times and in swarms Venom is protein based and has high affinity for causing allergic reaction that can be lethal in sensitive persons	*Local treatment:* Remove stinger if possible Apply ice pack to site(s) Use OTC antihistamine and NSAIDs routinely every 6 hr for 24 hr If person has more severe reaction, treatment may involve SQ epinephrine 0.1–0.5 cc of 1 : 1000 solution and IM or po corticosteroids

BITES	SIGNS AND SYMPTOMS	TREATMENT

	Local reactions:
	  Pain at site
	  Redness
	  Edema
	  Pruritus
	Systemic reactions:
	  N/V/D
	  Syncope
	  Headache
	  Seizures
	  Urticaria
	  Wheezing
	  Low B/P
	  Muscle spasms
	  Cardiopulmonary distress
	No correlation between
	  number of stings and
	  allergic reaction
	Can have delayed serum
	  sickness 10 days after being
	  stung
		Refer to emergency department if
		  reaction is not quickly resolved
		Prophylaxis:
		  Prescribe self-administered
		  Epi-Pen and encourage
		  person to obtain MedicAlert
		  bracelet

Scorpion stings
989.5
	Found mainly in warmer
	  desertlike climates
	Venom causes prolonged
	  firing of nerves that
	  eventually causes paralysis
	Severe pain at site of sting;
	  however, there is often no
	  sign of initial sting;
	  palpitation around the
	  sting area will elicit severe
	  pain
	Symptoms:
	  Muscle spasms
	  Drooling
	  Perioral numbness
	  Ptosis
	  Roving eye movements
	  Blurred vision
	  Slurred speech
	  Tongue fasciculations
	  Tachycardia
		No antivenin is available
		Treatment is supportive with
		  antihistamines, analgesics such
		  as morphine, and muscle
		  relaxants
		Monitor for anaphylaxis
		Treat tachycardia with beta-
		  blockers
		Td prophylaxis

Continued

BITES	SIGNS AND SYMPTOMS	TREATMENT
Fire ant sting 989.5	Aggressive ant resides in southern states, lives in underground burrows, swarms victims Site of sting is immediately painful with burning sensation Vesicle usually develops and may progress to pustule Extreme pruritus follows Generally localized symptoms, with en masse stings; may see systemic reaction Stings are more severe in young children	Supportive treatment is with ice and elevation of extremity Meat tenderizer applied immediately to bite may decrease local reaction Antihistamines for pruritus May need systemic support if anaphylaxis occurs; this can happen with multiple stings on young person
Marine hazards (fire coral) Marine 989.5	Marine animal delivers toxin via nematocysts on periphery of body Found mainly on coral reefs Symptoms include severe burning sensation and urticaria to site Patient may see erythema or hivelike lesions wherever skin is touched	Neutralize toxin immediately with acetic acid (vinegar), saline, or human urine Topical mid- to high-potency (see Table 4–1) steroids Antihistamines may help with local itching
Jellyfish stings 989.5	Marine fish delivers toxin on end of tentacles or with contact to body Symptoms (4 Ps): Pain Paresthesia Paralysis Pruritic rash	*Treatment includes* Immediately wash with acetic acid (vinegar) or saline for 30 min (jellyfish in Chesapeake Bay area are resistant to vinegar; use saline and baking soda) Apply shaving cream to facilitate removing fragments; carefully remove fragments of tentacle with double-gloved hands Use analgesics and antihistamines
Stingray 989.5	Found in warmer, coastal waters Wound is usually lacerated and may require debridement of fragments Wound is very painful, red, and hot to touch Person may experience N/V and weakness	Toxin is heat sensitive; immerse affected area in very warm water (113° F, 45° C) for 60–90 min Treat with antibiotic, usually third-generation cephalosporin or ciprofloxacin Td prophylaxis

BITES	SIGNS AND SYMPTOMS	TREATMENT
Dinoflagellate (red algae)	Increased urination, salivation, tonic paralysis and convulsions, cardiovascular collapse Algae starts in warm coastal water, and when bloom produce toxins, they may give water a red appearance Symptoms occur when there is an overabundance of algae Toxins are inhaled or eaten in contaminated fish Symptoms occur during strong winds and high waves Symptoms include 　Irritations to eyes, nose, and throat with tingling to lips and tongue 　Skin irritations and burning	Treatment is very simple: *go inside* Symptoms usually subside fairly quickly

NOTES

4

5

Respiratory and Related Ears-Nose-Throat Disorders

For complete history and physical examination, see Chapter 1.

Respiratory Tract Disorders

Ulcer of the Tongue	590.0
Ulcer of the Pharynx	478.29
Gingivitis	523.1

PRACTICE PEARLS
Aphthous Ulcer Treatments
- Labial or buccal: Kenalog in Orabase
- Multiple ulcers on tongue or pharynx: KVLBH (equal parts Kaopectate, viscous lidocaine, Benadryl, hydrocortisone, or triamcinolone) 1 tbsp; rinse, gargle, and spit out qid; may also use sucralfate (Carafate) suspension 1 to 2 tsp tid or qid, rinse and swallow (not approved by the Food and Drug Administration [FDA])
- Recurrent: try cimetidine (Tagamet) 400 to 800 mg before breakfast and supper, take until pain is gone
- PPI for 5–7 days

Gingivitis
- Cefadroxil 500 mg bid for 10 days
- Encourage patient to use Colgate Total toothpaste
- Perodex rinse bid (swish and spit out)
- May need pain medicine

Herbal Preparations (Not Exclusive)
- Echinacea: prophylaxis and treatment of respiratory infections, including flu symptoms; take 1 capsule bid for 10 days; **do not** use >8 weeks or at all in patients with autoimmune diseases
- Hyssop: use as expectorant; tea as needed, but **do not** take if pregnant
- Lobelia: expectorant and bronchial smooth muscle relaxant; take 200 mg capsule tid or 3 to 5 ml tid; **do not** exceed recommended dosage

- Slippery elm: to treat cough and sore throat; lozenges or 1 tsp powder, plus 1 tsp sugar, plus 2 cups boiling water (drink 1 to 2 cups daily)

Tinnitus

Tinnitus 388.30	Acoustic Neuroma 225.1
Subjective Tinnitus 388.31	Cerumen Impaction 380.4
Meniere's Disease 386.00	Otitis Media 382.9
Eustachian Tube Dysfunction 381.81	TMJ Disorder 524.60
Otosclerosis 387.9	Objective Tinnitus 388.32

CONDITION

- Any sound heard by the individual that is not attributable to external sound
  - Hissing, ringing, whining, buzzing
  - May be unilateral or bilateral sound
- Seems to increase with age until >70 years, then may diminish
- Subjective tinnitus (most common form) causes include the following:
  - Advancing age
  - Meniere's disease
  - Eustachian tube dysfunction
  - Otosclerosis
  - Change in blood pressure
  - Head and neck injuries
  - Acoustic neuroma
  - Chronic exposure to loud noise
  - Cerumen impaction
  - Otitis media (OM) with effusion
  - Allergies
  - Diabetes, thyroid disorder
  - TMJ disorder
- Common medications that can cause tinnitus:
  - ASA, NSAIDs
  - Macrolides, sulfa, quinolones
  - Antihistamines
  - Beta blockers (especially metoprolol)
  - Diuretics
  - ACE inhibitors
  - Tricyclic antidepressant, sedatives
  - Alprazolam
  - Calcium channel blockers
  - Narcotics
- Objective tinnitus can be heard by practitioner as clicking or humming vascular sound
  - May be pulsatile in synchrony with cardiac cycle
  - Is indicative of severe, possibly life-threatening vascular or mechanical problem and should be referred immediately

HISTORY

- Question person about localization of sound; pitch and frequency (constant or intermittent), subjective intensity of sound and progression of sound over time
- Has there been any change in hearing (either loss or hypersounds) or is there a change when head is repositioned?
- Has there been any pain, drainage, or fullness in ear(s)?
- Is there a history of trauma or vertigo associated with sounds?
- What is level of annoyance and has this changed lifestyle?

DIAGNOSTIC TESTING

- Routine examination with attention to vital signs and otoscopy with pneumatic otoscope and insufflation
- Weber's and Rinne test (see Figure 1–2)
- Cranial nerve testing (see Table 1–4)
- CBC, ESR, ANA titer, Lyme disease titer (if suspected), rheumatic factor, RPR (if suspect syphilis), TSH, FBS
- Audiology testing

TREATMENT

- May never find cause of tinnitus
- Regular exercise to increase circulation to head
- Avoid alcohol, nicotine, caffeine, and cheese; these may aggravate intensity of sound
- Decrease salt intake
- Avoid loud noises; play soft "white" noise, music, or ambient sounds
- Relaxation technique
- Medications that might help (but not proven to decrease sounds)
  - Anticonvulsants (carbamazepine [Tegretol], phenytoin [Dilantin]); these drugs suppress hyperactivity in auditory system
  - Ginkgo biloba (may improve circulation in head)
  - Antianxiety drugs to help manage stress
  - Melatonin (may improve sleeping for the person having trouble sleeping because of noise)
- Tinnitus maskers that resemble hearing aides but produce soft background noises; they are appropriate for "normal-hearing" person; they are open to the environment so person can still hear sounds
- Hearing aides for the person who has tinnitus due to hearing loss
- Biofeedback training to help person redirect circulation to head

Ocular Complaints

Pinguecula	372.51	Acute Angle-Closure Glaucoma	365.20
Acute Central Retinal Artery Occlusion	362.31	Sinusitis	473.9
Corneal Abrasion	918.1	Photophobia	368.13
Scleritis	379.00	Corneal Edema	371.20
Iritis	364.3	Red Eye	379.93

Practice Pearls

- Pinguecula is local conjunctival inflammation resulting from sun exposure and damage; treat with NSAID drops (ketorolac ophthalmic [Acular] 1 gtt qid × 5 days) and/or artificial tears as needed
- For complaint of sudden, painless total loss of vision in one eye:
  □ Acute central retinal artery occlusion
  □ Retina is pale and edematous with central macular cherry red spot
  □ Have patient breathe into paper bag (CO_2 retention causes vasodilatation) and immediately refer to emergency department or ophthalmologist
- For complaint of deep, intense pain, consider:
  □ Corneal abrasion
  □ Scleritis
  □ Iritis
  □ Acute angle-closure glaucoma
  □ Sinusitis
- For complaint of photophobia, consider:
  □ Corneal abrasion
  □ Iritis
  □ Acute angle-closure glaucoma
- For complaint of halo vision, consider:
  □ Corneal edema
  □ Acute angle-closure glaucoma
  □ Contact lens overuse

Upper Respiratory Tract Disorders

External Otitis Media 382.9	Serous Otitis Media 381.01	Allergic Rhinitis 477.9
Pseudomonas 041.7	Epistaxis 784.7	Pharyngitis 462.
Staphylococcus aureus 041.11	Sinusitis 473.9	Herpes virus 054.9
Streptococci 041.00	*Streptococcus pneumoniae* 481.	Rhinoviruses 079.3
Pneumococcal 041.2	Influenza 487.1	

CONDITION	SIGNS AND SYMPTOMS	DIAGNOSTICS
External Otitis Media	Pain in ear(s)	Usually none (NOTE:
Causative Agents	Itching and drainage	With pain or swelling
Bacterial	Pain around pinna and over	over mastoid process or
Pseudomonas (consider	lymph nodes	with chronic unresolving
especially if the	Pain with movement of	external otitis media,
drainage is purulent	pinna	follow up with an x-ray
green)	Ear canals may be swollen,	examination of the
Proteus	erythematous, and painful	mastoid)
Staphylococcus aureus	with exudate	
Streptococci	Tympanic membrane (TM)	
Fungal species	can be normal or	

- For complaint of blurred vision, consider:
  - □ Poor or abnormal tear production
  - □ Acute angle-closure glaucoma
- Topical anesthetic eye drops instilled in a red, painful eye will relieve corneal pain; pain will not be relieved if related to deep eye disease (e.g., glaucoma, sinusitis, migraine)

RED EYE

- Examining the patient's eyes can be a simple or complicated process depending on the history and examination performed; always record the patient's visual acuity in both eyes and in each individual eye whenever possible and ask the patient if his or her vision has been affected; if the patient is unable to cooperate with reading the eye chart, use any type of printed material and record whether the patient can see this material and at what approximate distance
- Determine the amount of inflammation involved; sit back and look at the patient's eyes; where is the inflammation in relation to the pupil? Is it localized or diffuse? Is it symmetric or asymmetric in one or both eyes? Are the eyelids swollen?
- Assess pupillary response for equality and reactivity to light and accommodation; failure of the pupils to react appropriately indicates a more serious problem
- Fluorescein uptake staining can be used in most offices easily and with minimal discomfort to the patient, especially if a topical anesthetic is used before staining; this simple test can determine if a serious condition exists and whether referral is needed
- For conditions affecting the eye, see Table 5–1 (p. 136)

TREATMENT	ADJUNCT THERAPY
Gentle irrigation of canal to remove debris	Counsel patient on care of ears
May instill ear wick into canal to help administer ear drops; leave in for 2–4 days	Do not put anything into the ears to clean them or to scratch
Ear Drops × 5 days	If the patient complains of itching in the ears, may try a mixture of 1:1 solution of white vinegar and rubbing alcohol after washing hair or after swimming
Polymyxin B sulfate combination (Cortisporin Otic Suspension) 4 gtts in ear qid *or*	Keep water out of ear canals for 2 wk with cotton balls impregnated with petroleum jelly gently placed into external ear canal.
Sulfacetamide and prednisolone sodium phosphate combination (Vasocidin Ophthalmic Solution) 2–3 gtts qid	Auralgan drops qh prn

Text continued on p. 134

Upper Respiratory Tract Disorders—cont'd

CONDITION	SIGNS AND SYMPTOMS	DIAGNOSTICS
	hyperemic and may have an exudative covering With repeated infection consider seborrhea, eczema, swimmer's ear, and undiagnosed diabetes	
Otitis Media *Causative Agents* Pneumococcal species *Haemophilus influenzae* *Moraxella catarrhalis* *Mycoplasma pneumoniae*	Pain in ear(s) Decreased hearing Fever Hyperemic, bulging TM with decreased mobility Perforation of the TM Bullae on the TM (often caused by *Mycoplasma pneumoniae*) Purulent fluid behind the TM	None
Serous Otitis Media	Hearing loss Feeling of fullness or pressure in ear(s) "Popping" sensation with yawning, swallowing, or nose-blowing TM retracted with yellowish or bluish colored fluid behind the TM Decreased mobility of the TM May follow an episode of URI, otitis media, or allergic rhinitis	None or tympanogram
Epistaxis	Bleeding from the nares or down the posterior nasopharynx Usually no related systemic symptoms Identify the localized area(s)	Monitor BP If chronic or frequent episodes with a potential or known bleeding disorder, monitor CBC and prothrombin time

TREATMENT	ADJUNCT THERAPY

Cortane-B Otic Aq. 3–4 gtts tid
ZOTO HC 3–4 gtts tid
Ciprofloxacin (Cipro Otic) 3 gtts bid
  (especially if *Pseudomonas* is suspected)
Ofloxacin (Floxin Otic) 10 gtt bid for 10
  days (may be used with perforated TM)
VoSol HC 4 gtts 3–4 times a day
  (coverage for bacterial and fungal
  infection)
 	
Recheck in 1 wk
Acetaminophen or ibuprofen prn for pain
	Prevention: after swimming, put a few
	  drops of vinegar, rubbing alcohol, or
	  peroxide in ears and immediately let it
	  drain out
	Auralgan (antipyrine/benzocaine) otic, if no
	  perforation, 2–4 gtts in ear canal every
	  1–2 hr until pain improves, then tid for
	  2–3 days

Antibiotic Therapy
Amoxicillin 500 mg tid or 875 mg bid ×
  5 days
TMP-SMZ DS (Bactrim) bid × 5 days
Cefaclor (Ceclor) 250 mg tid × 10 days
Cefuroxime (Ceftin) 250–500 mg bid
  5–10 days
Azithromycin (Z-Pak)
 	
Follow-up
4 wk	

If symptoms are mild or the patient is
  asymptomatic, the condition will usually
  spontaneously resolve in 2–3 wk
If symptomatic, use a topical decongestant
  such as oxymetazoline HCl (Afrin) 1–2
  sprays q12h (NOTE: Nasal sprays
  should only be used for 3 days because
  of nasal hypercongestion)
Hypertonic saline solution frequently
Oral decongestant and/or nonsedating
  antihistamine
Follow-up in 3 wk
	If associated with an allergy, may need to
	  refer to an allergist
	May try oral decongestants such as
	  pseudoephedrine HCl
	May try chewing gum to help relieve
	  blockage of the eustachian tube
	Autoinsufflation frequently (pinch nose
	  closed and swallow, trying to "pop" ears)
	Hearing testing, referral to ENT

Have the patient blow nose to remove clots
Have the patient hold pressure by pinching
  the nares closed for 10–15 min by the
  clock
Have the patient sit in upright position
If bleeding is not controlled and patient
	Advise the patient to use a humidifier in the
	  home, especially at night
	Use a small amount of a non-petroleum-
	  based product in the anterior nares at
	  night and during the day if the
	  environment is dry

Continued

Upper Respiratory Tract Disorders—cont'd

CONDITION	SIGNS AND SYMPTOMS	DIAGNOSTICS
	of bleeding in the anterior nares	Evaluate current medications
	Evaluate the septum for hematoma	
	If unable to identify area of bleeding in anterior nares, may be posterior bleeding (especially if bleeding is not controlled by conventional means of pressure)	
Sinusitis		
Causative agents	Cough	Percussion of sinuses
Streptococcus pneumoniae	Purulent nasal discharge	Transillumination of
Haemophilus influenzae	Fever	sinuses
Moraxella catarrhalis	Facial pain (when bending	Sinus x-ray
May be viral	forward, pain increases)	CT scan of sinuses
	Prolonged URI (usually longer than 3 wk)	*Classification*
	Nausea	Acute: symptoms last 10 days–3 wk
	Frequent clearing of throat	Chronic: symptoms last
	Halitosis	>3 wk
	Postnasal drip with sore throat	Recurrent: well between infections
	Pain in ethmoid, frontal, and sphenoid sinuses is greater in supine position	Persistent: some symptoms remain constantly
	Pain in maxillary sinus is greater in upright position	
	Nasal quality to speech	
	Nasal mucosa inflamed and boggy	
	Pain to palpation over mastoids and C2	
	Retracted TMs	
	Lymphoid hyperplasia ("erythremic cobblestone appearance") to posterior oropharynx	
Influenza		
Causative Agents	Sudden onset of malaise	Usually none
Influenza viruses A, B, and C	Fever	Can draw for serum influenza A and B titer or blood culture for virus
	Headaches	
	Myalgia	

*If high resistance to *S. pneumococcus* is suspected, give 3.0 to 3.5 g qd in divided doses.

TREATMENT	ADJUNCT THERAPY
status is questionable, refer to emergency department for an ENT consultation	Review methods to stop nose bleeding by pressure technique Use normal saline nasal spray frequently
Treatment regimens for sinusitis should last for 10–30 days: Amoxicillin 500 mg tid or 875 mg bid* Amoxicillin-clavulanate (Augmentin) 500 mg tid or 875 mg bid* Clarithromycin (Biaxin XL) 500 mg 2 tabs qd Clindamycin (Cleocin) 150 mg qid Cephalexin (Keflex) 250–500 mg qid Doxycycline (Vibramycin) 100 mg bid	Decongestants and expectorants combined: Guaifenesin and pseudoephedrine HCl Phenylephrine HCl and guaifenesin Topical steroid nasal spray same as allergic rhinitis Increase humidity in environment Saline sprays or washes Warm compresses to face Change toothbrushes because of contamination May refer to ENT or allergist if symptoms not resolved in reasonable time Consider giving pneumococcal vaccine q5y to patients with frequent or chronic sinusitis Probiotics 1–2 × day for entire antibiotic course and 10 days afterwards; 8 oz yogurt bid
If patient seen within first 72 hr for influenza A:	Analgesic Cough and cold preparations Rest Increase fluid intake

Continued

Upper Respiratory Tract Disorders—cont'd

CONDITION	SIGNS AND SYMPTOMS	DIAGNOSTICS
	Coryza Cough Sore throat Vomiting and diarrhea Elderly may exhibit lower grade fever (if any), lassitude, confusion, nasal obstruction	CBC with differential Quick screen nasal swab for influenza
Allergic Rhinitis *Causative Agents* Seasonal: pollens, grasses, and weeds Perennial: dust, mold, animal dander and saliva, and roach hair and excreta	Pruritus of nose, eyes, palate, and oropharynx Tearing Cough and nasal congestion Sneezing Allergic shiners, puffiness around eyes, and conjunctival injection Seasonal: worse in morning and improved by evening Perennial: vary day to day	Nasal smear for eosinophils Allergy skin tests
Pharyngitis *Causative Agents* Group A streptococcus *Staphylococcus aureus* *Haemophilus influenzae* *Moraxella catarrhalis* Adenovirus Enteroviruses Epstein-Barr virus Coxsackievirus A Herpes virus	Sore throat Tender, enlarged lymph nodes† (strep: often anterior cervical; mononucleosis: often posterior cervical nodes) Tonsillar exudate† (usually yellow with strep, and may be gray-white with mononucleosis), erythema, and enlarged tonsils Fever† No cough† Headache Strawberry tongue Rough, red, soft palate	Rapid strep test Monospot Throat culture Elevated to normal WBC with >10% atypical lymphocytes may indicate viral illness; increased sedimentation rate and decreased platelets are all indicative of viral illness

†With all four criteria, treat for strep with penicillin (or macrolide, if patient is allergic to penicillin); with two to three criteria, get a rapid strep test and treat only if results are positive; with one criterion, do not test for strep—treat for sore throat or fever.

TREATMENT	ADJUNCT THERAPY
Oseltamivir (Tamiflu) bid × 7 days; prophylaxis 1 tab daily, should be started within 48 hr of contact and continued for 10 days Zanamivir (Relenza) diskhaler, 2 inhalations bid for 5 days	Should last 7–10 days Acetaminophen, ibuprofen for fever/myalgia Humidifier Increased fluids Rest and stay home
Topical Steroid Nasal Spray Beclomethasone dipropionate (Beconase) 1–2 sprays each nostril bid Flunisolide acetate (Nasalide) 2 sprays each nostril bid Fluticasone propionate (Flonase) 1 spray each nostril qd ***Antihistamines (OTC)*** ***Antihistamines (Prescription):*** Cetirizine (Zyrtec) 10 mg/day Fexofenadine (Allegra) 60 mg bid Desloratadine (Clarinex) 5 mg/day Azelastine (Astelin) nasal spray 2 sprays in each nostril bid ***Other*** Montelukast (Singulair) 10 mg qd	Environmental modifications Avoidance of the allergen (see p. 142) Nasal cromolyn (Nasalcrom) started before symptoms arise and used through allergy season may prevent or decrease symptoms

Bacterial Treatment
Penicillin G benzathine and Procaine (Bicillin CR) IM single dose (if known strep +)
  <30 lb: 600,000 U
  30–60 lb: 900,000–1.2 million U
  >60 lb: 2.4 million U
Penicillin VK 500 mg bid × 10 days (if known strep +)
Amoxicillin 500 mg tid or 875 mg bid × 10 days
If the patient is allergic to penicillin:
Erythromycin 250–500 mg tid × 10 days
Azithromycin (Z-Pak)
Cefpodoxime proxetil (Vantin) 100 mg bid × 5 days
Antibiotics are not recommended with mono (unless there is co-existing strep infection); if tonsils and pharynx are severely swollen, tapered dosing of oral prednisone 30–50 mg over 10–14 days may be required
	Salt water gargles qid
	Benadryl, Maalox, and viscous xylocaine mixture as swish and spit for pain relief
	Analgesics (OTC or narcotic)
	Throat lozenges
	Topical anesthetic sprays
	Rest
	Increase fluid intake
	No contact sports if spleen enlarged

Continued

Upper Respiratory Tract Disorders—cont'd

CONDITION	SIGNS AND SYMPTOMS	DIAGNOSTICS
	Halitosis Dysphagia (worse with mononucleosis)	
Common Cold *Causative Agents* Rhinoviruses Parainfluenza virus Coronavirus	Mucoid rhinorrhea Scratchy throat Nonproductive cough Loss of taste and smell Sneezing Feeling "stuffed up"	None

Asthma

Asthma 493.90 Bronchospasm 519.1 CHF 428.0 Eczema 692.9 Persistent Cough 786.2 Episodic Wheezing 786.07 Chest Tightness 786.59 Dyspnea 786.09	Tachypnea 786.06 Mild, Diffuse 786.07 Shortness of Breath 786.05 Speaks in Short Sentences 784.5 Loud Wheezing 786.07 Can Only Speak in Short Phrases 784.5 Fatigue 780.79 Pulsus Paradoxus 374.43	Diaphoresis 780.8 Cyanosis 782.5 Respiratory Alkalosis 276.3 Hypoxemia 799.0 Community-Acquired Pneumonia 486. Cough with Sputum Production 786.2 Rigors 780.99

Asthma is defined as chronic inflammatory condition of the airways. Episodes are associated with widespread and variable airflow obstruction that is reversible either spontaneously or with treatment. Inflammation aggravates existing bronchial hyperresponsiveness from a variety of stimuli. Atopy may be a predisposing factor Symptoms can be induced from:

- Environmental allergens
- Exercise
- Drugs (aspirin, NSAIDs)
- Structural defects (polyps)
- Occupational conditions (chemical irritants)
- Bronchospasm from CHF
- Exposure to cold temperature and foods (e.g., ice cream)

SIGNS AND SYMPTOMS
- Persistent cough (may be only sign) occurring at night or with exercise, especially in cold and dry air
- Episodic, mild, diffuse wheezing
- Chest tightness

TREATMENT	ADJUNCT THERAPY
Cefaclor (Ceclor) 250–500 mg tid × 10 days	
Viral Treatment	
Supportive care unless symptoms change to bacterial	
Consider "burst" and "taper" steroid therapy for severe pain and/or swelling with mononucleosis	
No antibiotics unless secondary bacterial infection occurs	Decongestants
	Analgesics
	Rest
	Should last approximately 7–10 days
	Increase fluid intake
	Humidifier

- Dyspnea
- Tachypnea
- Prolonged expiratory phase
- Shortness of breath
- Speaks in short sentences with minor difficulty

More severe attacks
- Loud wheezing
- Use of accessory muscles
- Distant breath sounds
- Hyperresonance
- Intercostal retractions
- Can only speak in short phrases

Ominous signs
- Fatigue
- Pulsus paradoxus
- Diaphoresis
- Inaudible breath sounds with diminished wheezing
- Inability to lie flat
- Cyanosis (especially acral)
- Can only speak in words

DIAGNOSTICS
- CBC may show elevated WBC count, eosinophilia
- Peak expiratory flow rate decreased to <60% (see Appendix C)
- Respiratory alkalosis and mild hypoxemia on blood gases

Text continued on p. 142

Table 5-1   Red Eye Chart

Bacterial Conjunctivitis	372.30	Blepharitis	373.00	Acute Closed Angle Glaucoma	365.20
Allergic Conjunctivitis	372.14	Pterygium	372.40	Hordeolum	373.11
Viral Conjunctivitis	077.99	Subconjunctival Hemorrhage	372.72	Chalazion	373.2
Iritis	364.3	Zoster Ophthalmicus	053.20	Dacryocystitis	375.30
Keratoconjunctivitis	370.40	Corneal Abrasion	918.1		

CONDITION	SIGNS/SYMPTOMS	ADDITIONAL POINTS	TREATMENT
Bacterial conjunctivitis	Itching Tearing Moderate amount of yellow-green discharge Moderate conjunctival hyperemia No pain or vision disturbance No preauricular adenopathy Cornea clear	Bilateral or unilateral involvement Mucopurulent (yellow-green) discharge Red, shiny appearance to lower lids More common in winter and spring R/O sinusitis	***Broad-Spectrum Topical Antibiotics for 5 Days*** Sodium sulfacetamide 10% ophthalmic gtts (Bleph-10) 1-2gtts tid Gentamicin 3% ophthalmic gtts; 1-2gtts qid Ciprofloxacin 3.5% ophthalmic gtts (Ciloxan) 1-2gtts q2h while awake for 2 days then q4h (NOTE: Any of the above medications can be used as ointments also) ***General Measures*** Cold compresses to periocular area Artificial tears frequently Warn the patient and/or parents of the contagiousness of disease Child should not attend school or daycare until having received antibiotics for 24hr Use separate towels, frequently wash hands, avoid hand shaking Consider treating both eyes, even if unilateral infection

		Do not use topical steroids unless herpes simplex (dendritelike or shingles pattern on fluorescein staining) is ruled out Refer to ophthalmologist if not markedly better in 4 days
Allergic conjunctivitis	Bilateral itching Watery discharge May have history of atopy Conjunctiva and lids are swollen and reddened Intense itching of both eyes; if only one eye is involved, investigate further Seasonal occurrence May be accompanied by sneezing, rhinorrhea, "throat itching" Common in spring and fall	Avoid allergens Cold compresses Topical products to relieve itching and redness: Nedocromil 2% sol (Alocril) 1–2 gtts bid Olopatadine 0.1% sol (Patanol) 1–2 gtts bid Levocabastine 0.05% sol (Livostin) 1 gtt qid Artificial tears to decrease irritation
Viral conjunctivitis	Burning Itching Conjunctival injection Tearing Recent contact with another person with "red eye" Unilateral initial presentation followed by bilateral infection May find preauricular lymph node Often associated with URI Watery, mucoid discharge Moderate amount of mucous debris Transmission is from direct contact or from contaminated objects	Cold compresses Gently cleanse with water to remove debris (remember to wipe from inside of eye to outside) Artificial tears to decrease irritation Warn the patient of contagiousness of disease Frequently wash hands, use separate towels, avoid hand-shaking No antibiotic drops

Continued

5

Table 5-1 Red Eye Chart—cont'd

CONDITION	SIGNS/SYMPTOMS	ADDITIONAL POINTS	TREATMENT
Iritis	Redness in the area surrounding the cornea called "ciliary flush" Photophobia caused by movement of iris Pain with direct and indirect light Unilateral painful, red eye without discharge	*Caused by* Trauma Recent ocular surgery Ankylosing spondylitis Reiter's syndrome Arthritic psoriasis Herpes simplex or zoster	Urgent referral to an ophthalmologist
Keratoconjunctivitis (dry eye)	Inadequate tear film to cover and protect the cornea and conjunctiva Nonspecific irritation Burning Redness Dryness Foreign body sensation or gritty feeling	*Caused by:* Medications (antihistamines, Retin-A, beta blockers, atropine); ask also about dry mouth Lid deformities (scarring, blepharitis, incomplete closure with sleeping) Corneal deformities (pterygium) Rheumatic fever, SLE, Sjögren's syndrome Fluorescein staining reveals punctate staining on the cornea	Preservative-free artificial tears Lubricating ointment at night Humidifier when sleeping Investigation and elimination of the causes Referral to an ophthalmologist if condition persists
Blepharitis	Conjunctival redness and irritation Dryness, burning Dandifflike debris on lid margins and eyelashes	Associated with acne rosacea or seborrheic dermatitis May be due to overgrowth of *S. aureus* or *S. epidermidis*	Warm eyelid compresses and eyelid scrubs with baby shampoo 2–3 times per day; continue bid for 1 mo then daily after symptoms improve

		With chronic cases, may need antibiotic ointment (erythromycin [Ilotycin] ophthalmic ointment at hs or bacitracin ophthalmic ointment 3–4 times a day for 2–3 wk) Goal is to minimize symptoms because of the chronicity of disease If there is coexisting dandruff, treat condition
Pterygium	Conjunctival degeneration with resulting opacity partially covering the cornea Most commonly seen at the 3 o'clock or 9 o'clock position Conjunctival injection, tear filming	Usually grows slowly May obstruct vision Most commonly seen in persons with excessive exposure to ultraviolet light, windy conditions, or dusty surroundings	Surgical removal if visual disturbance occurs Artificial tears for irritation Protective eyewear when outside Consider ketorolac (Acular) ophthalmic 1 gtt qid until condition is improved
Subconjunctival hemorrhage	Blood loculated between bulbar conjunctiva and sclera	*Caused by:* Trauma Excessive straining Coughing Hypertension Vomiting	R/O bulbar rupture by following bleeding to posterior borders R/O hypertension No treatment necessary if no cause can be found; reassure person that symptoms usually resolve in 2–4 wk
Zoster ophthalmicus	Eye pain, tearing Photophobia Moderate conjunctival hyperemia Cornea may be clear or cloudy Mucoid discharge	Severe pain Vesicles may or may not be present Usually reactivation of old disease because of stress or infection Dendritic stain with fluorescein	Urgent referral to an ophthalmologist

Continued

Table 5–1 Red Eye Chart—cont'd

CONDITION	SIGNS/SYMPTOMS	ADDITIONAL POINTS	TREATMENT
Corneal abrasion	Pain and foreign body sensation Photophobia Tearing Conjunctival hyperemia	Usual history of scratching eye, feeling something hit eye, contact lens, or actual trauma Stain with fluorescein and use cobalt blue filter light to inspect eye for foreign objects or scratches	*Topical Antibiotic Drops or Ointment for 5 Days:* Sodium sulfacetamide (Bleph-10) 1–2 gtts tid Erythromycin (Ilotycin) small strip ointment to eye, 3–6 times a day Patching is usually necessary for 24hr except for contact wearers or for those patients with trauma from vegetative matter or fingernails (patching may mask infection) Remove contact lens until healing has occurred; use antipseudomonal drops (ciprofloxacin 2 gtts affected eye q4h or ofloxacin 1–2 gtts q1–6h × 7–10 days) Observe daily until resolved
Acute closed-angle glaucoma	Severe pain Constricted pupils Diffuse conjunctival hyperemia Corneal cloudiness	Sudden onset blurred vision and pain Nausea and vomiting Halos around light Fixed midpositioned pupils	Urgent referral to an ophthalmologist

Hordeolum	Swollen, tender, erythematous lesion located on eyelid margin Duration less than a few weeks	Caused by a blocked meibomian or Zeis gland; may be staphylococcal infection	Warm, moist compresses tid-qid for 20 min *Topical Antibiotic Ointment tid × 5 Days* Sodium sulfacetamide (Bleph-10) Erythromycin (Ilotycin)
Chalazion	Sterile, localized granuloma tissue on eyelid; gradual onset Firm, reddened nodule May be minimally painful, more irritating than painful Usually does not affect vision		May see spontaneous resolution over several years If visual disturbance or cosmetic problems occur, referral to an ophthalmologist is necessary
Dacryocystitis	Red, swollen painful medial canthus around the tear duct opening Tearing Discomfort May have fever	Obstruction of lacrimal sac due to infection or inflammation from overgrowth of normal skin flora, trauma, congenital obstruction, or nasal or sinus surgery Common pathogens are *S. aureus, S. pyogenes, S. epidermidis* May lead to cellulitis	Cultures of discharge *Topical Antibiotic Drops* Sodium sulfacetamide (Bleph-10) 1–2 gtt tid Erythromycin (Ilotycin) 1–2 gtt qid Ofloxacin (Ocuflox) 1–2 gtt q1–6h × 7–10 days Massage to ductal area Warm moist compresses Follow closely q24–48h

5

- CXR shows hyperinflation
- Pulse oximetry <90%

DEFINITION AND TREATMENT

See Tables 5–2 and 5–3

Practice Pearls

- Prevention of exposure to irritants or control of allergens is of utmost importance
- Early diagnosis and treatment are essential for maintaining normalcy
- Strength of attacks can be minimized with early treatment
- Treat any underlying illness or refer to allergist for testing
- Inhaled steroids DO NOT affect long-term growth in children
- Avoid less selective beta$_2$ agonists such as epinephrine, metaproterenol, and isoproterenol
- Albuterol liquid, which causes severe irritability, should be avoided if nebulized or inhaled beta$_2$ agonists can be used
- If more than two canisters are used per month, control of asthma is in question
- Albuterol can be used to control exercise-induced asthma (EIA) symptoms
- Tell patients not to trust the "float" test to determine how full their inhalers are; many of the new inhalers will float if they are full
- Patients with asthma should be instructed to perform peak flow testing daily and monitor their asthma symptoms based on peak flow "personal best" calculations; when exacerbations occur, there should be a plan in place to allow patient to start therapy immediately (see Appendix D)

ALLERGEN CONTROL MEASURES

- Because many patients with asthma have environmental stimuli that exacerbate their symptoms, allergen control is important; these measures can be beneficial for any persons who have allergy-induced rhinitis, sneezing, coughing, wheezing, or other respiratory symptoms that disrupt the person's daily activities; these are measures that must be instituted in the home and other places where the person spends a lot of time; the patient must be faithful in carrying out these measures daily
- Allergens usually fall into two categories: outdoor and indoor; the following are patient instructions for controlling allergens:

Outdoor Allergens

- Determine if there is a particular season that aggravates your asthma or allergies
- Keep your windows closed and use air-conditioning with ultra-sensitive filters
- When out driving, keep your windows up and use air-conditioning in car
- Limit your outdoor activity to early morning or late evening
- Limit number of houseplants in your home
- Wear mask when outdoors if you are going to mow the yard or rake leaves

Text continued on p. 148

Table 5-2 Definition and Treatment for Asthma

SYMPTOMS	PULMONARY FUNCTION*	LONG-TERM CONTROL	QUICK RELIEF
Mild Intermittent No more than 2 attacks per week Asymptomatic with normal PEF between exacerbations Exacerbations brief with variable intensity *Nighttime Symptoms* No more than 2 times a month	PEF 80% predicted with <20% variability Spirometry q2y	No daily medications required Patient education should be started continually reinforced with each visit Assess patient's knowledge of using inhalers initially and when changing types of inhalers Allergen control (see pp. 142, 148) Peak flow monitoring (see Appendix D for patient handout)	Short-acting bronchodilator such as inhaled beta$_2$ agonists (see Table 5-3)
Mild Persistent More than 2 episodes a week but <1 per day Exacerbations may inhibit activity *Nighttime Symptoms* More than 2 times a month	PEF 80% predicted with 20%-30% variability Spirometry q2y	Daily medications required Antiinflammatory inhaled corticosteroid (see Table 5-3) Patient education as with Mild Intermittent *Alternate Therapy* Sustained-release theophylline; must monitor closely for therapeutic levels *or* Leukotriene receptor antagonists (see Table 5-3)	Short-acting inhaled beta$_2$ agonist bronchodilator as needed for symptom control (see Table 5-3) Monitor number of exacerbations If beta$_2$ agonist used daily or frequency of use is increasing, may need additional long-term therapy Consult with physician for ongoing therapy
Moderate Persistent Daily symptoms Daily use of inhaled short-acting beta$_2$ agonists	PEF >60% but <80% predicted PEF >30% variability Spirometry q1-2y	Daily medication required Antiinflammatory agents for inhalation (same medication as for mild persistent asthma	Inhaled short-acting beta$_2$ agonist bronchodilator (see Table 5-3) should be used for symptom relief Daily use of inhaled short-acting

*See Appendix C.
PEF, Peak expiratory flow rate.

Continued

Table 5-2 Definition and Treatment for Asthma—cont'd

SYMPTOMS	PULMONARY FUNCTION*	LONG-TERM CONTROL	QUICK RELIEF
More than 2 exacerbations per week; activity affected *Nighttime Symptoms* More than one exacerbation a week		Antiinflammatory inhalation agent with a long-acting bronchodilator (see Table 5-3 for medications) Sustained-release theophylline can be used with antiinflammatory inhaler for relief of nighttime symptoms Leukotriene receptor antagonist (see Table 5-3) Patient education as with Mild Intermittent	beta$_2$ agonist is an indication for reevaluation of current therapy Consult with physician about referral if symptoms are not controlled
Severe Persistent Continual symptoms Limited physical activity Frequent exacerbations *Nighttime Symptoms* Frequent	PEF <60% with variability >30% Spirometer q1-2y	Daily medications include antiinflammatory inhaled corticosteroids *and* long-acting bronchodilators (see Table 5-3 for medications) May require sustained-release theophylline preparations *and/or* corticosteroids in a short-burst therapy or long-term therapy, depending on severity of disease and number of exacerbations Leukotriene receptor antagonist (see Table 5-3) Patient education as with Mild Intermittent	Short-acting beta$_2$ agonist inhaled bronchodilators (see Table 5-3) for immediate symptom relief If inhalers are being used daily, treatment may need to be reevaluated Refer to physician

*See Appendix C.
PEF, Peak expiratory flow rate.

Table 5–3 Drugs for Asthma

DRUG	ADULT DOSE	CHILD DOSE
Inhaled Short-Acting Beta$_2$ Agonist		
Albuterol nebulized solution (5 mg/ml)	2.5–5 mg q20 min × 3 doses, then 2.5–10 mg q4h prn	0.15 mg/kg q20 min × 3 doses, then 0.15–0.3 mg/kg q4h prn
Albuterol MDI (90 mcg/puff)	4 puffs q20 min up to 4 hr, then q4h prn	4 puffs q20 min × 3 doses, then q4h prn
Levalbuterol (Xopenex) nebulized solution: 1.25 mg/3 ml, 0.63 mg/3 ml, 0.31 mg/3 ml	0.63–1.25 mg solution q6–8h Do not mix with other drugs No dilution	6–11 yr = 0.31 mg nebulized solution tid >11 yr = 0.63 mg nebulized solution tid Do not mix with other drugs No dilution needed
Anticholinergics*		
Ipratropium bromide (Atrovent) solution for nebulizer: 500 mcg/vial	500 mcg q30 min × 3 doses then q2–4h prn Can be mixed with beta$_2$ agonists Not used first-line therapy	250 mcg q20 min × 3 doses then q2–4h Can be mixed with beta$_2$ agonists Not used first-line therapy*
Ipratropium bromide MDI (18 mcg/puff)	2–3 puffs q6–8h	1–2 puffs q6–8h Spacer with MDI will enhance therapy
Inhaled Corticosteroids†		
Beclomethasone dipropionate (QVAR) 40 and 80 mcg/spray MDI	40–80 mcg/spray bid (if patient is using bronchodilators alone) 40–160 mcg/spray bid (if patient is using other inhaled steroids)	5–11 yr = 40–80 mcg bid Start 40 mcg/spray bid and increase dose as needed
Budesonide (Pulmicort) DPI (dry powder inhaler) 200 mcg/dose	200–600 mcg/dose bid	200–400 mcg/dose bid
Budesonide (Pulmicort) 0.25, 0.5 mg/2 ml solution for nebulizer	0.25–0.5 mg/2 ml bid	1–8 yr = 0.25–0.5 mg 1–2 times a day if patient is using bronchodilator alone

*Contraindicated with soy or peanut allergy.
†Rinse mouth after use.

Continued

Table 5-3 Drugs for Asthma—cont'd

DRUG	ADULT DOSE	CHILD DOSE
Flunisolide (AeroBid) 250 mcg/puff	2 puffs bid	0.5 mg/day if patient is taking inhaled steroids 1 mg/day if patient is taking oral steroids 6–15 yr = 2 puffs bid
Fluticasone (Flovent) 44, 110, 220 mcg/puff	88–220 mcg bid	4–11 yr = 44–220 mcg bid
Fluticasone (Flovent Rotadisk) DPI 50, 100, 250 mcg/spray	100–1000 mcg bid Start at 100 mcg with bronchodilator alone bid Start 100–250 mcg if patient is taking inhaled steroids Start 1000 mcg bid if patient is undergoing long-term use of oral steroids	4–11 yr = 50–100 mcg bid > 12 yr = use adult dose
Triamcinolone (Azmacort) 100 mcg/spray	2 puff q6–8h or 4 puffs bid	6–12 yr = 1–2 puffs q6–8h >12 yr = use adult dose
Long-Acting Beta₂ Agonists Salmeterol (Serevent) MDI 21 mcg/spray DPI 50 mcg blister	1 puff q12h 1 blister q12h **Not for acute episodes**	<4 yr = 2 puffs q12h; use spacer if >8yr >12 yr for exercise-induced asthma (EIA); 2 puffs 30–60 min before exercise **Not for acute episodes**
Formoterol (Foradil) DPI 12 mcg/powder capsule	1 capsule DPI q12h 1 inhalation 15 min before exercise; may repeat in 12 hr **Not for acute episodes**	>5 yr = 1 DPI q12h >12 yr = 1–2 DPI inhalation 15 min before exercise; may repeat in 12 hr prn **Not for acute episodes**
Combination Long-Acting Beta₂ Agonist and Steroid Inhaler† Fluticasone/salmeterol (Advair) 100/50, 250/50, or 500/50 mcg DPI	1 inhalation bid Start with 100/50 mcg bid if patient is not taking any other steroids	12 yr = 1 inhalation bid No child dose

Medication	Adult	Pediatric
Other		
Theophylline comes in liquid, sustained release tablets and capsules	If patient is using steroids, start dose 250/50 mcg up to 500/50 mcg bid Starting dose 10 mg/kg/day not to exceed 900 mg/day	Elixophyllin 80 mg/15 ml 1–9 yr = 20–24 mg/kg/day 9–12 yr = 16 mg/kg/day 12–16 yr = 13 mg/kg/day Dosing is twice daily
Systemic oral steroids Prednisone: 1, 2.5, 5, 10, 50 mg Prednisolone: Pediapred 5 mg/5 ml Prelone 15 mg/5 ml	5–60 mg qd Usually given as "burst" therapy; start with high dose and taper over 5–10 days	1–2 mg/kg orally qd Usually given as "burst" therapy; short course starting with higher dose and taper quickly over 5–10 days
Leukotriene Modifiers		
Zafirlukast (Accolate): 10 mg or 20 mg tablet	20 mg bid Take on empty stomach	5–11 yr = 10 mg bid >12 yr = 20 mg bid Take on empty stomach
Montelukast (Singulair) 4 or 5 mg chew or 10 mg tablet	10 mg at hs	2–5 yr = 4 mg at hs 6–14 yr = 5 mg at hs
Zileuton (Zyflo) 300 mg or 600 mg tablet	600 mg qid with meals and at bedtime	None available
Cromolyn MDI 800 mcg/puff Nebulizer 20 mg/2 ml	2–4 puffs 3–4 times a day 20 mg/2 ml 3–4 times a day Initiate treatment before suspected symptoms	>2 yr 1–2 puffs 3–4 times a day 20 mg/2 ml 3–4 times a day Initiate treatment before suspected symptoms

*Contraindicated with soy or peanut allergy.
†Rinse mouth after use.

Indoor Allergens
- ☐ Wear mask when vacuuming or cleaning draperies or curtains
- ☐ Remove carpeting wherever possible
- ☐ Dust mite control should include:
  1. Covering or encasing mattresses and pillows with plastic covers
  2. Wash bedding weekly in hot water
  3. Replace bedroom carpets with hardwood floors or linoleum
  4. Vacuum bedroom carpets frequently using HEPA ultra-sensitive filters
  5. Remove any upholstered pieces of furniture and other dust collectors
  6. Decrease humidity in house and especially in bedroom
- ☐ Limit exposure to cockroaches and to the feces from cockroaches by:
  1. Prompt clean up after meals and remove and clean dishes
  2. Seal all food sources and dishes tightly
  3. Seal gaps around kitchen and bathroom pipes
  4. Either use some brand of roach bait stations or have cockroaches in house professionally exterminated
- ☐ Cat and dog allergens are another possible source of stimuli for asthmatics:
  1. If possible remove cat and/or dog from your environment
  2. If you cannot remove your pet from your environment, keep your pet out of your bedroom
  3. Minimize contacts with animals whenever possible
  4. Wash your pet weekly in water to decrease dander and loose hairs
  5. Keep pets off your furniture, especially chairs that you use frequently
  6. Vacuuming to remove dander and loose hairs is important and must be done weekly
  7. Make sure your pet has no fleas or ticks

Community Acquired Pneumonia (CAP)*

CONDITION
- Community acquired pneumonia is defined as acute infection of pulmonary parenchyma
- Caused by bacteria from the upper airway migrating to the lower airways
- See Table 5–4 for common pathogens

SIGNS AND SYMPTOMS
- Sudden onset and rapid progression of symptoms indicative of bacterial pneumonia
- General symptoms of CAP
  - ☐ Tachypnea, tachycardia, cyanosis
  - ☐ Fever, malaise, myalgia
  - ☐ Cough, exertional dyspnea, pleuritic chest pain

---

*Information adapted from IDSA/ATS guidelines.

Table 5-4 Common Pathogens in Community Acquired Pneumonia

Common pathogens associated with healthy persons	*Streptococcus pneumoniae* *Mycoplasma pneumoniae* *Chlamydia pneumoniae* *Haemophilus influenzae* *Respiratory virus* *Legionella pneumophila*
Common pathogen associated with elderly, communal exposure (daycare, long-term care facility), debilitated persons	*S. pneumoniae* *H. influenzae* *L. pneumophila* *Moraxella catarrhalis* *Pseudomonas* *Enterobacter*
Common pathogens associated with long-term disease (e.g., diabetes, alcoholism) or smoking	*S. pneumoniae* *H. influenzae* *Klebsiella* *L. pneumophila*
Common pathogens associated with altered sensorium and/or CNS impairment	*Staphylococcus acoreus* *M. catarrhalis* *Bacteroides*

- □ Anorexia, weight loss
- □ Decrease breath sounds, wheezing, rhonchi, rales
- □ Egophony ("e" to "a" sound) on auscultation, pleural friction rub, dullness to percussion
- Cough with sputum production
  - □ Bloody to rust colored may indicate streptococcal pneumonia
  - □ Green sputum may indicate pseudomonas, *H. influenzae,* or streptococcal pneumonia
  - □ Foul-smelling sputum may indicate anaerobes
  - □ Currant jelly consistency sputum may indicate *Klebsiella* or streptococcal pneumonia
- Rigors (severe shaking chills) followed by fever suggest streptococcal pneumonia
- H/A, malaise, N/V/D suggests infection with *Legionella*

DIAGNOSTICS

- CXR (AP and lateral views) should show frank consolidation in area of pneumonia and possible pleural effusion
  - □ False-negative results can occur with dehydration or very early onset of pneumonia

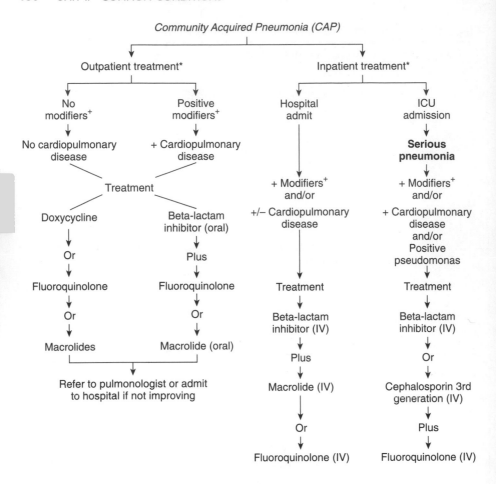

FIGURE 5–1 Community acquired pneumonia (CAP).

□ CXR is indicated in all symptomatic patients >40 years, current smokers or past smokers; a repeat CXR should be done in 4 to 6 weeks

□ If patient has consistent signs and symptoms of pneumonia but CXR does not show pneumonia, treat patient for pneumonia

- Pulse oximetry results should be >95% on room air and should not drop significantly with exertion
- If patient is >65 years, comorbidity exists or possible hospital admission; obtain CBC and complete metabolic profile
  - Leukocytosis with left shift may indicate bacterial infection; elderly may not have competent immune system to generate this response
  - Leukopenia (leukocytes <5000 mm^3) may indicate impending sepsis
  - Hgb <9 mg/dl and/or Hct <30% is indicative of higher mortality
- Sputum and/or blood cultures may be helpful in identifying pathogen(s) and using correct antibiotic
  - Disadvantage of sputum cultures
    1. Long incubation period of identification of pathogen
    2. Difficult to obtain a good specimen
    3. Findings may not change treatment

TREATMENT

- Determine how to treat based on patient's condition, suspected pathogen, and any modifying factors (Figure 5–1)
- Suggested antibiotic therapy (Table 5–5)

Table 5–5 Drug Therapy for Community Acquired Pneumonia

DRUG CLASS	DOSAGE*
Macrolides	Azithromycin (Z-Pak) 500 mg day 1; 250 mg days 2–5; in hospital: 500 mg IV qd, switch as soon as possible to oral zithromycin Erythromycin 333 mg 1 tab tid or 500 mg bid; 1 g IV q6h
Penicillins and beta-lactam inhibitors	Penicillin VK 500 mg q6h Amoxicillin 500–1000 mg tid Amoxicillin/clavulanate (Augmentin) 875 mg bid Nafcillin 1.5–2 g IV q4–6h
Tetracycline	Doxycycline 100 mg bid

Cephalosporin
  Second generation
  Third generation
	Cefaclor (Ceclor) 500 mg tid
	Cefprozil (Cefzil) 250–500 mg bid
	Cefuroxime (Ceftin) 250–500 mg bid
	Ceftriaxone (Rocephin) 500–1000 mg IM qd
	Cefpodoxime (Vantin) 200–400 mg bid
	Ceftazidime (Fortaz) 1 g IV/IM q8–12h

Fluoroquinolone (has antipseudomonal activity)	Levofloxacin (Levaquin) 750 mg po/IV qd Gatifloxacin (Tequin) 200–400 mg po/IV qd Moxifloxacin (Avelox) 400 mg po/IV qd; if started in hospital switch to oral medication as soon as possible
Other microbial agents	Vancomycin 1 g IV q12h Zyvox 600 mg po/IV q12h for 10–28 days

*Length of therapy usually 10 to 14 days.

- Suggested length of antibiotic therapy based on known or suspected cause of pneumonia
  - Streptococcal pneumonia: 7 days
  - *Mycoplasma, Chlamydia, Legionella*: 10 to 14 days
  - With long-term corticosteroid use, treat for >14 days
- Treat until afebrile and for at least 72 hours after fever resolves
- IV antibiotic therapy can be switched to oral antibiotic therapy (with same or similar class antibiotic) when patient can tolerate food and oral medications, has been afebrile for 24 hours, and shows obvious improvement in symptoms of cough and dyspnea
- Consider stopping PPI or switch to H_2 blocker (PPI may increase the chance of recurrent pneumonia) until antibiotic therapy is finished

Lower Respiratory Tract Disorders

| Acute Bronchitis | 466.0 |
| Mycobacterium Tuberculosis | 011.9 |

CONDITION	SIGNS AND SYMPTOMS
Acute Bronchitis An inflammatory process that involves the tracheobronchial tree, usually occurring after a URI Causative agents may involve rhinovirus, adenovirus, influenza, and other infectious agents Occurs more frequently in smokers and usually lasts longer; subsequent bacterial infections may occur more frequently in smokers	Increased mucus production with coughing, can be purulent or clear with varying amounts; the amount of mucus may indicate whether this is viral or bacterial, with more mucus produced if infection is bacterial Frequent paroxysms of coughing; smokers have longer periods of coughing Persistent dry cough May have wheezing and SOB Occasional fever (low-grade) Lung sounds: wheezing, scattered rales relieved with cough, rhonchi over large bronchi, early inspiratory rales Rhinitis pharyngitis, myalgias

- Patient may need oxygen support initially; if bronchitis is present, nebulizer treatment with beta agonist may help to decrease wheeze and cough; humidifier; increase fluid intake to 2 to 4 L a day

PREVENTION

- Encourage influenza and pneumococcal vaccines to all high-risk patients
- Stop smoking, stop IV drug use
- Keep teeth in good repair
- Non-leukopenic compromised patients (RA, SLE, alcoholism, DM, chronic high-dose steroid use, etc.) may not develop immunity when given pneumococcal or haemophylis vaccines

DIAGNOSTICS	TREATMENT

CXR usually normal or may show hyperinflation from new or old pulmonary disease and with long-term smoking
CBC usually normal
Sputum culture usually not indicated and not beneficial
	Symptomatic
	Stop smoking
	Increase fluids to 3000 ml/day
	Increase humidity
	Rest
	Acetaminophen for generalized discomfort
	Cough suppressants for nighttime coughing:
	    Benzonatate (Tessalon Perles) 1 tid–qid
	    Dextromethorphan 30 mg q6–8h prn
	    Codeine 15–30 mg q4–6h prn
	Expectorants can be useful
	If wheezing is present with SOB, nebulizer therapy with albuterol
	
	Consider the Following Modalities
	Healthy Adult:
	No antibiotics
	Use inhaler or nebulizer with albuterol routinely q4–6h for 3–5 days
	Cough suppressant
	
	Adult with Known COPD or Elderly with Underlying Disease:
	
	Antibiotic Therapy
	Clarithromycin (Biaxin) 500 mg 2 tabs qd × 7 days
	Azithromycin (Z-Pak)

Continued

Lower Respiratory Tract Disorders—cont'd

CONDITION	SIGNS AND SYMPTOMS
Mycobacterium Tuberculosis (TB)	
Primary lung infection acquired via droplets from contaminated persons	Fatigue
Under normal circumstances, the TB bacterium is inhaled and thus attracts the body's normal defense system; the bacterium is walled off without further incident; 90%–95% of TB bacteria are dormant	Weight loss (without trying)
	Fever (usually low-grade)
	Night sweats lasting longer than 1–3 wk
	Productive cough (initially dry; progresses to purulent; may see blood)
	Anorexia
TB becomes active when the body's defenses undergo periods of stress, fighting off current infections, corticosteroid therapy, or with aging of the immune system	
Common sites are the apices of the lungs, but disseminated TB can affect any body system	
Outbreaks of multi-drug resistant TB (MDR-TB) have doubled in the last 10 yr because of poor compliance with TB drug regimens, the advent of HIV drug therapy, and the increased number of immigrants	
When patient has a chronic disease or lives in a nursing home or a crowded home with poor hygiene, the possibility of TB is great	

DIAGNOSTICS	TREATMENT
	Amoxicillin-clavulanate 500 mg tid or 875 mg bid × 7 days
	Levofloxacin (Levaquin) 500 mg qd × 7 days
	Refer if no improvement seen in 3–5 days or if respiratory distress occurs
Mantoux skin test for TB: positive results if transverse diameter of the indurated area is as follows (use a ballpoint pen to lightly mark the skin in four directions toward the injection site; the pen will stop at the border of induration):	Refer to physician or health department for medications and follow-up
>5 mm if patient is HIV+, prior contact with TB+ person, abnormal CXR or child with symptoms of TB	
>10 mm if patient is foreign born, from high-risk countries, lives in medically underserved area, lives in long-term care facility, is drug abuser, health care worker, or a child <4 yr old	
>15 mm: all other persons	
Sputum culture for acid-fast bacilli	
Sputum culture for *M. tuberculosis*	
CXR may show old calcification in apex, pleural effusion	
Bronchoscopy with washings	

Chronic Obstructive Pulmonary Disease

Chronic Obstructive Pulmonary Disease	496.
Chronic Bronchitis	491.9
Emphysema	492.8

CONDITION	SIGNS AND SYMPTOMS
Chronic Bronchitis Causative agents are air pollution, airway infections, familial factors, allergy, and tobacco use Usually occurs in persons older than 35 yr	Excessive secretion of bronchial mucus with productive cough >3 mo Mild-to-moderate dyspnea Persistent-to-severe cough with mucopurulent sputum production History of multiple airway infections Rhonchi, wheezes, and central cyanosis Obesity Right ventricular failure common
Emphysema Results from excessive lysis of elastin or other structural proteins by lung neutrophils and macrophages Usually occurs in persons older than 50 yr Long-term tobacco use may be a cause	Abnormal permanent enlargement of air spaces distal to terminal bronchiole Has cough with mild-to-moderate sputum production SOB for >10 yr Cough occurs in mornings Dyspnea initially on exertion, then progresses to at rest Sputum is clear to mucoid Weight loss Person is usually thin and wasted appearing with hypertrophied accessory breathing muscles AP to lateral diameter increased Hyperresonant percussion and decreased breath sounds ***Acute Exacerbation*** Increased dyspnea, tachypnea Fatigue Tachycardia Use of accessory muscles Purulent sputum O_2 saturation <88% Fever (maybe)

5

DIAGNOSTICS	TREATMENT (FOR BOTH CHRONIC BRONCHITIS AND EMPHYSEMA)
CXR shows "dirty lungs" with increased markings Often heart is enlarged Diaphragm is asymmetric and rounded Elevated Hct Hypoxemia and hypercapnia *Pulmonary Function* (see Appendix C) Peak expiratory flow rate <60% normal Forced expiratory volume >3 sec	*Education* Avoid smoking, aspirin, beta blockers, and temperature extremes Assess work environment for irritants Liquefy secretions with oral hydration of at least 3000 ml/day (if not contraindicated because of CHF) Humidifier, especially at night Bronchial hygiene with pursed lip breathing and deep breathing before deep coughing Chest physiotherapy and postural drainage
Early Disease CXR shows decreased markings in periphery, hyperinflation Diaphragm is low or flat Sinus tachycardia on ECG ABGs are WNL *Progressive Disease* CXR has similar appearance but with bullae and blebs Enlarged heart Secondary polycythemia Supraventricular tachycardia on ECG Compensated respiratory acidosis *Pulmonary Function* (see Appendix C and p. 158) Total lung capacity increased (air cannot escape) and poor expulsion of air Increased respiratory volume	*Drug Therapies* Bronchodilator drugs (nebulizer better than inhaler) Ipratropium bromide (Atrovent) 2–4 puffs q6h Ipratropium and albuterol (Combivent) 2 puffs qid Albuterol 2 puffs q4–6h (as inhaler); or as nebulizer 0.25–0.5 ml in 3 ml normal saline q4–6h Inhaled steroids, for patient with medium-severe COPD who shows objective benefit with it (see Table 5–3) Theophylline is third-line drug now Oxygen as needed *Acute Exacerbation* Antibiotics for 7 days only with severe exacerbations Amoxicillin-clavulanate (Augmentin) 500 mg tid *or* 875 mg bid Doxycycline 100 mg bid Clarithromycin (Biaxin) 500 mg 2 tabs qd Levofloxacin (Levaquin) 500 mg qd Systemic corticosteroids 0.6–1.0 mg/kg/day; taper over 1–2 wk period; if no improvement in 24–48 hr, consider pulmonary consult or hospitalization

How to Read Pulmonary Tests Quickly

FUNCTION	NORMAL (%)	OBSTRUCTIVE	RESTRICTIVE	COMBINED
FVC	≥80	N to ↓	↓	↓
FEV$_1$	≥80	N to ↓	↓	↓
FEV$_1$/FVC	≥75	↓	N to ↑	↓
FEF	≥80	↓	↑, N, or ↓	↓
TLC	80–120	N to ↑	↓	↓
RV/TLC	25–40	↑	N	↑

FEF, Forced expiratory flow; *FEV$_1$*, forced expiratory volume in 1 second; *FVC*, forced vital capacity; *RV*, residual volume; *TLC*, total lung capacity.

Types of Pulmonary Disease

Emphysema 492.8	Bronchiectasis 494.0
Chronic Bronchitis 491.9	Cystic Fibrosis 277.00
Bronchial Asthma 493.90	Tracheobronchomalacia 519.1

OBSTRUCTIVE	RESTRICTIVE	OTHER RESTRICTIVE
Emphysema	Interstitial fibrosis	Thoracic deformities or surgery
Chronic bronchitis	Pulmonary edema	Pleural effusion
Bronchial asthma	Pneumonia	Pneumothorax or hemothorax
Bronchiectasis	Vascular congestion	Abdominal girth enlargement
Cystic fibrosis	Adult respiratory distress	Neuromuscular defects
Tracheobronchomalacia	syndrome (ARDS)	Respiratory center depression
	Sarcoidosis	Obesity
Treatment	*Treatment*	*Treatment*
May benefit from medication therapy for bronchodilation and secretion control	May be no particular treatment to correct disease	May need surgical correction for bone deformities or for fluid buildup
May need antibiotics at first sign of illness	Palliative treatment to enhance oxygen saturation	May be caused by surgery
Will need to monitor air flow quality with peak flow meter and PFT	Antibiotics if correctable illness such as pneumonia	Treat any cause aggressively
	Bronchodilators and diuretics may be needed	Monitor medications that patient is taking
	Consider referral to pulmonologist	Antibiotics for correctable conditions

NOTES

NOTES

6

Cardiovascular Disorders

For detailed history and physical examination, see Chapter 1.

HEART MURMURS

Heart Murmurs	785.2
Stenotic Valve	424.90
Regurgitant Valve	424.90
Septal Defect	745.9

Definition

Turbulent blood flow through the heart as a result of one or more of the following:
- Stenotic valve
- Regurgitant valve (i.e., one that does not stay closed)
- Septal defect
- Rapid blood flow (e.g., during pregnancy and in children)

Description of Murmurs
- Timing (i.e., systolic or diastolic)—systolic murmurs are synchronous with pulse and may or may not be normal; diastolic murmurs are *always* abnormal

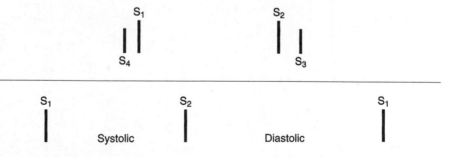

- Quality of sound (e.g., harsh, soft, blowing, or rumbling)
- Location best heard
- Radiation of murmur (e.g., to neck, left axilla, back, or across precordium), which will be in the direction of the blood flow
- Classification of murmurs (Table 6–1 and Figure 6–1)

Table 6–1 Classification of Murmurs

Systolic Murmurs	785.2	Diastolic Murmur	785.2
Aortic Stenosis	424.1	Aortic Regurgitation	424.1
Mitral Regurgitation	746.6	Mitral Stenosis	394.0
Mitral Valve Prolapse	424.0		

DESCRIPTION	ASSESSMENT	REFERRAL POINTS
Systolic Murmurs *Physiologic (Normal)* Grade 1-2/6, best heard with diaphragm Loudest at the middle to lower left sternal border No radiation	May be normal in children, or in adults with certain conditions (e.g., anemia, hyperthyroidism) No hemodynamic changes	Any previously undiagnosed murmur should initially be evaluated by a cardiologist; many nurse practitioners obtain an echocardiogram first
Aortic Stenosis Loud, harsh crescendo-decrescendo murmur Best heard at the second right ICS with the patient leaning forward but may be heard throughout precordium Frequently radiates to neck Often associated with a thrill	Fatigue, palpitation, DOE, dizziness, syncope, and angina Radial pulse diminished Pulse pressure may be narrow Sometimes patient has unexplained GI tract bleeding Often associated with aortic insufficiency	Initial evaluation by cardiologist; many nurse practitioners obtain an echocardiogram first Chest pain, dyspnea, or syncope is a critical referral point for valve replacement
Mitral Regurgitation Holosystolic, blowing, often loud Heard best at the apex in the left lateral position Decreases with inspiration Radiates to the left axilla and occasionally to back	Symptoms include fatigue, palpitation, dizziness, DOE, syncope, and angina; the symptoms range as to degree of regurgitation and CHF Left atrium usually markedly enlarged	Initial evaluation by cardiologist; many nurse practitioners obtain an echocardiogram first Antibiotic prophylaxis is recommended (see p. 192)

Mitral Valve Prolapse

Murmur may or may not be present; sounds like "whoop"	Symptoms include dysrhythmias, chest pain, and anxiety	Initial evaluation by cardiologist; many nurse practitioners obtain an echocardiogram first
A midsystolic click is best heard over the apex with the diaphragm	Most commonly found in white, Anglo-Saxon women	Antibiotic prophylaxis is recommended in some cases (see p. 192)
The click and murmur are best heard while the patient is in the sitting or squatting position or with Valsalva's maneuver	Prognosis for most people is excellent, and treatment may not be indicated	Encourage patients to remain well hydrated, have adequate salt intake, and to avoid caffeine and decongestants
	Diagnosis is made only with echocardiogram; not all clicks are significant	

Diastolic Murmurs

Aortic Regurgitation

Faint and high-pitched, decrescendo, often starts simultaneously with S_2	Minor symptoms for years, then rapid deterioration	Initial evaluation by cardiologist; many nurse practitioners obtain an echocardiogram first
Heard best with diaphragm pressed firmly at the left third ICS, with the patient leaning forward and breath held in deep expiration	May have associated head bobbing, diaphoresis, carotodynia, and a quick rise, flip, or collapsing arterial pulse	Must be referred early for repair
Radiates down	Pulse pressure is often widened	Antibiotic prophylaxis is recommended (see p. 192)
	Apical impulse displaced down and to left	
	Fingernail-bed pressure reveals a pulsating red color	

Mitral Stenosis

Diastolic rumble, best heard at apex with patient in left lateral position	DOE is common	Initial evaluation by cardiologist; many nurse practitioners obtain an echocardiogram first
Best heard with bell of stethoscope		Poorly tolerated in pregnancy
Often associated with an opening snap, and the S_1 may be louder than usual		

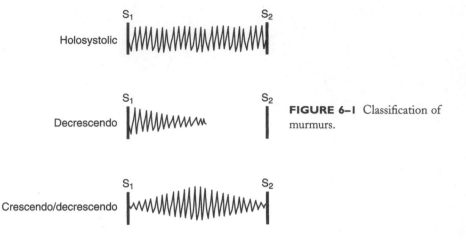

S_1 S_2

Holosystolic

S_1 S_2

Decrescendo

FIGURE 6–1 Classification of murmurs.

S_1 S_2

Crescendo/decrescendo

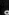

• Grading

1/6	Barely audible
2/6	Audible but soft
3/6	Easily audible, same loudness as S_1 and S_2
4/6	Same as 3/6 but with a thrill palpable
5/6	Audible with only a rim of the stethoscope on the chest; thrill palpable
6/6	Audible with the stethoscope lifted just barely off the chest; thrill palpable

Practice Pearls

• To differentiate a heart murmur from a carotid bruit, simultaneously palpate the cardiac apex while listening to the bruit; a radiating murmur will be synchronous with the apical impulse, whereas a carotid bruit occurs somewhat later
• A new murmur found during a sports physical examination should be evaluated by a physician before allowing the patient to participate in sports
• A new murmur in the setting of an acute MI may indicate a ruptured papillary muscle and impending cardiogenic shock; *it is a surgical emergency*
• If the murmur starts with S_1, it is probably associated with mitral or tricuspid valves; if it does not, think aortic or pulmonic stenosis

ANGINA

Angina 413.9	Prinzmetal's Angina 413.1	CAD 414.00
Acute Coronary Syndrome 411.1	Non Q Wave MI 410.70	ECG Changes 794.31
Variant Angina 413.1	Q-Wave MI 410.70	

Classification (Table 6–2)

Stable angina occurs at predictable times (e.g., with exercise or at stressful times).

Table 6–2   Classification of Angina

CLASS	ACTIVITY/ONSET	LIMITS TO NORMAL ACTIVITY
I	Prolonged exertion	None
II*	Walking >2 blocks	Slight
III*	Walking <2 blocks	Marked
IV	Minimal or rest	Severe

*A practical differentiation between class II and III is the ability to walk two blocks or climb one flight of stairs.

ACUTE CORONARY SYNDROME

Immediate referral
- Class III or IV angina (new or increasing)
- Rest angina
- Variant or Prinzmetal's angina (reversible ST segment elevation on ECG)
- Non–Q-wave and Q-wave MIs

Risk Stratification for Significant Disease
- High likelihood
  - History of CAD
  - Men older than 60 years; women older than 70 years
  - Changes in hemodynamics
  - ECG changes: ST increase or decrease of more than 1 mm, marked symmetric T wave inversion in multiple precordial leads (V_1 through V_6), or bipolar T waves in leads II, III, and aVF
- Moderate likelihood
  - Significant CAD risk factors (especially diabetes)
  - Extracardiac vascular disease
  - ECG changes: ST depression of 0.5 to 1 mm or T wave inversion of more than 1 mm in leads with dominant R waves
- Low likelihood
  - One risk factor (not diabetes)
  - No changes in ECG (NOTE: One half to one third of patients with angina have normal ECG readings)

Diagnostics
- Initial
  - ECG, obtained before administration of nitrates or calcium channel blocker if possible
  - Cardiac enzymes with isoenzymes, including troponin
  - Chemistry profile (be sure it includes serum magnesium)
  - Fasting lipid profile
  - Low-level stress test in men and cardiolyte nuclear stress in women (regular stress test is only 42% accurate in women)
  - Echocardiogram

- Definitive workup
  □ Cardiac catheterization
  □ Thallium studies or chemical (e.g., dipyridamole or dobutamine) stress test

Treatment

- Consult with a physician if angina is new onset or changing in characteristics
- Medications (Table 6–3)
  □ Nitrates are used for acute treatment and prevention
  □ If necessary, practitioner may prescribe beta blocker, calcium channel blocker, or both for prevention
  □ ASA 81 mg qd to reduce risk of MI or CVA
- Dietary therapy: after a review of the lipid profile, select an appropriate diet; consider calorie reduction for the overweight or obese patient
- Exercise: after clearance by a physician, exercise to 65% to 75% of maximum for age
- Smoking cessation
- Consider a statin (see Table 6–10) to reduce risk of MI and CVA, even if cholesterol level is not elevated

Practice Pearls

- Teach the patient about medication(s) and the expected side effects
- Teach the patient how to read labels and calculate fat intake
- Have the patient keep a diary of symptoms and precipitating events; refer if the patient continues to have symptoms, even with a normal treadmill
- Do not give isosorbide mononitrate (Imdur, ISMO, or Monoket) in q12h dosing (see Table 6–3); it is designed with an abstinence period to prevent tachyphylaxis
- Encourage family CPR training
- Teach the family when to call 911 or emergency medical system
- Women usually have atypical angina—vague, but descriptive; unexplained SOB; exhaustion; "full" feeling or discomfort; indigestion; profound fatigue; disturbances in sleep or thinking; it often occurs with arm activities
- MI prevention—primary: 81 mg ASA qd for all males and females >65 years; with *very* high-risk patients: 81 mg ASA and low-dose warfarin (INR 1.5); subsequent: 160 to 325 mg ASA qd
- Omega-3 fatty acids can decrease triglycerides, inhibit blood clotting, and may decrease dysrhythmias associated with sudden cardiac death; encourage two to three capsules a day or three servings of fish (primarily salmon, tuna, mackerel, herring, or sardines) weekly

CHEST PAIN

786.50

Practice Pearls

- Consult with a physician regarding patients with chest pain
- If possible, try to obtain a 12-lead ECG while the patient still has chest pain or discomfort before administering nitrates or calcium channel blockers

Table 6-3 Medications for Angina

MEDICATION	ADVANTAGES AND DISADVANTAGES	EXAMPLES
Nitrates	Reduce angina and improve exercise tolerance in stable angina Prevent AMI in unstable angina Most require a 6- to 8-hr period of abstinence to prevent tachyphylaxis Disadvantages include tolerance, H/A, hypotension, and need to regularly space doses	Nitroglycerin sublingual 0.4 mg (range 0.3–0.6 mg) q5min until pain free, up to 3 tabs or 3 sprays Nitroglycerin sustained release (Nitro-Bid) 2.5–18 mg bid–qid Nitroglycerin ointment (2%, 15 mg/in) $^1/_2$–3 in q8h Nitroglycerin transdermal (Nitro-Dur, Transderm-Nitro) 0.2–0.8 mg worn for 12 hr qd Isosorbide dinitrate (Isordil Titradose) sustained release 40–80 mg q8–12h Isosorbide dinitrate (Isordil sublingual) 2.5–1.0 mg prn Isosorbide mononitrate (Monoket 10–20 mg or ISMO 20 mg) given bid, 7 hr apart or (Imdur 60–120 mg) given once daily
Antiplatelet agents	Prevent AMI in stable and unstable angina Reduce mortality in unstable angina Disadvantage is bleeding; monitor Hgb and platelets yearly	ASA 81–325 mg qd Enteric-coated ASA 325–500 mg qd Clopidogrel (Plavix) 75 mg qd
Beta blockers	Improve exercise tolerance and reduce angina in stable angina Reduce angina and prevent AMI in unstable angina Particularly helpful if patient has exercise-associated tachycardia with angina Disadvantages include bronchoconstriction, AV block, reduced contractility (may induce CHF), and changes in blood lipids	*Noncardioselective Agents* Propranolol HCl (Inderal) 20–80 mg tid–qid *or* Inderal-LA 80–320 mg qd Nadolol (Corgard) 40–240 mg qd *Cardioselective Agents* Atenolol (Tenormin) 50–100 mg qd Metoprolol tartrate (Lopressor) 50 mg bid *or* extended release (Toprol XL) 100 mg qd maximum dose for both is 400 mg qd
Calcium channel blockers	Improve exercise tolerance and reduce angina in stable angina Reduce angina in unstable angina Particular promise has been seen with amlodipine and felodipine Disadvantages include hypotension, AV block, reduced contractility (may induce CHF), and tachycardia with some agents	Nifedipine (Procardia XL) 30–90 mg qd Diltiazem HCl (Cardizem CD) 120–480 mg qd Nicardipine (Cardene) 20–40 mg tid Verapamil HCl (Calan or Isoptin) 80–120 mg qd Amlodipine (Norvasc) 5–10 mg qd

- Do not obtain a stress test with unstable angina (acute coronary syndrome)
- A constant aching pain that might be in the substernal area and lasts all day or a pain that is present only in one position and not in others is usually not caused by heart disease
- Pain over the apical region of the heart or over the right anterior chest region is not typical of coronary artery pain
- The fleeting, momentary pain in the chest described as a needle jab or stick, lasting only 1 or 2 seconds, is not heart pain
- A BP cuff left on and inflated too long may mimic the left arm pain of a patient with a cardiac disorder
- Look for associated symptoms with chest pain; patients with AMI frequently complain of feeling unusually tired for the months or weeks preceding the MI
- If the patient is able to localize the pain with a finger or two to a small region, it is usually not cardiac in nature; cardiac pain tends to be diffuse
- NTG sublingual tablets are good until the expiration date on the bottle, as long as they are kept in the original bottle, tightly capped, and at room temperature
- For chest pain differential diagnoses, see Table 6–4

Table 6–4 **Chest Pain Differential Diagnoses**

Acute Myocardial Infarction 410.90	Pneumothorax 512.8	Esophagitis 530.10
Aortic Dissection 441.00	Pneumomediastinum 518.1	Biliary Colic 574.50
Pericarditis 423.9	Pneumonia 486.	Acute Pancreatitis 577.0
Acute Coronary Artery Insufficiency 411.89	Esophageal Spasm 530.5	Peptic Ulcer Disease 533.9
Pulmonary Embolism 415.1		

DESCRIPTION	CONFIRM BY	EXCLUDE BY
Acute MI		
Severe, oppressive, constricting retrosternal discomfort; often radiates to left shoulder and down left arm (on inside of arm)	ECG evolution Serial cardiac enzymes	Usually by normal serial ECGs or observation in hospital Normal serial cardiac enzymes
Onset is usually at rest		
Lasts >30 min		
Often accompanied with anxiety, restlessness, diaphoresis, or dyspnea		
Prior history of angina or MI		
Levine's sign		
Possible dysrhythmias or CHF		
Aortic Dissection		
Very abrupt, tearing pain in anterior or posterior chest, frequently	May be found in echocardiogram or abdominal U/S	Normal mediastinum on CXR

Table 6–4 Chest Pain Differential Diagnoses—cont'd

DESCRIPTION	CONFIRM BY	EXCLUDE BY
between shoulders; often migrates to arms, abdomen, and legs	Usually found with angiography, CT scan, or MRI	
Pulse deficits		
Shocky but hypertensive		
Possible neurologic changes (especially in legs)		
Diastolic HTN with aortic diastolic murmur		
Pericarditis		
Pleuritic chest pain, often worse in supine position, better when sitting up; referred to trapezius ridge	Typical ECG evolution Pericardial friction rub Echocardiography	Normal ECG Normal echocardiogram Absence of friction rub
Pericardial friction rub		
Often associated disease (e.g., viral infection, connective tissue disease)		
Acute Coronary Artery Insufficiency		
Severe, oppressive, constricting, retrosternal discomfort	Clinical findings with transient ECG ischemic changes	Normal ECG ($\frac{1}{2}$–$\frac{1}{3}$ may be normal despite presence of CAD)
Lasts >30 min	Normal cardiac enzymes	Observation in hospital
Often accompanied with anxiety, restlessness, diaphoresis, or dyspnea	Stress test or angiography, or both	Normal stress test or angiography when stable
Prior history of angina or MI		
Ischemic ECG changes		
Levine's sign		
Possible dysrhythmias or CHF		
Pulmonary Embolism		
Pleuritic chest pain or sudden dyspnea, apprehension, and palpitations	V/Q scan or pulmonary angiography or both ECG changes typical of PE (right ventricular strain)	Normal V/Q scan Observation in hospital
Occasionally, acute nonpleuritic chest "pressure" with hemoptysis		
Clinical signs of DVT		
Factors predisposing to venous thrombosis (e.g., postpartum, use of OCs, prolonged bedrest, CHF)		
Pneumothorax or Pneumomediastinum		
Sudden dyspnea or retrosternal pain, cough, and lateral chest pain	CXR	Normal CXR (including lateral view)

Continued

Table 6–4 Chest Pain Differential Diagnoses—cont'd

DESCRIPTION	CONFIRM BY	EXCLUDE BY
Diminished breath sounds with possible mediastinal shift Possible history of asthma, COPD, or chest trauma Possible subcutaneous emphysema (skin "crackles" to touch)		
Pneumonia Usually pleuritic chest pain with cough and fever Dull to percussion A to E changes	CXR	Normal CXR (>24 hr after symptom onset)
Esophageal Spasm Substernal constricting pain, often at time of swallowing History of dysphagia Pain related to cold and carbonated drinks or food	Barium swallow Endoscopy Esophageal manometry	Normal esophageal manometry
Esophagitis Heartburn and acid brash Worse when bending over or supine Better with antacids	Endoscopy Biopsy UGI series	Normal endoscopy and biopsy or UGI series
Biliary Colic Constant epigastric or right upper quadrant pain Lasts 15 min–6 hr Associated with N/V; possible fever	Clinical history Abdominal U/S or biliary scan	Absence of gallstones
Acute Pancreatitis Severe epigastric or periumbilical pain, radiating to the back Clinically, looks very sick Associated with N/V Tender epigastrium History of alcohol use or gallstones; may be associated with high triglycerides and DM	Elevated serum amylase and lipase	Normal amylase and lipase
Peptic Ulcer Disease Epigastric postprandial discomfort Usually relieved with antacids or food May respond to antacid or H_2 antagonist trial	Upper GI series or endoscopy	Normal GI series or endoscopy

CONGESTIVE HEART FAILURE

Congestive Heart Failure 428.0	Aortic Stenosis 424.1	Heart Failure 428.9
Ischemia 459.9	Mitral Regurgitation 746.6	Systolic Dysfunction 428.2

Definitions

- CHF is the failure of the heart to keep up with the metabolic demands of the tissues; possible etiologies include the following:
- Ischemia
- Valvular
  - □ Aortic stenosis
  - □ Mitral regurgitation
- Toxins
  - □ Alcohol
  - □ Chemotherapy
- Infections/Metabolic
- Congenital
- Rheumatologic
- Heart failure is a chronic illness that is characterized by progressive deterioration punctuated by periodic symptomatic exacerbations; as a result of the initial "event," the heart undergoes structural changes characterized by dilatation, hypertrophy, fibrosis, and altered shape; these lead to progressive systolic and diastolic dysfunction, arrhythmias, increased myocardial oxygen demand, and secondary mitral and tricuspid regurgitation
- Systolic dysfunction occurs when the heart muscle is dilated and thin walled; there are low ejection fractions (e.g., less than 45%) because of reduced contractility of the weakened muscle; it often results from CAD or MI
- Diastolic dysfunction is associated with a hypertrophied myocardium with elevated filling pressures; the ejection fraction is higher than 45%; diastolic dysfunction is often the result of HTN; it is found also with diabetes and chronic kidney disease
- Left ventricular versus right ventricular failure: left ventricular failure is associated with reduced cardiac output to the system and associated pulmonary congestion; right ventricular failure is associated with systemic congestion; right ventricular failure is usually the result of left ventricular failure and may also be associated with pulmonary HTN or COPD (called *cor pulmonale*)

Clinical Findings

- Symptoms
  - □ Exertional dyspnea
  - □ Exercise intolerance
  - □ Cough, worse in recumbent position

- □ Nocturnal symptoms
  Orthopnea: difficulty breathing beginning less than 1 minute after lying down
  Paroxysmal nocturnal dyspnea: occurs 2 to 4 hours into sleep
- □ Edema of legs and feet
- □ Abdominal discomfort
- □ Fatigue or altered mental status
- Signs
  - □ Rales (specific but not very sensitive finding; clear lung fields tell very little about the fluid status of the heart)
  - □ Increased JVP (best physical finding for determining the fluid status) (see p. 9)
  - □ Laterally displaced PMI
  - □ Peripheral edema
  - □ Hepatomegaly and ascites
  - □ Decreased carotid upstrokes

Diagnostics

- To determine the degree and type of CHF and if there is a reversible cause; for suggested evaluation, see also Table 6–5

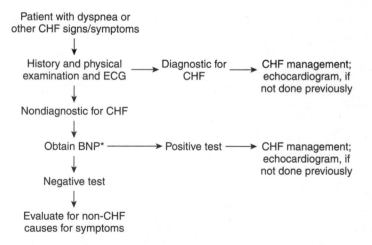

*B-type natriuretic peptide: peptide secreted mainly by ventricles, in response to stretch and increased volume in the ventricles; it facilitates the diagnosis of CHF and can be used as a prognostic marker

| Table 6–5 | Recommended Testing for Heart Failure Signs and Symptoms |

TEST	FINDING	POSSIBLE DIAGNOSIS
ECG	Acute ST-T changes	Ischemia
	Atrial fibrillation	Thyroid disease
	Bradycardia	CHF due to slow rate
	Previous MI	Depressed LV function
	LVH	Diastolic dysfunction
CBC	Anemia	Decreased O_2 carrying capacity
UA	Proteinuria	Nephrotic syndrome
	Casts	Glomerulonephritis
Serum creatinine	Elevated	Renal failure
Serum albumin	Decreased	Increased extravascular volume
TSH	Abnormal	Hypothyroidism or hyperthyroidism
Echocardiogram	Abnormal	Systolic or diastolic dysfunction
		Valvular heart disease
		Pulmonary HTN

Classification

- NYHA classification describes the severity of symptoms; ejection fraction (EF) does not correlate with class

I	No limitations to physical activity
II	Symptoms with usual activities
III	Symptoms with minimal activities
IV	Inability to carry out physical activity without discomfort; symptoms at rest

- ACC/AHA* guidelines classify patients at risk for having CHF

STAGE		PATIENT DESCRIPTION
A	High risk for developing heart failure	HTN
		CAD
		DM
		Family history of cardiomyopathy
B	Asymptomatic heart failure	Previous MI
		Left ventricular systolic dysfunction
		Asymptomatic valvular disease
C	Symptomatic heart failure	Known structural heart disease
		Shortness of breath and fatigue
		Reduced exercise tolerance
D	Refractory end-stage heart failure	Marked symptoms at rest despite maximal medical therapy

*American College of Cardiology/American Heart Association.

| Table 6–6 | Medications for the Treatment of Heart Failure |

STAGE	SUGGESTED MEDICAL THERAPY
B	ACE inhibitor*
	Patient with recent or remote MI, regardless of EF
	All patients with decreased EF (<45%)
	Beta blocker
	Patient with recent MI, regardless of EF
	All patients with decreased EF (<45%)
	Carvedilol (Coreg) 3.125 mg bid, doubling q2wk, to 25 mg bid, if tolerated
	Metoprolol extended release (Toprol XL) 12.5–25 mg qd, doubling q2wk, to 200 mg qd, if tolerated
C	ACE inhibitor*: all patients
	Beta blocker: all patients
	Carvedilol (Coreg) 3.125 mg bid, doubling q2wk, to 25 mg bid, if tolerated
	Metoprolol extended release (Toprol XL) 12.5–25 mg qd, doubling q2wk, to 200 mg a day, if tolerated
	Digoxin: symptomatic patients; not over 0.125 mg/day; aim for serum level of 0.5 to 0.8 ng/ml
	Diuretics*: only as needed to correct or maintain fluid balance
	Spironolactone: patients with NYHA Class III–IV symptoms; monitor serum K^+ and creatinine monthly for 9 mo, q3mo for 9 mo, and then periodically
	Alternative vasodilators (e.g., hydralazine): as needed
D	Referral to heart failure center or cardiologist for management

*See Tables 6–11 to 6–13 for dosing and precautions.

Treatment
- CHF should be managed in conjunction with a physician
- Risk reduction
  - Weight reduction if the patient is obese
  - Control lipids, HTN, and DM
  - Maintain fluid balance: sodium less than 3 g/day and daily weights
  - Stop smoking and ETOH consumption
- Encourage regular exercise (e.g., walking) to tolerance
- Take medications (according to the ACC/AHA* guidelines) (Table 6–6)

12-LEAD ECG
See Figure 6–2 for normal 12-lead ECG.

Ischemia, injury, and infarct of the ventricle are reflected in the 12-lead ECG; each area of the ventricle is reflected in certain leads. In infarction, there is a strong correlation between the leads showing changes and the location of actual disease.

*American College of Cardiology/American Heart Association.

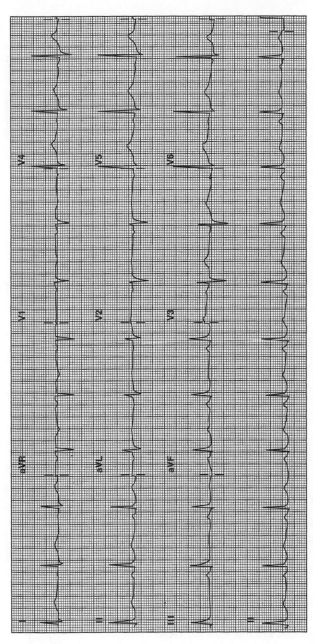

FIGURE 6–2 12-Lead ECG. Because 12-lead ECG tracings do not look alike, it is important to know the criteria for "normal":

- Sinus rhythm
- Normal measurements (i.e., PR 0.12–0.2 seconds, QRS 0.04–0.1 seconds, and QT 0.32–0.44 seconds)
- All ST segments level with baseline (i.e., no depression or elevation)
- All T waves upright except aVR; also may be inverted in lead III or V_1
- QRS complex in leads I, II, and aVF upright
- Normal R wave progression: in looking at leads V_1 through V_6, the QRS complex becomes more positive than negative in either V_3 or V_4

Any deviation from these criteria will create an abnormal ECG, which is not necessarily life threatening.

Acute Changes on the 12-Lead ECG

	LEADS	ARTERY INVOLVED
Left Ventricle		
Anterior	V_1, V_2, V_3, V_4	Left anterior descending coronary artery
Inferior	II, III, aVF	Usually RCA but may be left circumflex
Lateral	I, aVL, V_5, V_6	Left circumflex
Posterior	V_1, V_2 (acute changes include tall R wave and ST depression)	RCA
Right Ventricle		
Right ventricular MI (associated with inferior MI)	V_4 on the right side of chest (V_4R) (acute change is ST elevation >1 mm)	RCA

Acute Changes on the 12-Lead ECG

Ischemia	ST segment depression of more than 1 mm and T wave inversion (if the inversion is deeply symmetric, it is more significant)
Injury	ST segment elevation of more than 1 mm is generally significant
Necrosis	Q waves are signs of necrosis; to be diagnostic of an MI, the Q wave must be at least 0.04-second wide or more than one quarter of the total height of the QRS complex

- Generally, progressive changes on the ECG tracing indicate acute MI
  - ◻ T waves initially heighten and become peaked
  - ◻ ST segments elevate
  - ◻ T waves become inverted
  - ◻ Q waves form, and R waves lose some of their height (subendocardial [non–Q-wave] MIs do not develop Q waves)
- **It is important that the nurse practitioner treat the patient and not the ECG. Refer for clinical symptoms. Do not wait for ECG changes.**

Emergency Treatment of Suspected AMI
- Administer oxygen
- Start IV line (if equipment is available)
- Give 81 or 325 mg of ASA (R/O aortic dissection or peptic ulcer disease)
- Transport to the hospital by advanced life support means immediately

AMBULATORY DYSRHYTHMIAS

| 427.9 |

As a general rule, significant dysrhythmias require oxygen therapy.
For classification, see Table 6–7.

Table 6–7   Ambulatory Dysrhythmias

Fast Rhythms   **427.9**
Sinus Tachycardia   **427.89**
Atrial Fibrillation   **427.31**
Paroxysmal Supraventricular Tachycardia   **427.89**
Sinus Bradycardia   **427.89**
AV Blocks   **426.10**
Premature Ventricular Contractions   **427.69**

DESCRIPTION	TREATMENT	REFERRAL
Fast Rhythms		
Sinus Tachycardia		
Normal components with rate >100/min	Treat the cause	If unable to detect and treat the cause
May be normal in children but never found in adults without a cause (e.g., fear, pain, anxiety, fever, CHF, hypoxia, hyperthyroidism, hypotension, AMI)	Requires appropriate diagnostic workup after an analysis of history and possible causes	
Atrial Fibrillation		
Irregular ventricular rhythm with absence of P waves	Depends on the ventricular rate and if the rhythm is acute (new onset) or chronic	Any new onset of atrial fibrillation should be referred for evaluation
May be acute or chronic rhythm	With rapid rate, digoxin, diltiazem HCl, or beta blockers may be tried	All new medications should be initiated by physician
Increased risk with CAD, COPD, AMI, hypoxia, holiday heart syndrome (associated with excessive alcohol bingeing), hyperthyroidism, hypomagnesemia, obstructive sleep apnea	With excessively slow rate, atropine may be tried. Consider emergency transfer if the patient is hemodynamically unstable	Consider warfarin with high-risk patients (over 75 years, HTN, poor left ventricular function, or prior CVA or TIA); INR goal is 2–3
Paroxysmal Supraventricular Tachycardia		
Sudden onset of regular rhythm with narrow QRS complexes and a rate usually >150/min	Rhythm may terminate spontaneously or require therapy to stop	New onset should be referred for evaluation and treatment plan

Continued

Table 6–7	Ambulatory Dysrhythmias—cont'd	
DESCRIPTION	TREATMENT	REFERRAL
Causes include CAD, medications, mitral valve prolapse, hyperthyroidism, digoxin toxicity, and excessive stimulants (e.g., caffeine, ETOH, nicotine, drugs such as cocaine)	Simple measures to try include Valsalva maneuver and cough. Possible medications include adenosine, verapamil HCl, diltiazem HCl, propranolol HCl. Electrical cardioversion may be indicated if the patient shows signs of hemodynamic instability. Consider emergency transfer if the patient is hemodynamically unstable	All new medications should be initiated by physician
Slow/Irregular Rhythms		
Sinus Bradycardia or AV Blocks		
Ventricular rate <60/min; if <40/min, consider presence of AV block. Causes include medications, athletic heart, hypothyroidism, vagal response, and AMI	Attempt to treat the cause if possible. If the patient is symptomatic (e.g., hypotensive, altered mentation, SOB, chest pain), consider giving IV atropine 0.5–1.0 mg rapidly	If unable to detect and treat the cause, refer. If associated with syncopal episode or if ventricular rate is <40/min, refer to physician or emergency department
Premature Ventricular Contractions (PVCs)		
Wide QRS complexes interspersed in the normal rhythm (may be occasional to frequent). Causes include AMI, CAD, electrolyte imbalance, hypoxia, and medications	Often do not require treatment, but a concern is development of ventricular tachycardia (three or more PVCs in a row at rate >100/min). PVCs should not be treated unless determined to be significant by a physician. Verify normal serum potassium and magnesium levels	If ventricular tachycardia develops (even brief runs of it), transfer to a hospital via emergency transport

HYPERLIPIDEMIA

272.4

Hyperlipidemia is a leading cause of mortality and morbidity, especially when it is associated with coronary heart disease.

Screening Recommendations

- Adults >20 years: fasting lipoprotein profile (total, LDL, and HDL cholesterol, and triglyceride levels) every 5 years

- There is no consensus on screening in pediatrics; consider in obese child with other risk factors (e.g., strong family history of DM, CVD, or HTN)

Secondary Causes of Hyperlipidemia

- Need to be ruled out before beginning lipid-lowering therapy
- Diseases
  □ Hypothyroidism
  □ DM
  □ Obstructive liver disease
  □ Chronic renal failure
- Medications that can elevate LDL or lower HDL cholesterol levels
  □ Hormones (estrogen or progestin)
  □ Steroids (anabolic or corticosteroids)
  □ Thiazide diuretics
  □ Beta blockers

Following are four types of hyperlipidemia and their treatments (according to the Adult Treatment Panel III [ATP III] guidelines)

LIPID TYPE	TREATMENT
Total cholesterol >200 mg/dl	Treat actual component changes
	Encourage therapeutic lifestyle changes (see p. 180)
LDL cholesterol	Encourage therapeutic lifestyle changes (see p. 180)
>160 mg/dl with zero-one risk factor*	Drug therapy (Table 6–8)
>130 mg/dl with ≥ two risk factors*	Statins are usually tried first, but bile acid sequestrant or nicotinic acid can be used
>100 mg/dl with CAD, other known PVD, DM	If the initial dose does not achieve the LDL goal, increase the statin dose or add a bile acid sequestrant or nicotinic acid
	Refer to cardiologist if unable to achieve the LDL goal with this therapy
HDL cholesterol <40 mg/dl	After the LDL cholesterol goal is met, emphasize: Weight reduction, if applicable
	Increased physical activity (e.g., walking 30 min 5 times a week)
	May use nicotinic acid or a fibrate (see Table 6–8)
Elevated triglycerides >150 mg/dl (high)	Most often found in patients with metabolic syndrome (see p. 182)
100–149 mg/dl (borderline)	If >500 mg/dl, patient is at risk for the development of acute pancreatitis

*See p. 180 for risk factors.   *Continued*

LIPID TYPE	TREATMENT
	Treatment depends on the severity and cause of the elevation; for all patients, a main goal is to achieve the target goal for the LDL
	With borderline triglycerides, emphasize:
	Weight reduction, if applicable
	Increase physical activity (e.g., work up to walking 30 min 5 times per week)
	Little or no alcohol, concentrated sweets
	With high triglycerides, also add drug therapy (see Table 6–8):
	Statin to lower LDL cholesterol *or*
	Nicotinic acid or fibrate (fibrates are often more helpful than statins)
	May use nicotinic acid if cholesterol is also elevated

Risk Factors

- Major (other than elevated LDL cholesterol level)
  - Men aged 45 years or older or women aged 55 years or older
  - Family history of premature CHD (male first-degree relative younger than 55 years or female first-degree relative younger than 65 years)
  - Low HDL cholesterol level
  - BP of 140/90 mm Hg or more *or* taking antihypertensives
  - Cigarette smoking
- Other risk factors
  - Lifestyle/habit: obesity, physical inactivity, and atherogenic diet
  - Emerging risk factors: lipoprotein(a), homocysteine, prothrombotic and pro-inflammatory factors; impaired fasting glucose (pre-DM); and evidence of subclinical atherosclerotic disease

Practice Pearls

- Therapeutic lifestyle changes include the following:
  - Diet therapy—should be tried for 3 months before medications are started (unless CAD exists or the patient is diabetic); the suggested diet follows; the patient may benefit from consultation with a dietitian
  - Total fat less than 35% of total calories
    Less than 7% total calories from saturated fats

    Up to 10% total calories from polyunsaturated fats

    Up to 20% total calories from monounsaturated fats

  - Cholesterol less than 200 mg/day
  - Increased soluble fiber (approximately 20 to 30 g/day)
  - Encourage regular exercise (e.g., walking 30 minutes 5 times a week)
  - Weight loss, if applicable
- If triglycerides are elevated, the LDL is small and dense, regardless of its value; trigs ÷ HDL >3 means insulin resistance

Table 6–8 Medications for Hyperlipidemias

MEDICATION	INITIAL DOSE	MONITORING
Statins—take at hs, except lovastatin (taken with the evening meal) or atorvastatin (does not matter when taken)		
Atorvastatin (Lipitor)	10 mg qd	With all statins, monitor LFTs
Fluvastatin (Lescol)	20–40 mg qd	before starting therapy, and then
Lovastatin (Mevacor)	20 mg qd	periodically (e.g., every 6–12 mo
Lovastatin (Altocor [extended release])	60 mg qd	thereafter); stop drug if levels are 3 times normal; simvastatin dose
Pravastatin (Pravachol)	10–20 mg qd	not to exceed 40 mg qd.
Rosuvastatin (Crestor)	10–20 mg qd	
Simvastatin (Zocor)	5 mg qd	
	40 mg qd for patient with CHD or DM	
Bile Acid Sequestrants		
Cholestyramine (Questran, Cholybar)	4 g tid–qid	With bile acid sequestrants, monitor lipids periodically during
Colestipol (Colestid)	6 g qd	therapy. It is not necessary to
Colesevelam (Welchol)	3 tablets bid or 6 tablets qd with food	monitor LFTs. Marked hypertriglyceridemia may be exacerbated with these medications.
Fibric Acid Derivatives (Fibrates)		
Gemfibrozil (Lopid)	600 mg bid ac	Monitor LFTs and lipids at start of
Fenofibrate (Tricor)	67–200 mg qd	therapy, at 12 wk, and periodically
Clofibrate (Atromid-S)	2 g qd	thereafter; stop if ALT greater than 100 units/L.
Nicotinic Acid		
Niacin (nicotinic acid)	1–3 g tid with or after meals	Monitor blood glucose, LFTs (with large doses, prolonged therapy, or in combination with a statin), and cholesterol periodically.
Niacin, extended release (Niaspan)	500 mg hs, adjust dose by 500 mg qd at 4-wk intervals	
Miscellaneous Medications		
Lovastatin and Niacin (Advicor)	20 mg lovastatin and 500 mg niacin qd	Monitor according to components.
Ezetimibe (Zetia)	10 mg qd	Monitor lipids periodically.
Omega-3 capsules (Lovaza)	4 caps qd	Monitor lipids periodically.

- In patients being treated to prevent complications, start drug therapy only after lifestyle changes have been made
- Pharmacologic therapy
  □ Controlled trials have shown that HMG-CoA reductase agents ("statins") decrease overall mortality when used for primary and secondary prevention in hyperlipidemia; use cautiously with patients who consume substantial amounts of alcohol or have a history of liver disease
  □ Do not use bile acid sequestrants or statins in the treatment of isolated elevations of VLDL because both may increase VLDL levels
  □ Do not use the statins with fibrates because rhabdomyolysis may occur
  □ Constipation resulting from bile acid sequestrants can be reduced by increasing the dose slowly and by the concomitant administration of psyllium (Metamucil) or methylcellulose (Citrucel)
  □ Administer ASA or NSAIDs (see Appendix E) 30 to 60 minutes before nicotinic acid (niacin) to reduce the uncomfortable side effects
  □ Administer statins bid if insomnia occurs
  □ With high LDL or total cholesterol levels, patient may try cod liver oil one to two capsules daily, or 4 g of fresh bulb garlic, or 4 to 12 mg of allicin (Kwai) daily
  □ Omega-3 fatty acids can lower lipids; patient can take two servings of fish per week (salmon, tuna, mackerel, herring, or sardines) or two omega-3 fatty acid capsules qd
- Also treat HTN; patients with known CAD or DM should take ASA 81 mg/day
- Women usually require a calorie-restricted diet and exercise to lower lipids

METABOLIC SYNDROME

This condition is characterized by insulin resistance and prothrombotic and proinflammatory states.

Diagnosis

Metabolic syndrome is diagnosed when three or more of the following symptoms are present:
- Abdominal obesity (waist circumference)
  □ Men more than 40 inches (102 cm)
  □ Women more than 35 inches (88 cm)
- Triglycerides: 150 mg/dl or more
- HDL cholesterol level
  □ Men less than 40 mg/dl
  □ Women less than 50 mg/dl
- BP of 130/85 mm Hg or higher, or on medication for hypertension
- FBS level of 110 mg/dl or higher

Management

- Reduce underlying causes; encourage weight reduction and increased physical activity (e.g., work up to 30-minute walks 5 times a week)

- Treat HTN
- ASA 81 mg/day for patient with CHD
- Treat specific dyslipidemias

HYPERTENSION

401.9

Definition

Diagnosis is made after three or more elevated readings at different times; at each visit, check the BP at least two times with the patient sitting for at least 5 minutes. Average the readings and classify by the highest reading—systolic or diastolic (Table 6–9).

Initial Workup

- Specific history questions
  - Past medical history

    Cardiovascular, cerebrovascular, or renal diseases

    Diabetes

    History of HTN (what level, any treatment, and results)

    Current medications (prescription and OTC)

    Cardiovascular risk factors (e.g., smoking, hyperlipidemia, microalbuminuria, or estimated creatinine clearance less than 60 ml/min (see p. 297)
  - Sleep apnea
  - Social factors: sexual function, exercise, work schedules, how to pay for medications, and alcohol intake
  - Family history: HTN, CVA, CAD, CHF, renal disease (including polycystic kidneys), DM, pheochromocytoma, cardiomyopathy, and sudden death

Table 6–9 Classification of Hypertension

CLASSIFICATION	SYSTOLIC READING	DIASTOLIC READING	FOLLOW-UP
Normal	<120 mm Hg	<80 mm Hg	—
Prehypertension	120–139 mm Hg	80–89 mm Hg	Recheck in 1 yr
High blood pressure			
Stage I	140–159 mm Hg	90–99 mm Hg	Recheck in 2 mo
Stage II	≥160 mm Hg	≥100 mm Hg	Treat and recheck in 1 mo
Diagnosis in pregnancy	>30 mm Hg above base or >140 mm Hg	>15 mm Hg above base or >90 mm Hg	Refer to high-risk obstetrician

Data from the *Seventh Report of the Joint National Committee on Prevention, Detection, Evaluation, and Treatment of High Blood Pressure (JNC 7)* (2003). National High Blood Pressure Education Program; National Heart, Lung, and Blood Institute; National Institutes of Health.

- Specific examination
  - General appearance, including calculation of body mass index (BMI) (see Appendix A)
  - Funduscopic examination
  - Neck: thyroid and presence or absence of JVP or bruits
  - Cardiovascular: heart sounds, PMI, breath sounds, edema, and peripheral pulses
  - Abdomen: liver and presence or absence of bruits in abdomen and femoral areas, and presence or absence of abnormal aortic pulsation
  - Neurological: cranial nerves, DTRs, and sensory changes
- Diagnostic tests
  - Laboratory values: CBC, BUN, creatinine, electrolytes, glucose, calcium, LFTs, lipid profile (see p. 179), and UA
  - ECG
  - Consider CXR, captopril renal scan to rule out renal stenosis

Treatment

- Goals: BP less than 120/80 mm Hg; if the patient is >85 years, goal is 140–160/80–90
- With "white coat" HTN, if BP is not normal in office after 3 to 6 months of observation, treat according to office BP readings, despite readings elsewhere, especially with other risk factors (e.g., hyperlipidemia or obesity)
- Patients with prehypertension are twice as likely to develop HTN as those with normal BP; strongly encourage lifestyle modifications for those patients
- Initiate lifestyle changes
  - Weight reduction if overweight
  - Diet: see Table 6–10 for DASH diet
  - Exercise: regular physical activity; try 30-minute walk at rate of 2 to 3 mph 5 times weekly
  - Smoking cessation
  - Alcohol: 2 oz of whiskey, 10 oz of wine, or 24 oz of beer daily; women and thin patients should consume half of these amounts
- If lifestyle changes are unsuccessful, try any of the following (see Tables 6–11 to 6–13 for drug information), although a thiazide should be used first, unless a compelling reason for another agent exists (e.g., ACE-I for patient with DM)
  - Diuretics (especially thiazides: proven to reduce mortality and morbidity)
  - Beta blockers (proven to reduce mortality and morbidity); use first in patient with HTN, or after myocardial infarction
  - ACE inhibitors and angiotensin II receptor blockers; use first in patients with HTN or DM or heart failure or chronic kidney disease
  - Calcium channel blockers; use as alternative to beta blocker in a patient with stable angina
  - Alpha receptor blockers
  - Alpha-beta blockers
  - Arterial vasodilators

Text continued on p. 191

Table 6–10 DASH Diet*

FOOD GROUP	DAILY SERVINGS	1 SERVING EQUALS	EXAMPLES
Grains and grain products	7–8	1 slice bread ½ cup dry or cooked cereal, pasta, or cooked rice	Whole-grain breads, pita, English muffin, bagel, grits, oatmeal
Vegetables	4–5	1 cup raw leafy vegetables ½ cup cooked vegetables 6 oz vegetable juice	Tomatoes, potatoes, carrots, peas, squash, broccoli, turnip greens, kale, collards, spinach, artichokes, sweet potatoes
Fruit	4–5	8 oz fruit juice 1 medium fruit ¼ cup dried fruit ½ cup fresh, frozen, or canned fruit	Apricots, bananas, dates, grapes, oranges, grapefruit, mangoes, melons, peaches, pineapples, prunes, raisins, strawberries, tangerines
Low-fat and nonfat dairy products	2–3	8 oz milk 1 cup yogurt 1½ oz cheese	Skim or 1% milk, low-fat buttermilk, nonfat or low-fat yogurt, part-skim mozzarella cheese, nonfat cheese
Meat, poultry, fish	2 or fewer	3 oz cooked meats, poultry, or fish	Lean cuts with visible fat and skin removed; broiled, roasted, or boiled
Nuts and legumes	1	¾ oz or ⅙ cup nuts 1 tbsp seeds ½ cup cooked legumes	Almonds, filberts, mixed nuts, peanuts, walnuts, pecans, sunflower seeds, kidney beans, lentils

*The DASH (Dietary Approach to Stop Hypertension) diet is low in fat and cholesterol; high in fiber, potassium, calcium, and magnesium; and moderately high in protein. It provides about 2000 kcal a day.

Table 6–11 Suggested Initial Antihypertensive Agents*

PATIENT PROFILE	SUGGESTED AGENT*	AGENTS TO AVOID
Acute MI	Beta blocker without ISA†	
Asthma, COPD	Calcium channel blocker Alpha blocker Central alpha agonist	Beta blocker (not cardioselective)
Black race	Diuretic Calcium channel blocker	Beta blocker and ACE inhibitor less effective
BPH	Alpha blocker	

*Also see Table 6–12 for cautions and Table 6–13 for dosing guidelines.
†Intrinsic sympathomimetic activity (i.e., blocks beta$_1$ receptors while mildly stimulating beta$_2$ receptors).

Continued

Table 6–11 Suggested Initial Antihypertensive Agents—cont'd

PATIENT PROFILE	SUGGESTED AGENT*	AGENTS TO AVOID
CHF, diastolic	Calcium channel blocker ACE inhibitor or angiotensin II receptor blocker	Alpha blocker Beta blocker with ISA† Direct vasodilator Diuretic
CHF, systolic	ACE inhibitor or angiotensin II receptor blocker, with diuretic Carvedilol	Beta blocker (except carvedilol) Most calcium channel blockers and alpha-beta blockers
Depression		Beta blockers Central alpha agonist
Diabetes, type 1	ACE inhibitor Diuretic (thiazide) Central alpha agonist	Beta blocker with ISA† Alpha blocker
Diabetes, type 2	ACE inhibitor Calcium channel blocker	Diuretic at high dose
Elderly	Diuretic Calcium channel blocker	Alpha blocker (use cautiously because of postural hypotension)
Hyperlipidemia	ACE inhibitor or angiotensin II receptor blocker Calcium channel blocker Beta blocker with ISA† Alpha blocker	Beta blocker without ISA† Diuretic without ACE inhibitor Methyldopa
Ischemic heart disease	Beta blocker without ISA† Calcium channel blocker	Beta blocker with ISA† Vasodilator
Isolated systolic HTN	Diuretic Calcium channel blocker	
Left ventricular hypertrophy	ACE inhibitor or angiotensin II receptor blocker Calcium channel blocker	Beta blocker with ISA† Direct vasodilator
Obesity	ACE inhibitor or angiotensin II receptor blocker Alpha blocker Calcium channel blocker	Beta blocker
Peripheral vascular disease	Calcium channel blocker Alpha blocker	
Renal insufficiency	Loop diuretics usually needed with advanced renal disease ACE inhibitor or angiotensin II receptor blocker (depends on cause)	Beta blocker
Tachycardic	Calcium channel blocker (especially verapamil or diltiazem)	
Young or with hyperdynamic circulation	Beta blocker ACE inhibitor or angiotensin II receptor blocker	

*Also see Table 6–12 for cautions and Table 6–13 for dosing guidelines.
†Intrinsic sympathomimetic activity (i.e., blocks beta$_1$ receptors while mildly stimulating beta$_2$ receptors).

Table 6–12 Cautions and Contraindications for Antihypertensive Agents

ANTIHYPERTENSIVE AGENT	MONITOR	CAUTIONS	CONTRAINDICATIONS
ACE inhibitors	Serum potassium Serum BUN and creatinine at baseline and after dose increases	Reduce or discontinue use of diuretic before initiating therapy Captopril and moexipril should be given 1hr ac Discontinue therapy if the patient develops swelling of hands or face, sore throat, or fever (of undetermined origin)	Hypertrophic cardiomyopathy Bilateral renal artery stenosis or stenosis of a solitary kidney Pregnancy (consider urine or serum HCG prior to use)
Angiotensin II receptor blockers	Serum potassium and BUN/creatinine at baseline	Use cautiously if patient is volume depleted	Pregnancy (consider urine or serum HCG prior to use) Renal artery stenosis (as above) Hypertrophic cardiomyopathy
Alpha blockers	Postural BP changes Heart rate	Elderly patients Type 1 DM	Asthma Overt CHF Severe bradycardia AV block greater than first degree
Alpha-beta blockers	Postural BP changes	Hepatic impairment Pregnancy Children	
Beta blockers	Heart rate for bradycardia	Peripheral vascular disease Type 2 DM Hyperlipidemia (may increase triglycerides and decrease HDL) May be less effective in African Americans	Type 1 DM Asthma/COPD Severe CHF AV blocks Severe PVD Raynaud's phenomenon
Beta blockers with ISA*		Taper slowly because of rebound HTN May accelerate ischemia in CAD Taper slowly because of rebound HTN	Pregnancy (atenolol)

*Intrinsic sympathomimetic activity (i.e., it blocks beta$_1$ receptors while mildly stimulating beta$_2$ receptors).

Continued

Table 6–12 Cautions and Contraindications for Antihypertensive Agents—cont'd

ANTIHYPERTENSIVE AGENT	MONITOR	CAUTIONS	CONTRAINDICATIONS
Calcium channel blockers	Heart rate for bradycardia	May aggravate CAD and CHF	Bradycardia AV blocks
Central alpha agonists	Postural BP changes	Concomitant depression Taper slowly because of rebound HTN	
Direct vasodilators		May precipitate angina in CAD Concomitant treatment with diuretic or beta blocker may be indicated	Hypertrophic cardiomyopathy Hyperdynamic circulation Following MI
Diuretics: loop	Electrolyte panel plus Mg^{++} Weight	May develop tolerance; using staggered dosing may decrease tolerance Ototoxicity may occur with high doses of furosemide Hypokalemia†	Preeclampsia Mitral valve prolapse Hypertrophic cardiomyopathy
Diuretics: potassium sparing	Electrolytes Weight	Renal insufficiency or failure Concomitant use of NSAIDs	Preexisting hyperkalemia Concomitant use of ACE inhibitors
Diuretics: thiazide	Electrolyte panel plus Mg^{++} and Ca^{++} Weight	Hyperlipidemia Type 2 DM Hypokalemia†	Sulfa allergy Serum creatinine >2.5 mg/dl Hypertrophic cardiomyopathy Preeclampsia Poorly controlled gout Mitral valve prolapse

†See Table 6–13 for treatment.

Potassium Supplementation

Dosing	
Prevention	16–24 mEq qd
To correct depletion	40–100 mEq qd
Suggested Products	
8 mEq	Klor-Con 8 or Slow-K
10 mEq	K-Dur 10, K-Tab, Kaon 10, Klor-Con 10
20 mEq	K-Dur 20, 15 ml of Kaochlor 10% liquid
25 mEq	K-Lyte/Cl effervescent
50 mEq	K-Lyte/Cl 50 effervescent

Table 6–13 Antihypertensive Medication Dosing Guidelines

MEDICATION	INITIAL DOSE	MAINTENANCE MAXIMUM
ACE Inhibitors		
Benazepril HCl (Lotensin)*	10 mg qd	80 mg qd
Captopril (Capoten)*	25 mg bid–tid	450 mg qd
Enalapril maleate (Vasotec)*	2.5 mg qd (with diuretics) 5 mg qd (without diuretics)	40 mg qd
Fosinopril (Monopril)*	10 mg qd	80 mg qd
Lisinopril (Zestril, Prinivil)*	10 mg qd	40 mg qd
Quinapril (Accupril)*	10 mg qd	80 mg qd
Ramipril (Altace)	2.5 mg qd (may be opened and mixed with applesauce, water, or apple juice)	20 mg qd
Moexipril HCl (Univasc)*	7.5 mg qd 1 hr ac	30 mg qd
Trandolapril (Mavik)	1 mg qd	8 mg qd
Perindopril (Aceon)	4 mg qd	8 mg qd
Angiotensin II Receptor Blocker		
Candesartan (Atacand)	16 mg qd (lower dose if volume depleted or on other antihypertensive agents)	32 mg qd
Irbesartan (Avapro)*	150 mg qd	300 mg qd
Losartan potassium (Cozaar)	50 mg qd (25 mg with volume depletion or hepatic impairment)	50 mg bid *or* 100 mg qd
Losartan potassium/ hydrochlorothiazide (Hyzaar)	50/12.5 mg qd	2 tab qd
Telmisartan (Micardis)*	40 mg qd	80 mg qd
Valsartan (Diovan)*	80 mg qd	320 mg qd
Eprosartan mesylate (Teveten)	600 mg qd	800 mg qd
Alpha Adrenergic Blocker†		
Prazosin HCl (Minipress)	1 mg bid–tid	15 mg qd
Terazosin HCl (Hytrin)	1 mg hs	20 mg qd
Doxazosin mesylate (Cardura)	1 mg qd	16 mg qd

*Also comes in combination with hydrochlorothiazide.
†Give initial dose at bedtime to decrease syncopal episodes; not a first-line BP medication.

Continued

Table 6–13 Antihypertensive Medication Dosing Guidelines—cont'd

MEDICATION	INITIAL DOSE	MAINTENANCE MAXIMUM
Alpha Agonist (Central)		
Clonidine (Catapres)	0.1 mg bid	2.4 mg qd
Guanabenz acetate (Wytensin)	4 mg bid	64 mg qd
Methyldopa (Aldomet)*	250 mg bid–tid	3000 mg qd
Alpha-Beta Blocker		
Carvedilol (Coreg)	6.25 mg qd *or* bid	50 mg qd
Labetalol HCl (Normodyne, Trandate)	100 mg bid	1200 mg qd
Beta Blocker		
Atenolol (Tenormin)	25–50 mg bid	100 mg qd
Metoprolol tartrate (Lopressor),* metoprolol succinate (Toprol XL)	50–100 mg qd	450 mg qd
Nadolol (Corgard)	40 mg qd	320 mg qd
Propranolol HCl (Inderal)*	40 mg bid	640 mg qd
Propranolol HCl (Inderal LA)	80 mg qd	640 mg qd
Bisoprolol fumarate*	5 mg qd	20 mg qd
Beta Blocker with ISA‡		
Acebutolol HCl (Sectral)	400 mg qd	1200 mg qd
Pindolol (Visken)	5 mg bid	60 mg qd
Calcium Channel Blockers		
Diltiazem HCl		
(Cardizem SR)	60–120 mg bid	360 mg qd
(Cardizem CD, Tiazac)	120–240 mg qd	360 mg qd
(Cardizem LA)	180–240 mg qd	540 mg qd
Verapamil HCl		
(Calan SR, Isoptin SR)	120–240 mg qd	480 mg qd
(Verelan)	120–240 mg qd	480 mg qd
Calcium Channel Blockers (Dihydropyridines)		
Amlodipine (Norvasc)	2.5–5 mg qd	10 mg qd
Felodipine (Plendil)	5 mg qd	10 mg qd
Isradipine (DynaCirc)	2.5 mg bid	20 mg qd
Nicardipine (Cardene SR)	30 mg bid	120 mg qd
Nifedipine		
(Procardia XL)	30–60 mg qd	120 mg qd
(Adalat CC)	30–60 mg qd	90 mg qd
Nisoldipine (Sular)	20 mg qd	60 mg qd
Calcium Channel Blocker/ACE Inhibitor (Not recommended for initial therapy)		
Amlodipine and benazepril HCl (Lotrel)	2.5 mg/10 mg qd	10 mg/40 mg qd

*Also comes in combination with hydrochlorothiazide.
‡Intrinsic sympathomimetic agent.

Table 6–13 Antihypertensive Medication Dosing Guidelines—cont'd

MEDICATION	INITIAL DOSE	MAINTENANCE MAXIMUM
Enalapril and diltiazem maleate (Teczem)	5 mg/180 mg qd	10 mg/360 mg qd
Thiazide Diuretics		
Chlorothiazide (Diuril)	500–1000 mg qd	1000 mg qd
Hydrochlorothiazide (HydroDIURIL, Esidrix, Microzide)	6.25–50 mg qd	50 mg qd
Indapamide (Lozol)	1.25 mg qd	5 mg qd
Metolazone (Zaroxolyn)	2.5–5 mg qd	5 mg qd
Loop Diuretics		
Bumetanide (Bumex)	0.5–2 mg qd	10 mg qd
Torsemide (Demadex)	5 mg qd	10 mg qd
Furosemide (Lasix)	40 mg bid	80 mg qd
Direct Vasodilator		
Hydralazine HCl (Apresoline)	10 mg qid	300 mg qd

- If there is inadequate response to initial drug therapy (BP still more than 20/10 mm Hg above goal)
  - □ Increase drug dose *or*
  - □ Substitute another drug *or*
  - □ Add a second agent (thiazide, if not already on one)
- If response to the these changes is inadequate, add a second or third agent; consult with a physician if the patient requires more than two drugs for therapy. Most patients will require two or more antihypertensive agents
- Resistant HTN is diagnosed when the BP goal is not met, despite patient adhering to full doses of a three-drug regimen that includes a diuretic; consultation with hypertensive specialist should be considered

Practice Pearls
- Follow up every 1 to 2 months, depending on status, until BP goal is reached. Once stable, follow-up visits can be at 3- to 6-month intervals. In patients older than 50 years, systolic HTN is a more important CVD risk factor than diastolic HTN
- Treat with decongestants cautiously; pseudoephedrine HCl has the lowest cardiovascular risk profile
- Coughing could be due to the ACE inhibitor; if bronchospasms occur, consider the effect of beta blockers; if the patient currently smokes, choose a cardioselective beta blocker
- Evaluate for secondary HTN with the following (often, a captopril renal scan is done to rule out renal artery stenosis):
  - □ Very severe HTN that is resistant to therapy

- □ Onset before age 25 or after age 65 years
- □ Clinical findings that suggest a secondary cause

  Muscle weakness or polyuria: primary aldosteronism

  Palpitations, H/A, or diaphoresis: pheochromocytoma

  Anxiety and weight loss or gain: hyperthyroidism or hypothyroidism

  Flank pain or trauma: renal cause
- With difficulty controlling BP, ask about herbs (e.g., ginseng can decrease efficacy of many antihypertensive agents)
- Diuretics can elevate serum cholesterol and triglyceride levels and decrease HDL levels in diabetics
- Thiazides are more effective than loop diuretics in HTN, except when serum creatinine levels are more than 2.5 mg/dl
- For emergency treatment of HTN in office, consider nitroglycerin spray sublingually or nitroglycerin paste or captopril 6.25 to 25 mg po or clonidine 0.1 to 0.2 mg initially and then 0.05 to 0.1 mg qh to the maximum of 0.7 mg; use with caution if patient is tachycardic or has cardiac decompensation; start routine medication (e.g., calcium channel blocker or clonidine) and recheck every 1 to 2 days until BP stabilizes
- NSAIDs may interfere with the effects of ACE inhibitors, beta blockers, and diuretics
- Sexual or erectile dysfunction may occur with alpha blockers, beta blockers, and central alpha agonists
- Edema with amlodipine is not fluid related, so diuretics do not help; try decreasing the dose or add ACE/ARB or change to a different medication

ANTIBIOTIC PROPHYLAXIS AGAINST ENDOCARDITIS[*]
High Risk (Always Pretreat)
- Prosthetic valve
- History of endocarditis
- Congenital heart disease defects
- Heart transplant that develops problems in a heart valve

Negligible Risk (Do Not Need to Pretreat)
- Surgically repaired congenital heart defects
- History of coronary artery bypass graft surgery
- Calcified aortic stenosis
- MVP
- Rheumatic heart disease
- Bicuspid valve disease

---

[*]For dental, oral, respiratory tract, or esophageal procedures.

- Physiologic, functional, or innocent murmurs
- Previous rheumatic fever without valve damage
- Pacemakers or implanted defibrillators

PATIENT STATUS	AGENT	REGIMEN
Not allergic to penicillin and able to take oral medication	Amoxicillin	*Adult:* 2 g 1 hr before procedure *Child:* 50 mg/kg 1 hr before procedure
Not allergic to penicillin but unable to take oral medication	Ampicillin	*Adult:* 2 g IM or IV within 30 min of procedure *Child:* 50 mg/kg IM or IV within 30 min of procedure
Allergic to penicillin	Clindamycin	*Adult:* 600 mg 1 hr before procedure *Child:* 20 mg/kg IV 1 hr before procedure
	Azithromycin	*Adult:* 500 mg 1 hr before procedure *Child:* 15 mg/kg 1 hr before procedure
Allergic to penicillin and unable to take oral medication	Clindamycin	*Adult:* 600 mg IV within 30 min of procedure *Child:* 20 mg/kg IV within 30 min of procedure

MARFAN SYNDROME

759.82

Characteristics
- Tall, with arm span exceeding height
- Waist-to-crown measurement is less than waist-to-floor measurement
- Long, thin fingers and toes

Possible Complications
- Associated with aortic dilation and dissecting aortic aneurysm
- Pneumothorax

Evaluation
- Obtain measurements above (e.g., arm span and height)
- Echocardiogram: possible valvular findings

     Aortic insufficiency and regurgitation

     Mitral valve prolapse and insufficiency

Treatment
- Refer to cardiologist for further evaluation

NOTES

7

Vascular and Blood Disorders

Chronic Peripheral Vascular Disease

Chronic Venous Insufficiency **459.81**
Varicose Veins **454.9**
Chronic Peripheral Arterial Disease **443.9**
Thromboangiitis Obliterans (Buerger's Disease) **443.1**
Raynaud Disease **443.0**

DESCRIPTION	SIGNS AND SYMPTOMS	DIAGNOSTICS AND TREATMENT
Chronic Venous Insufficiency Venous incompetence due to valve destruction when valve leaflets become contracted and are incapable of preventing retrograde flow of blood Results from ischemia in vasculature, skin, and supporting tissue	Edema progresses from distal to proximal May be unilateral or bilateral Tiredness or heaviness in legs after prolonged standing or sitting Hemosiderin staining (bronzing) of skin Scaly skin with cutaneous atrophy Skin warm with normal color when elevated; cyanotic when dependent for prolonged periods Usually a history of DVT Tingling, itching, "hot legs"	*Diagnostics* Doppler U/S Venogram ABI *Treatment* Decrease edema Four to six 30-min rest periods during the day Graduated compression hose With ulcer >2 × 2 in or not healed after 2 mo, compression therapy; add pentoxifylline (Trental) 400 mg tid or cilostazol (Pletal) 50–100 mg bid Gradual exercise Meticulous skin care Refer if ulcer continues to worsen
Varicose Veins Occurs when valve damage permits backflow of blood, thus causing an engorgement of veins Greater and lesser saphenous system is most commonly affected Age of onset ~20 yr	Tortuous, dilated, superficial vessels Heaviness and fatigue in legs Diffuse calf aching without exercise Elevation of legs produces rapid relief of symptoms Affected limb may be edematous	*Diagnostics* Doppler U/S Venogram *Treatment* Elevate legs periodically Avoid prolonged standing Support hose should be used daily and put on

Continued

DESCRIPTION	SIGNS AND SYMPTOMS	DIAGNOSTICS AND TREATMENT
Affects women more than men Caused by increased abdominal pressure due to obesity, pregnancy, prolonged standing, or heredity		before getting out of bed in the morning Avoid restrictive clothing, especially around the waist and groin Avoid OCs and HRT Refer for surgical consultation if severe

Chronic Peripheral Arterial Disease

DESCRIPTION	SIGNS AND SYMPTOMS	DIAGNOSTICS AND TREATMENT

Occurs commonly in the terminal aorta, iliac, superficial femoral, and popliteal arteries; begins as stenosing lesions that progressively narrow to complete obstruction
It is related to hypertension, cigarette smoking, lack of exercise, obesity, and hyperlipidemia
Diabetics are at higher risk for loss of the extremity
Primarily affects men over 50 yr of age
Gluteal and thigh pain related to aortoiliac obstruction
Calf pain related to femoral artery obstruction
	Symptoms have a gradual onset, unless thrombosis is present
	Intermittent claudication (reproducible pain that occurs with exercise, relieved by rest)
	Claudication severity:
	  Mild—can walk >2 blocks; little interference with ADL
	  Moderate—pain with walking 1–2 blocks; some interference with ADL
	  Severe—pain with walking $<^1/_2$–1 block; significant interference with ADL
	Rest pain at night
	Sleep with feet hanging off bed (aids circulation)
	Severe, intolerable pain without exertion
	Pain is seldom completely relieved
	Coldness of extremity and clear demarcation of warmth to coolness
	No edema unless disease is severe
	Hair loss distal to occlusion with muscle atrophy and paresthesia, ulcers, and gangrene
	Color changes:
	Dependent = red
	Elevated = pallor
		Diagnostics
		Check pedal pulses both at rest and after walking to rule out arterial insufficiency
		Perform ABI (see p. 198)
		Doppler ultrasound
		Arteriography
		
		Treatment
		Smoking cessation is the most important factor
		Exercise programs that encourage collateral circulation formation (see p. 198)
		Control HTN
		Meticulous foot care
		Observation of feet for development of ulcers
		Antiplatelet agents (e.g., ASA, warfarin, clopidogrel (Plavix) 75 mg qd should be used to decrease risk of MI or CVA (warfarin therapy, p. 199)
		Ginkgo biloba 60–80 mg bid–tid
		Cilostazol (Pletal) 100 mg 1–2 times a day may help with pain (not if patient has CHF)
		Refer to a vascular surgeon for invasive treatment

Thromboangiitis Obliterans (Buerger's Disease)

DESCRIPTION	SIGNS AND SYMPTOMS	DIAGNOSTICS AND TREATMENT
Inflammatory reaction of small blood vessels	Legs are most often affected Pain may be severe in	*Diagnostics* Arteriography

DESCRIPTION	SIGNS AND SYMPTOMS	DIAGNOSTICS AND TREATMENT
Probably directly related to excessive nicotine use More common in men younger than 40 yr May have a genetic component Highest incidence among Jewish and Asian persons	affected leg and may be worse at rest Rubor is noted from dilated capillaries in addition to cyanosis with shiny, tight, thin skin Coldness, numbness, tingling, and burning sensation in the affected extremity Intermittent claudication noted in the arch of foot Because of the decrease in circulation, presence is often noted with poorly healing ulcers especially in distal portions of digits Paroxysmal "electrical shock" pain is indicative of ischemic neuropathy	***Treatment*** Refer to a vascular specialist for treatment Teach the patient to protect the extremity from trauma and eliminate exposure to hot and cold temperatures Smoking cessation helps decrease the symptoms
Raynaud's Disease Characterized by paroxysmal digital ischemia induced by cold or emotional stress Extreme vasospasm leads to insufficient blood flow to digits and may cause gangrenous lesions Most common in women who smoke and are between the ages of 20 and 40 yr Associated with preexisting autoimmune or connective tissue disease Frequent co-morbidity with migraine headache	Usually bilateral and symmetric Usually involves fingers more often than toes Pain may be severe Three-phase color change occurs in response to a "trigger": 1. Pallor with digits turning absolutely white 2. Cyanosis from slow return of blood flow 3. Rubor from reactive hyperemia	***Diagnostics*** Cold stimulation test ***Treatment*** Refer to a vascular specialist or rheumatologist for initial treatment Smoking cessation Dress warmly and avoid unnecessary cold exposure Gloves, hat, and heavy socks, especially in winter Calcium channel blockers may be used in severe cases Review the patient's medications to determine any use of drugs that might aggravate the symptoms (e.g., beta adrenergic blocking agents, ergot preparations, amphetamines, appetite suppressants, imipramine, clonidine)

CALCULATION OF THE ANKLE-BRACHIAL INDEX (ABI)

Definition. The ABI is a diagnostic determination for lower-extremity arterial ischemia.

Procedure. A handheld Doppler transducer is placed over either the dorsalis pedis or the posterior tibialis artery. The BP cuff is inflated at the ankle until the signal stops; systolic pressure is recorded when the signal reappears during cuff deflation. Brachial systolic pressure is recorded in a similar manner.

Calculation. The ABI is calculated as the ankle pressure divided by the brachial pressure.

Interpretation. Normal ankle systolic pressure exceeds arm systolic pressure. Ankle pressure does not begin to change until the diameter of the artery is reduced by at least 50%. The ABI normally does not fall after exercise.

ABI	DISEASE SEVERITY
>1	Normal (no disease)
0.9–1	Mild occlusive disease; may have intermittent claudication
0.5–0.8*	Moderate to severe occlusive disease; wound healing impaired
<0.5*	Severe occlusive disease, ischemia, rest pain

*Refer to vascular surgeon.

EXERCISE PROGRAM FOR PERIPHERAL ARTERIAL DISEASE

Peripheral Arterial Disease	443.9

- Exercise therapy allows patients with peripheral arterial disease to walk farther and reduces the severity of the symptoms through development of collateral circulation; most patients who participate in a regular exercise program increase the distance they are able to walk without claudication in 6 to 12 months
- A standard walking program involves walking 2 to 4 times daily to the point of claudication (patients must understand that the pain does not indicate that any damage is occurring and that it is not harmful); an optional mode of exercise is the stationary bicycle with no resistance (adjust the revolutions per minute with claudication pain); this is helpful with overweight patients for non–weight-bearing exercise
- The goal is to exercise 45 to 60 minutes daily; instruct patients to stop exercising if claudication occurs and resume exercise as soon as the symptoms resolve
- With peripheral disease there may also be concomitant coronary artery disease; consider obtaining a stress test before initiating an exercise program

Warfarin (Coumadin) Anticoagulation Therapy

INDICATION	DOSING	MONITORING	CAUTIONS
DVT Atrial fibrillation (AF) Dilated cardiomyopathy Thrombotic CVA After valve replacement Selected AMI patients Valvular heart disease Pulmonary emboli	Begin with 2–5 mg qd po for 2–3 days; measure PT-INR on day 3 and estimate maintenance dose Use 1 dose and vary multiples, fractions, or alter doses according to days of the week (Monday thru Sunday) When making adjustments, increase or decrease the dose by 10%–20% considering the total weekly dose	May do initial screening of PT-INR before beginning therapy to rule out any underlying bleeding disorders When initiating therapy, do serial monitoring q3–7d until patient is stable, then weekly for 2–3 wk, then monthly When adjusting dosages, do PT-INR q7d to determine dosage adjustment needed ***Therapeutic Goals*** Low: PT 16–19 sec INR 2–3 Low goal for DVT, AMI, AF, PE, and tissue heart valves High: PT 19–22 sec INR 3–3.5 High goal for mechanical heart valves	Many medications interact with warfarin; review the patient's medications and any new medications Avoid vitamin K supplements and foods that are high in vitamin K (see Appendix B) Avoid alcohol Teach the patient to monitor for S/S of bleeding Use electric razor Use soft toothbrush Increase fluids Patient should inform other health care providers or dentists that he or she is taking warfarin; doses are usually stopped about 4–5 days before any invasive procedure (does not have to stop for dental procedure if INR is therapeutic) Avoid falls

Practice Pearls

- There are no absolute contraindications to warfarin therapy; the patient's benefit vs. risk ratio should be thoroughly evaluated before therapy is begun and then monitored closely
- Some patients are not candidates for warfarin therapy due to lifestyle, age, or disease process; the practitioner must establish an alliance with the patient to ensure adequate monitoring before starting warfarin therapy
- Warfarin should be discontinued if active bleeding occurs or if the patient becomes pregnant or refuses close monitoring
- With initial idiopathic DVT (i.e., no history of cancer, recent surgery, or trauma) give warfarin for 13 months
- With recurrent DVT, warfarin should be given indefinitely (often over lifetime)
- With an INR greater than 3 but less than 5, hold warfarin for 1 to 2 days; recheck INR (INR will decrease in 24 to 48 hours) and then restart at appropriate dose
- With INR greater than 5 and with high risk for bleeding (INR will decrease in 24 to 48 hours), do one of the following and recheck INR every 24 hours until <5:
  □ INR 5 to 9: hold warfarin and give vitamin K 1 to 2 mg po or IM
  □ INR greater than 9: hold warfarin and give vitamin K 3 to 5 mg po or IM

Acute Peripheral Vascular Disease

| Thrombophlebitis 451.9 |
| Acute Arterial Occlusion 444.9 |

PREDISPOSING FACTORS	SIGNS AND SYMPTOMS	DIAGNOSTICS AND TREATMENT
Thrombophlebitis		
Estrogen therapy, which increases platelet adhesiveness	Aching in calf or thigh unilaterally, aggravated by muscle activity	***Diagnostics*** Doppler flow study Contrast venography (this is considered gold standard)
Immobility (any reason) decreases blood flow in legs by 50%, leading to stasis	Swelling in affected limb, usually unilateral	Impedance plethysmography Duplex U/S
Long bone trauma or crushing injury	Localized tenderness to palpation, which is most marked at site of occlusion	***Treatment*** *DVT*
Postoperative hip surgery or open prostate manipulation	Increased warmth to touch Erythema Tender, cordlike vein (uncommon)	Refer to a collaborating physician for initial treatment
Pregnancy and first postpartum month (because of hyperfibrinogenemia)	Positive Homans' sign (accurate less than 30% of the time)	May be treated as outpatient if no PE: give enoxaparin (Lovenox) 1 mg/kg SC q12h (use actual body weight to
Increases in blood viscosity due to extreme high		

Acute Peripheral Vascular Disease—cont'd

PREDISPOSING FACTORS	SIGNS AND SYMPTOMS	DIAGNOSTICS AND TREATMENT
altitude changes, nephrotic syndrome, and polycythemia vera Cancer Deficiencies of endogenous anticoagulants Varicose veins leading to stasis Heart disease leading to decompensation (e.g., CHF)		calculate dose) for 5–7 days; warfarin is usually begun within 72 hr of diagnosis; or fondaparinux (Arixtra) SC dose dependent on weight; or rivaroxaban (Xarelto) 15 mg bid for 21 days, then 20 mg daily for 6 mo Follow-up care for monitoring anticoagulant therapy Discontinue use of OCs/HRT Avoid crossing legs Avoid prolonged sitting or standing Smoking cessation Do not massage affected limb Use antiembolic hose/stockings to decrease future incidences of thrombosis and to provide support to venous system *Superficial thrombophlebitis* Apply heat Elevate extremity NSAIDs for pain (see Appendix E) Consider antibiotic therapy No smoking Bed rest except for bathroom for 3–5 days Follow-up in 24–48 hr and in 1 wk
Acute Arterial Occlusion Atherosclerotic heart disease Atrial fibrillation Arterial injury occurring after insertion of arterial lines Arteriosclerosis obliterans Collagen vascular disorders DIC Hypercoagulability	Sudden onset pain, coldness, numbness, and pallor to affected limb Loss of peripheral pulses distal to occlusion After the occlusion, cutaneous sensation is lost in first hour Bruit is common if arterial plaque is source of embolus	*Diagnostics* Doppler flow study Arterial angiography Digital subtraction angiography *Treatment* Refer to a collaborating physician or to emergency department immediately

7

ANEMIA

285.9

Anemia is a symptom of a disease and usually results from a decrease in circulating RBC mass. Anemia can be caused by overdestruction of RBCs by the spleen, inadequate production of RBCs by the bone marrow, or massive loss of RBCs (Table 7–1). Whatever the reason, there is a significant decrease in the oxygen-carrying cells available to the tissues. Anemia is defined as a Hgb/Hct of less than 13.5 g/dl and 40% in men and less than 12 g/dl and 37% in women. Additional RBC indices include MCV (the cell size), MCH (the cell color), and RDW (the amount of variation in cell width). The reticulocyte index reflects the body's production of immature RBCs and is used to determine whether the origin of the anemia is within or outside the bone marrow. Below is the calculation for the reticulocyte index:

$$\text{Reticulocyte count (\%)} \times \frac{\text{Patient's hematocrit}}{\text{(Normal hematocrit)}} + 2 = \text{Reticulocyte index}$$

RETICULOCYTE INDEX >2	RETICULOCYTE INDEX <2
Hemolytic anemia:	Abnormal RBC production:
G6PD	Anemia of chronic disease
Sickle cell	End-stage renal disease (decreased erythropoiesis)
Vasculitis	Vitamin deficiency (B_{12}, folate)
Mechanical destruction:	Hypoplastic/aplastic anemia
Mechanical heart valve	Iron deficiency
Dialysis anemia	
Hypersplenism	
Blood loss	

Signs and symptoms depend on the suddenness of the onset of anemia. The severity of adult anemia does not reliably indicate the origin or the clinical significance. Symptoms can be slow to manifest and often only become noticeable when there is an increased demand for oxygen. Patients with mild anemia are often asymptomatic and may only complain of fatigue, SOB, or palpitations after exercise or exertion. If anemia continues to progress the patient may have more marked symptoms.

When the Hgb value falls below 7.5 g/dl, resting cardiac output rises with an increase in both heart rate and stroke volume. This results in tachycardia and widened pulse pressure. Patients with severe anemia often exhibit symptoms at rest. The following symptoms are suggestive of an anemia:
- Dizziness
- Headache
- Irritability
- Difficulty concentrating or sleeping
- Syncope or vertigo
- Hypersensitivity to cold from decreased blood flow to skin

- Anorexia, indigestion, and nausea from shunting of blood away from the GI system
- Amenorrhea or increased bleeding with menses
- Impotence or decreased libido in males
- Pallor to skin, especially to creases on palms of the hands; note if creases are as pale as the surrounding skin (usually noted with Hgb value <7 g/dl)
- Chest pain, especially with chronic conditions (e.g., CRF)
- SOB

Patients with anemia associated with vitamin B_{12} or folate deficiency may exhibit similar symptoms of low volume but will also have the following:

- Mentation changes, such as confusion, slow or deteriorating memory or thought processes, or agitation
- Paresthesia in extremities
- Weakness or faintness
- Stomatitis or a sore, smooth tongue
- Anorexia, weight loss, or diarrhea

Refer patients with anemia:

- For colonoscopy if there is a positive Hemoccult result
- If transfusion is required
- For genetic counseling with inherited hemoglobinopathy
- To rule out bone marrow failure in folate deficiency, especially if patient has been compliant but is unresponsive to therapy
- If hemolytic condition is suspected or present

VASCULAR WOUND CARE AND TREATMENT

Wounds neither develop nor heal overnight. Measure wound(s) accurately and note the color, odor, and general appearance. Monitor treatments weekly and do not change them quickly (Table 7–2).

Practice Pearls

- Heel ulcers with dry eschar and without evidence of infection (e.g., edema, redness, or exudative discharge) should be left alone and monitored weekly; use protective wraps to minimize any type of pressure while the patient is out of bed and use air pressure beds and cutout heel protectors while in bed
- Protect a fragile elderly person's lower extremities by using sheepskin wraps with Velcro to surround the leg from knee to ankle; these wraps are warm and nonconstricting
- If an extremity shows evidence of edema, use diuretic therapy and elevation of the extremity to decrease the edema; edema will decrease healing in the wound bed; supportive stockings or Ace wraps can be used if a member of the staff or patient's family is skilled in applying these therapies; monitor for complications with every application
- Rule out venous thrombosis if a single extremity is edematous
- Protein-rich fluid retains a "pit" when depressed >1 mm, suggesting cardiac disease (CHF); protein-poor fluid will "spring-back" quickly when depressed, suggesting hepatic or renal disease or malnutrition

Text continued on p. 209

Table 7–1 Classification of Anemia

Iron Deficiency Anemia   280.9
Thalassemia   282.4
Anemia of Chronic Disease   285.2
Folate Deficiency   281.2
Vitamin B$_{12}$ Deficiency   266.2
Sickle Cell Anemia   282.60

CLASS	AT RISK	PHYSICAL FINDINGS	
Iron Deficiency Anemia (IDA)			
Commonly caused by blood loss and occasionally by dietary deficiency	Infants Pregnant women Menstruating women Persons with GI bleeding ASA/NSAID use Patients with cancer Persons with lead poisoning Older persons Impoverished	Easily fatigued Tachycardia with mild exertion Shortness of breath Palpitations Brittle hair Koilonychia (spoon-shaped nails) Palmar crease, circumoral, and conjunctival pallor Symptoms usually start occurring with Hgb less than 10 g/dl	
Thalassemia			
Congenital abnormality of Hgb synthesis	Persons of Southeast Asian descent, including Vietnamese and Chinese; Pacific Islanders; and those of Mediterranean descent	*Minor:* FH of mild anemia, not identified until later in life during an acute illness Symptoms similar to IDA with mild pallor, splenomegaly, and bronzing of skin	*Major:* Identified in early childhood with *severe* symptoms of anemia, growth retardation, and jaundice
Anemia of Chronic Disease (ACD)			
Normocytic anemia usually caused by bone marrow disorders (e.g., aplasia, cancers of bone marrow, malnutrition, and other metabolic problems)	Persons with chronic disease conditions such as cancers, chronic infections, early iron deficiency, chronic renal or liver failure, aplastic anemia, and hemolytic anemia	Same symptoms as with IDA but usually milder Patient may have hepatosplenomegaly and jaundice Autoimmune hemolytic anemia presents with rapid onset anemia with fever, chills, H/A, back and abdominal pain, jaundice, and hepatomegaly	

LABORATORY VALUES	TREATMENT
↓ Hgb ↓ Hct ↓ Ferritin <20 ng/ml ↓ Fe ↓ TIBC ↑ RDW ↓ MCV ↓ RBC N ↓ Reticulocyte index	Correct the underlying cause Begin oral iron replacement therapy with ferrous sulfate 300 mg tid between meals or Niferex-150 bid between meals Recheck Hgb and ferritin in 1 mo Continue iron replacement for 6 mo after normal lab values reached Diet should be high in iron-rich foods (see Appendix B) Refer to specialist if unresponsive to therapy

Minor:	Major:	TREATMENT
↓ Hgb ↓ Hct N ↑ Ferritin N Fe N TIBC N RDW ↓ MCV N ↑ RBC Reticulocyte index <2 Hgb electrophoresis to determine type of thalassemia	↓ Hgb ↓ Hct ↑ Ferritin ↑ Fe N ↓ TIBC ↑ RDW ↓ MCV ↓ RBC Hgb electrophoresis to determine type of thalassemia	Treatment aimed at identifying type of thalassemia Supportive care is needed initially if symptoms are mild; may need transfusions if symptoms are severe Iron supplements are not indicated because patient is not deficient Genetic counseling should be given if individual is of childbearing age

LABORATORY VALUES	TREATMENT
N ↓ Hgb N ↓ Hct N Ferritin N ↓ Fe N ↓ TIBC N MCV ↑ RDW N ↓ Reticulocyte index Hct not <24%; if Hct <24% check for other causes	Treat the underlying cause Prevent rapid progression of an underlying disease state Maintain adequate nutrition with iron-rich foods (Appendix B) and oral iron supplements in the beginning (see IDA treatment) Patients may need erythropoietin (must not have IDA) or transfusions; monitor patient for volume overload with any replacement therapy

Continued

Table 7–1   Classification of Anemia—cont'd

CLASS	AT RISK	PHYSICAL FINDINGS
Screen for IDA, hemolytic anemia, and vitamin deficiency		
Folate or Vitamin B$_{12}$ Deficiency		
Caused by failure to absorb vitamin B$_{12}$ and folate from the stomach mucosa; can be caused by chronic PPI use	Malnutrition commonly seen in the elderly, the poor, and persons with increased alcohol use Persons with chronic gastritis and loss of intrinsic factor, which diminishes absorption of folate and vitamin B$_{12}$ Persons with chronic renal and liver failure Persons with hypothyroidism Persons with autoimmune disorders (e.g., Hashimoto's thyroiditis or vitiligo)	Symptoms similar to other anemias with: Glossitis, angular cheilitis, pica Brittle hair Diarrhea, anorexia Peripheral paresthesias Difficulty with balance Romberg's and Babinski's signs Changes in mentation with mild confusion, apathy, depression, and memory loss
Sickle Cell Anemia		
Autosomal recessive disorder of Hgb precursor A resulting in misshapen and unstable RBCs, which in turn result in early cell destruction or poor ability of cells to carry oxygen	Predominantly found in American and Central African blacks Usually found in infancy through screening Can have few episodes of varying degrees of severity, but usually have long history of anemia with recurrent episodes of pain	Symptoms same as IDA, along with vaso-occlusive crisis in microvascular beds, microvascular infarcts, abdominal pain, bone and joint pain, chest pain and stroke, splenomegaly, and hypovolemic shock

LABORATORY VALUES	TREATMENT

N ↓ Hgb
N ↓ Hct
N Ferritin
N Fe
N TIBC
↑ MCV
↑ RDW
Reticulocyte index <2
↓ Folate or ↓ vitamin B_{12} (diagnosis determined by deficiency)
MCV between 95 and 110 usually indicative of alcohol excess; MCV >115 usually indicative of vitamin deficiency; increased MCV with normal folate and vitamin B_{12}, consider drug therapies that interfere with nucleic acid synthesis and leukemias
	Replace deficient vitamin:
	  Folic acid 1 mg qd;
	  Cyanocobalamin 100 µg
	  SC/IM qd for 5–10 days, then 1000 µg every month
	Replacement is for life
	Levels return to normal within 2 mo
	Recheck vitamin level in 4 wk and then again in 8 wk
	Symptoms will resolve quickly if deficiency has been of a short duration
	Increase dietary sources of deficient vitamin (see Appendix B)
	Start iron replacement therapy for 1 mo (see IDA treatment); monitor for hypokalemia as volume improves
	Advise patient of increased risk of esophageal, pancreatic, and rectal cancer risks associated with vitamin B_{12} deficiency

Laboratory values usually low to normal, except when person is in crisis Hgb electrophoresis for disease or trait Reticulocyte index >2	No specific treatment and no cure Yearly influenza immunizations and pneumococcal vaccine q5y are recommended to reduce incidence of infection Identify factors that can precipitate a crisis Use oxygen at high concentrations for hypoxia Aggressive pain therapy Antibiotics for infections Maintain good hydration at all times Well-balanced diet Genetic counseling Folic acid supplementation Transfusions may be needed periodically Psychiatric counseling Monitor for drug abuse

| Table 7–2 | Differentiation of Venous, Arterial, and Diabetic Ulcers |

Arterial Ulcer	447.2
Venous Ulcer	707.9
Diabetic Ulcer	250.8

ARTERIAL	VENOUS	DIABETIC
History Intermittent claudication Rest pain usually present Atrophy of skin, hair loss over extremity	No claudication or pain at rest Ankle or leg edema Chronic nonhealing ulcer Reddish-brown discoloration	Diabetes mellitus Peripheral neuropathy No claudication
Pain and Temperature Acute pain, worse at night Sharp or burning Cool or cold foot Reddens with dangling; turns pale white with elevation	Moderate discomfort Aching Warm foot	Painless Warm or cold foot
Ulcer Location End of toes Between toes Heels Lateral malleolus Distal foreleg Phalangeal heads	Medial malleolus (most common) Over any bony prominence May initially mimic an abscess formation	Plantar area of foot Metatarsal heads Any area of stress or pressure Heel
Ulcer Appearance Deep with even edges Grayish base with nonerythematous borders Base is dry Little granulation tissue Shiny, thin skin around ulcer	Superficial with uneven edges Pink base with granulation tissue Base is moist with moderate to heavy drainage	Deep Pale with even edges Little granulation tissue Light to moderate drainage
Pulses and Neurologic Decreased or absent pulses Paresthesia	Normal pulses No paresthesia	Usually normal pulses May or may not have paresthesia
Treatment* Long-term wound care Prevent infection Meticulous foot care Whirlpool therapy daily to improve circulation and cleanliness	Long-term wound care Prevent infection Staging to determine treatment needed Gentle massage to surrounding tissue and frequent turning to relieve pressure Keep area elevated to decrease swelling and improve circulation	Control DM Prevent infection Meticulous foot care and monitoring by the patient, family, or health care workers Whirlpool therapy bid–tid Refer to podiatrist Patient education handout (see Appendix D)

*For wound staging and treatment protocols see p. 210.

- Treat infection promptly with antibiotics that cover gram-negative, gram-positive, and anaerobic bacteria; pseudomonal infection usually has a sweet odor and may respond to Dakin's solution applied daily; a rapidly regressing wound in which epithelium seems to be melting is typical of MRSA, and this may respond to vancomycin topically and intravenously; a strong odor of decay and a wound that will not heal may be associated with gangrene (especially if the person is diabetic) and will need referral
- Wounds will heal faster if the eschar is removed and the wound bed is kept moist and clean; the type of debridement will depend on the size of the wound and the comfort level of the practitioner; petroleum jelly (Vaseline) gauze dressings work well, are inexpensive, and can be changed daily; gentle scrubbing with Bactistat or a similar product will facilitate removal of debris and keep the wound clean
- Silverlon dressings can be used every 1 to 5 days without being changed; the Silverlon fabric dressing can be reused until the color starts to dim; if this therapy is going to work, you will see a positive change in the wound within 6 days; Silverlon does seem to decrease pain in the wound
- Oxygen therapy can be used to heal wounds without damaging tissue; wrap the leg with light-weight gauze or a stockinette, and then cut a window out over the wound; tape a plastic bag to the gauze and over the wound (do not tape to the skin) and cut a small hole in the bag; insert oxygen tubing; start oxygen at 5 to 8 L/min for 15 to 20 minutes daily; use a petroleum jelly gauze dressing over the wound bed to keep it moist between treatments; you should begin to see results in 5 to 7 days but may take extended time for total healing
- Check for peripheral pulses when an ulcer is found on a lower extremity; use Doppler ultrasound if indicated to determine vascular status; cilostazol (Pletal) may be helpful to increase circulation to distal extremities
- Refer patients with wounds that are enlarging, are tunneling, have a foul odor, and are not responding to therapy in a reasonable amount of time, depending on specific protocols

Defining the Wound

Although the underlying disease process is important, the color of a wound can be a significant tool in determining treatment modalities. The following colors relate to progression of wounds:

Red	Clean, healthy granulation tissue. Initial layers of tissue begin as pink tissue then proceed to beefy red
Yellow	Sloughing tissue, indicating microorganisms at work and the need for cleaning. Exudate can be whitish yellow, greenish yellow, or beige.
Black	Eschar or necrotic tissue. This should be removed as soon as possible, because it is an excellent medium for bacterial proliferation.

Staging of Wounds

The staging of wounds gives a good indication of the ulcer formation and the stage of healing or deterioration:

STAGE	DEFINITION
1 (early, localized erythema)	Nonblanching erythema of intact skin The heralding lesion of skin ulceration
2 (red to yellow ulcer)	Partial-thickness skin loss involving epidermis, dermis, or both The superficial ulcer that presents clinically as an abrasion, blister, or shallow crater
3 (yellow ulcer)	Full-thickness skin loss involving damage to or necrosis of subcutaneous tissue that may extend down to, but not through, underlying fascia The ulcer at presentation is a deep crater, with or without undermining of adjacent tissue
4 (black ulcer)	Full-thickness skin loss with extensive destruction, tissue necrosis, or damage to muscle, bone, or supporting structures Undermining and sinus tracts also involved

Treatment Algorithm for Stage I Wounds

Definition.   Nonblanching erythema of intact skin with discoloration, warmth, or hardness of skin. Skin is unbroken but may be inflamed and painful. Texture is spongy to firm with a red ulcer.

Treatment.   Relieve pressure and friction with frequent turning and gentle massage to the area. Keep the area clean and dry, the extremity elevated, and bed linens off the affected area. Evaluate shoes and socks for constrictions or areas of friction. With each dressing change, gently clean the area with normal saline or mild, hypoallergenic soap and dry thoroughly. Start a daily multivitamin regimen with zinc (220 mg bid) and vitamin C (500 mg tid) until the wound heals. Provide a high-protein diet (unless contraindicated). Arginine Intensive Drink (Arginaid) made by Novartis, is a useful protein drink to enhance healing;

and

Apply protective ointment, moisturizing lotion, or lubricating sprays to surrounding areas that are in danger of breakdown. Examples include Aloe Vesta protective ointment, Granulex spray, Dermagran Ointment, and triple antibiotic ointment;

or

Apply skin sealants or transparent films to protect skin from mechanical stripping or maceration due to contact with body fluids (Table 7–3). Examples include Hollister Skin Gel, Sween Prep, OpSite, Tegaderm, and Vaseline gauze;

or

Apply hydrocolloids to pressure and friction areas for added protection, especially if these areas are over a bony prominence or are not healing with above measures (see Table 7–3). Examples are DuoDerm Extra Thin, Epilock Dressing, and Comfeel Ulcer Care Dressing.

Table 7–3 Wound Care Dressing Description

DRESSING	DESCRIPTION
Alginates (seaweed)	Absorbent, conforms to wound shapes
	Interacts with wound exudate to form gel that enhances healing
	Indicated for wounds with moderate to heavy exudate or with tunneling wounds
Composites	Combination products with moisture-retention and absorbent properties
	Indicated for open wounds with moderate to heavy drainage
Foam	Semipermeable, nonadherent dressings that form a moist environment for wound healing and insulation
	Indicated for open wounds with minimal to heavy drainage and as secondary dressings to further absorb drainage
Hydrocolloids	Nonpermeable adhesive dressings used to assist clean wounds to form granulations and necrotic wounds to self-debride
	Indicated for wounds that are necrotic or have light to moderate drainage
Hydrogels	May be water- or glycerin-based gels, gauze, or other types of dressings
	Indicated for open wounds with light drainage
Skin protectants	Creams or sprays that toughen skin that has been compromised from friction or skin over bony prominences
	Application of protectant usually involves some type of massage to apply; this enhances circulation to damaged area
	Indicated for intact skin
Skin sealants	Form barriers over tissue to protect tissue from mechanical friction or maceration
	Indicated for intact skin

WOUND WITH LIGHT TO MODERATE DRAINAGE	WOUND WITH HEAVY DRAINAGE
Composites*	**Alginates***
Alldress	Kaltostat
Epilock	Sorbsan Topical
Telfa Dressing	Curasorb
Hydrogels*	**Composites***
Carrasyn Gel	Transorb
Wound Dressing	

*Not inclusive of all products.

Continued

DuoDerm Hydrogel	Sofsorb Wound
SAF-Gel	Veritex Wound
Hydrocolloids*	**Foams***
DuoDerm Extra Thin	Lyofoan
Comfeel Contour Dressing	Hydrasorb
CarraSmart	
Restore Extra Thin Dressing	
Transparent Films*	
AcuDerm	
Poly Skin	
OpSite	
Blisterfilm	
Tegaderm	
Foams*	
Mitraflex	
Epiloci	
3/4 Foam Dressing	

*Not inclusive of all products.

and

Continue close monitoring to prevent progression or recurrence of ulcer or wound. Establish treatment plan with caregivers for monitoring and prevention.

Treatment Algorithms for Stage 2 Wounds

Definition.   Partial-thickness skin loss involving epidermis or dermis. Ulcer is superficial and presents as an abrasion, blister, or shallow ulcer. Ulcer may have drainage and may be red to yellow.

Treatment.   Use the same supportive therapies as with Stage 1 wounds. Objectively assess the area by determining its size, depth and the amount, color, and odor of the drainage. Document the location of the ulcer. A photograph of the site can be beneficial for long-term evaluation. Clean with normal saline or Bactistat cleanser, using gentle irrigation (e.g., with a 35-ml syringe with a 19-g needle or angiocatheter) and/or scrubbing daily and with each dressing change. There may be a need for debridement, depending on the depth and appearance of the ulcer (see p. 213). Prompt treatment with topical antibiotic ointment or oral antibiotics is recommended if infection is present. Antibiotics used for infection should have antibacterial effectiveness against gram-negative, gram-positive, and anaerobic organisms.

and

Use a dressing that promotes healing (see Table 7–3).

and

Prevent further deterioration of surrounding skin by decreasing peripheral edema (e.g., use diuretic therapy, elevate the extremity, use compression dressing, and avoid constricting clothing, shoes, and socks). Avoid smoking if possible. Avoid prolonged sitting or standing; have the patient lie down for a while in the morning and afternoon. Consider cilostazol (Pletal) to enhance circulation in lower extremities. Daily oxygen therapy directly to the wound or a Silverlon dressing may improve healing.

Debridement Modalities

Sharp surgical debridement	Use of scalpel for superficial removal of necrotic tissue; can also score or cross-hatch eschar over wound before enzymatic debridement; debride immediately if wound infection is present; may need to hospitalize patient and excise larger area under anesthetic
Mechanical debridement	Wet-to-dry dressings Hydrotherapy Wound irrigation Dextranomers (not highly recommended)
Autolytic debridement	Involves using synthetic dressings to cover a wound and allow devitalized tissue to self-digest with normally present wound fluids Examples: OpSite, Tegaderm, wound filler, and hydrating dressings
Enzymatic debridement	Application of topical debriding agent to devitalized tissues Good option if patient cannot tolerate surgery or if no infection is present Examples Collagenase Santyl, Elase ointment, Panafil, and Granulex spray If eschar is thick may need to cross-hatch it to allow debriding agent to be absorbed

Treatment Algorithm for Stage 3 and 4 Wounds

Definition. Stage 3 wounds involve full-thickness skin loss, with subcutaneous tissue damage or necrosis that may extend to the fascia. The wound appears as a deep crater extending to underlying tissue. The color may be white to black with foul-smelling drainage. Pain may not be present except in surrounding tissue.

Stage 4 wounds involve deep underlying skin loss with massive destruction to underlying tissue, including muscle, bone, and supporting structures. Tunneling or sinus tracts are usually found with these wounds. Drainage is usually moderate to heavy and foul smelling. Osteomyelitis is a possibility if bone is involved.

Treatment. Use the same supportive therapies as with Stage 1 wounds. Objectively assess the area for the location, size, and depth of the wound and for the presence of tunneling. Also, assess the drainage for color and odor. Record the presence of infection and whether the infection is localized or systemic. Promptly start antibiotic therapy if infection is suspected. Remove any wound crust or eschar. If the wound is not healing after 2 to 4 weeks of optimum care obtain a deep culture of the wound by aspirating wound contents. Start systemic antibiotics as indicated by the culture. Consult with a physician for treatment modalities needed. Some modalities that might be used are whirlpool therapy, packing with alginates daily, or other recommended packing procedure, and debridement of the area.

NOTES

NOTES

NOTES

8

Abdominal Disorders

For complete history and physical exam, see Chapter 1.

DIFFERENTIAL DIAGNOSIS OF ABDOMINAL PROBLEMS BASED ON PAIN LOCATION

Epigastrium

AMI	Peptic ulcer
Pneumonia	Gastritis
Pleurisy	Pancreatitis
Esophagitis	Cholecystitis

Right Upper Quadrant
Pleurisy
Cholecystitis
Perforated duodenal ulcer
Appendicitis
Ectopic pregnancy
Perforated colon
Splenic rupture
Pancreatitis
Hepatitis

Left Upper Quadrant
Pleurisy
Splenic rupture
Perforated gastric ulcer
Pancreatitis
Diverticulitis
Ectopic pregnancy
Perforated colon
Aortic aneurysm
Fecal loading

Periumbilicus

Regional enteritis	Perforated duodenal ulcer
Appendicitis	Aortic aneurysm
Leaking aortic aneurysm	Diverticulitis

Right Lower Quadrant
Appendicitis
Acute regional enteritis
PID
Ectopic pregnancy
Ovarian torsion/cyst
Incarcerated inguinal hernia
Perforated duodenal ulcer
Colon cancer
Pancreatitis
Cecal diverticulitis

Left Lower Quadrant
Sigmoid diverticulitis
PID
Ectopic pregnancy
Ovarian torsion/cyst
Incarcerated inguinal hernia
Perforated gastric ulcer

Hypogastrium

Regional enteritis	Ulcerative colitis
PID, UTI	Colon cancer

Practice Pearls

- With abdominal complaints, keep the focus broad initially; symptoms inconsequential to the patient may be important
- Colon cancer screening guidelines (>50 years or <40 years if close relative had polyps or colon cancer):
  - □ Three fecal occult blood tests annually *or*
  - □ Flexible sigmoidoscopy q5y *or*
  - □ q5–10y *or*
  - □ Colonoscopy q10y: if no history of colon cancer in immediate family; if colon cancer in immediate family, colonoscopy is recommended 5 years before the youngest case identified for all family members; if polyps noted, recommend follow-up per gastroenterologist
- Constipation relief suggestions:
  - □ Warm together 60 ml prune juice and 30 ml milk of magnesia (MOM) and drink while it is warm
  - □ PBA: mix together 1 cup prune juice, 1 tbsp unprocessed bran, and applesauce to desired consistency; start with 30 ml a day with breakfast and if necessary increase weekly to total of 90 ml tid
  - □ Miralax daily (may take 3 days to see results initially)
  - □ Stool softeners: docusate sodium (Colase) up to 2 capsules bid (these soften stools but do not increase peristalsis)
  - □ Lactulose 15 ml bid (adult); 1 mg/kg/day in divided doses (children)
  - □ Consider lubiprostone (Amitiza) for chronic idiopathic constipation
  - □ Consider other medications as a cause (e.g., anticholinergics, narcotics, laxatives)
  - □ Daily use of psyllium or methyl cellulose as bulk fiber (can use 2–3 times daily)
  - □ Increase water intake to 2 to 4 L daily
- Monitoring liver function:
  - □ The ALT/AST ratio can help differentiate alcohol-induced liver damage from infectious hepatitis (ALT > AST = infectious hepatitis; AST > ALT = alcohol-related damage)
  - □ Albumin level: albumin controls osmotic pressure, which maintains vascular fluid in vessels; decreased albumin leads to edema seen in cirrhosis, liver failure, and malnutrition; increased albumin may indicate dehydration
  - □ Total bilirubin is a function of the breakdown of hemoglobin and evaluates the liver's ability to dispose of this substance; with obstructive jaundice, stones, or damaged liver cells, total bilirubin is increased
- Acute abdominal pain persisting longer than 6 hours is probably a surgical problem
- Pain followed by nausea and vomiting is probably a surgical problem
- Nausea and vomiting followed by pain is probably a medical problem
- For hemorrhoids try this compounded product, used up to qid: NTG ointment 2%, mixed 50/50 with petroleum jelly (Vaseline) for 1% concentration, then mixed with an equal amount of cortisone cream 1% for NTG ointment 0.5%
- Possible studies for diarrhea lasting >1 week
  - □ Stool specimens for:
    1. Ova and parasites (O&P), C&S, and *Clostridium difficile* (infectious disease)

2. Blood

3. pH (carbohydrate metabolism)

4. Fecal fat (fat malabsorption syndrome)

5. Fecal alpha-2 antitrypsin (protein malabsorption)

6. Electrolyte and osmolarity (secretory versus osmotic diarrhea)

- Radiographs:
  1. Abdominal films (flat and upright)
  2. UGI with small bowel follow-through
  3. Barium enema
- Colonoscopy
- Other laboratory tests:
  1. Electrolytes, liver profile, and amylase
  2. Protein and albumin
  3. CBC, ESR, and immunoglobins

• Travelers' diarrhea does not require antibiotics unless diarrhea is severe. Prompt control of symptoms is the treatment of choice. Use antidiarrheal medications such as loperamide (e.g., Imodium) if no fever or bloody stools. Try Pepto-Bismol 2 tablets qid for relief of diarrhea. Save antibiotics for the more severe episodes of diarrhea with fever or bloody stools. Antibiotics of choice are:
- Ciprofloxacin 500 mg bid for 3 to 5 days
- Ofloxacin 300 mg bid for 3 to 5 days
- Norfloxacin 400 mg bid for 3 to 5 days

Text continued on p. 236

Common Abdominal Problems

PROBLEM	SIGNS AND SYMPTOMS	DIAGNOSTICS AND TREATMENT
UPPER ABDOMINAL PROBLEMS		
Gastroesophageal Reflux Disease 530.81 Peptic Ulcer Disease 533.9 *Helicobacter pylori*–Induced Gastritis 041.86 Cholecystitis 575.10 Acute Gastroenteritis 558.9 Pancreatitis 577.0		
Gastroesophageal Reflux Disease Reflux of gastroduodenal contents into the esophagus because of relaxation of the lower esophageal sphincter (LES) Common in all ages Incidence in men equal to that of women Multiple causes: Foods that relax LES: Chocolate Peppermint High-fat foods Irritating foods Citrus fruits Spicy foods Tomatoes	Heartburn usually occurs about 1 hr after a large meal and is made worse by lying down Metallic, acid taste in mouth Belching Regurgitation of fluids or foods Pain increases when lying down at night or when bending forward Pain decreases with antacids Anterior chest pain or burning; can have radiation to jaw or neck Recurrent pneumonia or bronchospasm Laryngitis, hoarseness Chronic, nonproductive cough Throat clearing Dental erosion	*Diagnostics* Clinical history good indicator of disease CBC Barium swallow *Helicobacter pylori* testing if unresponsive to therapy *Treatment* If no alarming symptoms and clinical history indicates GERD is probable diagnosis, initiate therapy with the following: *Diet Modification* Do not eat meals or drink carbonated beverages 2–3 hr before bedtime Decrease the amount of fried, fatty, and spicy foods Raise the head of the bed using 4–6 in blocks Decrease weight if patient is obese

8

Hiatal hernia
Cigarette smoking
Coffee
Medicines that relax LES:
  Theophylline
  Anticholinergics
  Progesterone
  Calcium channel blockers
  Alpha adrenergic agents
  Diazepam
Medicines that aggravate:
  Tetracycline
  Quinidine
  Potassium tabs
  Iron salts
  NSAIDs, ASA
  Bisphosphonates

Peptic Ulcer Disease

Includes both gastric and duodenal ulcers
Common features of gastric and duodenal ulcers:
Occurs between 40 and 60 years of age
Prior history of *H. pylori* infection
Chronic NSAID use
History of long-term dyspepsia
Incidence of occurrence equal between men and women

Not to Be Missed
Anorexia
Unintentional weight loss
Blood in stools
Dysphagia or painful swallowing
Pulmonary disorders
Barrett's esophagus (high risk in obese patients, white male >50yr)
Anemia

Gastric Ulcer
Chronic recurrent upper abdominal pain
Burning, gnawing, aching, and "hunger pains"
N/V
Symptoms occur after eating, usually within about 1 hour
Feeling of fullness during eating is common
Pain in left subcostal area, epigastric tenderness, voluntary muscle guarding
Pain is usually relieved by antacids

Monitor the medication regimen
Decrease use of caffeine, nicotine, and alcohol
Avoid foods that relax the LES

Drug Therapy
Use antacids whenever symptoms are present
If symptoms are predictable, use antacids 1hr pc and hs *or* OTC H_2 blocker ac meals
If symptoms are intense and predictable, use prescription H_2 blocker or proton pump inhibitor (PPI) (see chart on p. 231)
Refer to gastroenterologist if no response to therapy
Refer for gallbladder U/S; if negative and still symptomatic, consider HIDA*

Diagnostics
Diagnostic studies are usually the same for identifying which type of ulcer is being treated:
CBC with differential
UA
Liver enzymes
Amylase
Barium swallow
Stool for occult blood
Endoscopy with biopsy
H. pylori testing

Continued

*U/S first to rule out stones.

Common Abdominal Problems—cont'd

PROBLEM	SIGNS AND SYMPTOMS	DIAGNOSTICS AND TREATMENT
	Duodenal Ulcer Chronic, recurrent midline epigastric distress or pain near the xiphoid; usually occurs 45–60 min after a meal or awakens the person in the middle of the night, not near breakfast time Nausea with emesis of acid-tasting gastric juices without food in emesis Pain relieved by food, milk, antacids, or vomiting; however, eating may increase pain Epigastric pain with palpation and guarding **Not to Be Missed** Recurrent vomiting Dysphagia Unintentional, rapid weight loss GI bleeding Anemia	**Treatment** Treatment therapies areaimed at both gastric and duodenal ulcers Review all medications, including OTC and herbal products *Acute Phase* Diet Modification Nutritious meals on a regular schedule with snacks between meals Avoid cigarette smoking and alcoholic beverages Avoid any foods known to irritate the patient's stomach *Drug therapy* Initiate for 4–8 wk; any of these can be effective, but PPIs are most effective*: Antacids: 2–4 tbsp before and after meals and hs (magnesium causes diarrhea; aluminum causes constipation; use combination product to offset side effects) Sucralfate: 1 g 30–60 min before meals and hs (especially useful with NSAID-induced ulcer) H₂ blocker (see chart on pg. 231) Proton pump inhibitor (PPI) (see chart on pg. 231) *Maintenance Phase* If symptoms resolve with the above therapy, instruct the patient that there is a high probability for recurrence; if the patient is at

high risk for recurrence (e.g., previous ulcer history, positive *H. pylori*, ETOH abuse, high stress environment), use acute phase medication at half the dose, indefinitely

Helicobacter pylori-Induced Gastritis

Can occur at any age

Infection may last years because of difficulty in eradicating bacteria

Injury is to mucosal lining and is caused by urease, a bacterial by-product of *H. pylori*

H. pylori is present in ~90% of duodenal ulcers and ~80% of gastric ulcers

Same as ulcer disease

Suspect infection if patient complains of feeling "sick" with constitutional symptoms

Diagnostics

Serum for *H. pylori* (serum may remain positive for life; if treatment is successful, symptoms resolve)

Endoscopy for tissue urease/biopsy or recurrent symptoms after treatment with antibiotic

Treatment

Symptom relief is the goal of therapy; treat with one of the following suggested regimens:

Dosing regimens, 10-day therapy:
Amoxicillin 1 g po bid
Clarithromycin (Biaxin) 500 mg po bid *and*
PPI of choice (see chart p. 231)

Metronidazole (Flagyl) 500 mg po bid
Clarithromycin (Biaxin) 500 mg po bid
PPI of choice (see chart p. 231)

Bismuth subsalicylate 525 mg qid
Metronidazole (Flagyl) 250 mg qid
Tetracycline 500 mg qid
PPI of choice (see chart p. 231)

Dosing regimen, 14-day therapy:
Prevpac 1 dose bid.
Helidac plus H₂-blocker (see chart p. 231)

Continued

Common Abdominal Problems—cont'd

PROBLEM	SIGNS AND SYMPTOMS	DIAGNOSTICS AND TREATMENT
Cholecystitis	RUQ pain radiating to right shoulder or scapula area; pain usually occurs after ingestion of a large or fatty meal; pain occurs suddenly and is severe and subsides slowly; tenderness usually follows pain in same area N/V occurs after ingestion of large or fatty meal Inability to consume normal amounts of food because of "full" feeling Regurgitates bitter fluids Heartburn	*Diagnostics* CBC shows leukocytosis and a shift to left ECG to R/O AMI CXR to R/O pneumonia U/S of gallbladder; if negative and no improvement in symptoms, order HIDA HIDA scan, if indicated Serum amylase (may be elevated) Serum alkaline phosphatase (may be elevated) Total bilirubin (may be mildly or markedly elevated) *Treatment* Refer to a surgeon for further evaluation and monitoring
Acute Gastroenteritis Primarily a self-limiting disease Viral gastroenteritis occurs more often in the winter Bacterial gastroenteritis occurs in groups of people who have eaten contaminated food	Acute onset N/V Flatulence with explosive diarrhea Crampy, abdominal pain Headache, myalgia Fever 101°–103°F (38.3°–39.4°C) Malaise Diffuse tenderness to abdomen with hyperactive bowel sounds	1 dose Helidac qid for 14 days plus H$_2$-blocker for 28 days Refer to gastroenterologist if no response to two trials *Diagnostics* CBC usually normal; leukocytosis with bacterial infection Stool for occult blood usually negative *Treatment* *Immediately refer if* Obvious dehydration Positive neurologic signs

8

	Neurologic symptoms indicate botulism and immediate referral to emergency department	Severe abdominal pain with N/V

General Care

Monitor closely if patient is elderly or very young
Bed rest
Cracked ice chips with N/V; follow with clear liquids for 24hr; if N/V abates, progress to a BRATY diet (refer to Appendix B)
Monitor for progressing dehydration
Teach good hand washing and preparation of food
Follow-up in 24–72hr if symptoms continue or worsen
Diarrhea may continue for weeks with *Salmonella*
Antidiarrheals may help but may also prolong symptoms
Antiemetic if needed
Stool-bulking agents (e.g., FiberCon) can slow diarrhea
Lactobacillus (Lactinex) 2 capsules bid–qid to reestablish normal bowel flora

Pancreatitis
Usually caused by chronic ingestion of alcohol for long periods
Other causes:
Biliary tract disease
Trauma from surgery or blunt trauma
Hypertriglyceridemia
Renal failure
Viral infection

Generalized, marked abdominal pain and distention
Severe epigastric pain radiating to midback
N/V, dehydration
Low-grade fever
May have signs of intraabdominal bleeding with ecchymosis in flanks or periumbilical area

Diagnostics

CBC, usually with leukocytosis and hemoconcentration
Electrolytes with low Ca^{++} and Mg^{++}
Liver enzymes are usually elevated
Ultrasound or CT of pancreas usually definitive test
Lipid profile
Amylase

Treatment

Refer to physician immediately

Continued

8

Common Abdominal Problems—cont'd

PROBLEM	SIGNS AND SYMPTOMS	DIAGNOSTICS AND TREATMENT
LOWER ABDOMINAL PROBLEMS		

Irritable Bowel Syndrome 564.1
Diverticulitis 562.11
Appendicitis 541
Colon Cancer 154.0
Crohn's Disease (Regional Enteritis) 555.9
Ulcerative Colitis 556.9
Acute Infectious Diarrhea 009.2

PROBLEM	SIGNS AND SYMPTOMS	DIAGNOSTICS AND TREATMENT
Irritable Bowel Syndrome ≥3 mo of continuous or recurrent abdominal pain/discomfort relieved with BM, or associated with change in frequency or consistency of stool; not usually diagnosed initially in person >40yr	Symptoms worse with stress Crampy lower abdominal pain Abdominal distention, gas, and bloating Pain relieved with passage of flatus or stool Pain often associated with meals Symptoms do not disturb sleep Diarrhea or constipation with small volume stools No bleeding or weight loss Abdominal examination shows mild tenderness to abdomen with hyperactive bowel sounds Rectal examination normal	*Diagnostics* CBC, comprehensive chemistry panel, TSH Stool is negative for blood and pathogens Barium enema shows decreased motility Colonoscopy is normal *Treatment* *Lifestyle Changes* Stress reduction and management techniques Increase physical exercise Dietary changes (vary with each patient); lactose-free; no caffeine; avoid flatulence-producing foods (e.g., beans, brussels sprouts, cabbage, grapes, raisins, wine, beer); avoid large meals as well as spicy, fried, or fatty foods. Increase bulk or fiber up to 20g qd Increase fluids Encourage annual rectal examination especially after age 40yr

Drug Modalities

Bulk laxatives such as psyllium-based products or methylcellulose

For cramping:

Dicyclomine HCl 20–40 mg qid

Hyoscyamine sulfate 1 tab tid ac

Clidinium and chlordiazepoxide (Librium) 1–2 caps ac and hs

Hyoscyamine, atropine, scopolamine, and phenobarbital (Donnatal) 1–2 caps or tabs tid

For diarrhea use:

Loperamide 2 mg, initially 4 mg followed by 2 mg after each stool up to 16 mg qd; only for severe cases

For urgency and chronic diarrhea after meals: PPI or H_2 blocker at prescription dose (see chart on p. 231); should see results in 3 days

For constipation (short-term use in women):

Tegaserod 6 mg bid ac meals for 4–6 wk

Paxil 10 mg qd; titrate up to 40 mg qd and decrease if diarrhea occurs

Avoid narcotics and depressants

Refer with:

Anemia

Nocturnal symptoms

Fever

Unintentional weight loss

Persistent diarrhea or constipation

Rectal bleeding

Steatorrhea

Symptom onset after age 40 yr

Continued

8

Common Abdominal Problems—cont'd

PROBLEM	SIGNS AND SYMPTOMS	DIAGNOSTICS AND TREATMENT
Diverticulitis Common complication of diverticulosis caused by microperforation of the diverticulum from trapped food particles Usually involves only one diverticulum Perforation is walled off and becomes an abscess	Abdominal pain can be steady and severe or crampy and intermittent Usually found in LLQ but can be generalized to lower abdomen Constipation more often than diarrhea Pain increased with bowel movements Increased flatulence N/V Fever (low grade) Abdominal guarding, rebound with positive peritoneal signs if abscess occurs (usually left side) Rectal examination may show tenderness or a mass	*Diagnostics* CBC shows mild leukocytosis ESR is elevated Stool for occult blood is positive No x-ray studies during acute phase except flat and upright films CT abdomen After acute phase: barium enema, which will confirm diverticula Sigmoidoscopy may show reddened mucosa *Treatment* *Severe Disease* Consult with a physician for admission to hospital IV fluids for hydration and bowel rest CT abdomen and pelvis Cipro 400 mg IV q12h and metronidazole 500 mg IV q6-8h *Outpatient Treatment* Clear liquids, progress slowly to soft, bland foods Avoid laxatives, enemas, and bulk additives such as psyllium products in acute phase Antibiotics × 7 days Amoxicillin-clavulanate 500 mg tid *or* TMP-SMZ DS 1 tab bid *plus* metronidazole 250-500 mg bid *or*

Appendicitis

Abdominal pain can vary: midline, RLQ, periumbilical area, epigastric area
N/V follows pain
Anorexia
Pain with guarding
Positive peritoneal signs
Low-grade fever (maybe)
Symptoms may be vague
Pain worsens with movement
Stooped appearance when walking
Positive Markel's sign (heel jar test) good predictor for peritoneal irritation

Ciprofloxacin 250–500 mg bid
and/or metronidazole 250–500 mg bid

Generalized Measures
Bed rest
High-fiber diet along with psyllium or cellulose products when infection resolved
May use stool softeners

Diagnostics
CBC may show leukocytosis and shift to left (generally)
UA is normal
Flat and upright abdominal x-ray examinations may show a fecalith
CT scan

Treatment
Refer to a surgeon if symptoms suggest appendicitis

Colon Cancer
Increased risk:
>40 years old
FH colon CA
Adenomatous polyps
Inflammatory bowel disease
Sedentary lifestyle
Fiber-deficient diet

Right-Sided Involvement
May be asymptomatic
Unintentional weight loss
Anemia
Positive occult blood in stool
Crampy, colicky, intermittent abdominal pain

Left-Sided Involvement
Diarrhea or constipation
Shape of stool changes

Diagnostics
CBC may show anemia
Positive stool for occult blood
Barium enema shows lesion/mass
Colonoscopy shows lesion and biopsy can be done

Treatment
Refer to a surgeon for management

Continued

8

Common Abdominal Problems—cont'd

PROBLEM	SIGNS AND SYMPTOMS	DIAGNOSTICS AND TREATMENT
	Bright red bleeding mixed with normal stool Fullness after defecation Generalized lower abdominal pain Anemia ***Sigmoid/Rectal Involvement*** Obvious rectal bleeding Mucoid drainage from anus Pain with defecation	
Crohn's Disease (Regional Enteritis) Occurs in young and older adults Increased risk of colon CA	Abdominal pain, colicky or steady, usually found in RLQ or periumbilical area Intermittent diarrhea followed by constipation Recurrent attacks of mucoid diarrhea Anorexia, flatulence, malaise, and weight loss Low-grade fever, never shaking chills Abdominal mass in RLQ Perianal disease with fistula Milk products and coarse foods may irritate bowel	*Diagnostics* Macrocytic anemia Positive occult blood Barium enema shows fissures or deep ulcers UGI tract series with small bowel follow-through shows irregularity, ulceration, and luminal narrowing Colonoscopy *Treatment* Refer to a physician and co-manage Stop smoking *Diet* Nonresidue, well-balanced diet high in protein, vitamins, and calories; avoid raw fruits and vegetables Vitamin supplement

8

Ulcerative Colitis

Primarily in young adults
Increased risk for colon CA greater than for Crohn's disease

Stools are frequent with blood and mucus; may occur without feces
Diarrhea can occur any time
Cramping, abdominal pain is usually mild
Anorexia, malaise, weight loss, and fatigue
No signs of peritoneal irritation
Abdominal tenderness is mild
Does not involve small bowel
Rectal tenesmus
Intolerance to dairy products

Diagnostics
Microcytic anemia
ESR increased
Stools positive for occult blood, mucus, and pus
Barium enema shows size of colon decreased and shortened lumen; barium enema should not be performed with active disease
Colonoscopy

Treatment
Refer to a physician and co-manage after acute phase
Stop smoking

Diet
Avoid dairy products

*H_2-blockers and PPIs can be used 12 hr apart. Antacids and H_2-blockers can be used in the same day, but not at the same time.
Medication doses (prescription strength)
H_2 blockers
Ranitidine, 150 mg bid or 300 mg hs
Cimetidine, 400 mg bid or 800 mg hs
Nizatidine, 150 mg bid or 300 mg hs
Famotidine, 20 mg bid or 40 mg hs
Proton Pump Inhibitors (PPI)
Omeprazole, 20–40 mg qd
Lansoprazole, 15–30 mg qd
Rabeprazole, 20 mg qd
Esomeprazole, 20–40 mg qd
Pantoprazole, 40 mg qd
Omeprazole + sodium bicarbonate (Zegerid) OTC, 20 mg qd × 4 wk and give 1 hr before meals

8

Acute Infectious Diarrhea*

AGENT	ONSET	FEVER	EMESIS	ABDOMINAL PAIN	WATERY DIARRHEA	BLOOD	MUCUS	FOUL ODOR	TRANSMISSION	TREATMENT
Staphylococcus aureus	1–6hr	—	++	+	–/+	—	—	—	F	Supportive care and rehydration
Escherichia coli "travelers diarrhea"	2–5 days	+/–	+/–	++	++	—	—	—	F or W	Supportive care and rehydration; May need antibiotics (fluoroquinolone) if diarrhea is severe
Shigella	1–7 days	—	+/–	+/–	+	+/–	+/–	—	P–P, F–O, W	Monitor environment for poor sanitation; antibiotics: tetracycline, ciprofloxacin, erythromycin; Found in salads, raw vegetables, dairy products, poultry; Report to health department
Salmonella	1–3 days	+	+ @ onset	+	+	+/–	+/–	—	P–P, Pets	Supportive care and rehydration; Antibiotics (if life-threatening): TMP-SMZ, ciprofloxacin, ampicillin; antibiotics may prolong shedding of salmonella

								Comments
Campylobacter	2–5 days	+/−	+/−	++	+	+	F-O, Pets, P-P	Can be found in contaminated powdered eggs, poultry, turtles, fresh produce, and foods fertilized with animal feces Report to health department Supportive care and hydration Antibiotics (unless mild case): erythromycin, tetracycline, ciprofloxacin
Rotavirus	Acute onset	+@ onset	++	++	+	−	−	Found in unpasteurized milk, poultry, fresh produce Report to health department Supportive care and rehydration; dehydration can be severe
						−	F-O, P-P	

Continued

*Diarrhea lasting <1wk. For diarrhea lasting >1wk, see p. 218.

—, Absent; +, present; ++, severe; +/−, may be present; F, food; F–O, fecal-oral route; N, nosocomial; P–P, person-to-person route; W, water.

Acute Infectious Diarrhea—cont'd

AGENT	ONSET	FEVER	EMESIS	ABDOMINAL PAIN	WATERY DIARRHEA	BLOOD	MUCUS	FOUL ODOR	TRANSMISSION	TREATMENT
Clostridium difficile	1–21 days after antibiotics started	+/–	–	+/–	+	–	–	++	N/P-P	Common in children younger than 5 yr and attending day care Supportive care, rehydration Usually occurs days to weeks after antibiotic therapy Discontinue use of antibiotic if currently taking one Usual antibiotic to stop infection is vancomycin HCl or metronidazole Avoid anti-motility agents Probiotics daily and 1 mo after symptoms resolve
Giardia lamblia	1–3 days	–	+	++	++	–	–	–	W	Supportive care, rehydration Antibiotics: quinacrine HCl or metronidazole Report to health department

	Incubation							Transmission	Comments
Ascariasis	Weeks to years after infestation occurs; symptoms occur depending on amount of worm infestation	—	+/–	+/–	+	—	—	F–O, dirt	Diarrhea stool will contain worms until all worms are expelled. Anthelmintic: mebendazole or pyrantel pamoate
Clostridium perfringens	8–16 hr	—	+	++	++	—	—	F	Supportive care, hydration, and rehydration
Norwalk-like virus	24–48 hr	+	+	+	++	—	—	Aerosol, F, P–P	Supportive care, hydration, and rehydration. Can be found in salads, sandwiches, and fruit (food handlers)

—, Absent; +, present; ++, severe; +/–, may be present; *F*, food; *F–O*, fecal-oral route; *N*, nosocomial; *P–P*, person-to-person route; *W*, water.

Hepatitis

573.3

Hepatitis is growing in prevalence across the world (Table 8–1). More and more people are discovering they have acquired hepatitis years ago through receiving contaminated blood transfusions or having high-risk lifestyles (e.g., multiple sex partners, IV drug use, or sharing needles). Hepatitis can remain dormant for up to 20 years and may be completely asymptomatic.

To prevent spread of the illness, the practitioner needs to be able to identify the type of hepatitis and how infective the patient is at the initial visit. The progression of hepatitis is difficult to predict, and laboratory testing is sometimes slow and cumbersome. The exact test needed to identify the type of hepatitis can be difficult to decide on, and then the interpretation of each test can be very confusing.

Following are tests that can be ordered initially to give the practitioner the most useful information, given the circumstances. Be aware that because laboratories often have different panels and protocols, these tests may not be available as suggested below.

1. Patient presents to office saying, "I had hepatitis, but I don't know what kind and I want to know which one I had." Patient is asymptomatic and doesn't know if she/he has had hepatitis immunization.

   Order Hepatitis Panel (screening), which usually includes antibody for hepatitis A, hepatitis B, and hepatitis C. Further testing will be needed if any positives noted.

2. Patient appears in office, asymptomatic, with high-risk behaviors (either in the past or currently), and partner has had unspecified hepatitis in the past.

   Order total anti-HAV, HBsAg, total anti-HBc, and anti-HCV antibody.

3. Patient has acute symptoms of jaundice, hepatomegaly, and constitutional symptoms.

   Order: LFTs, IgM anti-HAV, HBsAg, IgM anti-HBc, and anti-HCV.

4. Patient has positive hepatitis C report from the blood bank but is asymptomatic. Patient reports he was given blood transfusion in 1989.

   Order: HCV RNA quantitative with reflex to genotype by PCR, CBC, LFT, PT/PTT, albumin, hepatitis A and B antibody, and HIV if history of high-risk behaviors (either now or in the past).

INTERPRETATION OF HEPATITIS LEVELS

HAV

- IgM anti-HAV: an acute marker of infection, peaks in first week, and disappears in about 8 wk
- IgG anti-HAV: remote infection, is not contagious, peaks after 1 mo, and may persist for years
- Anti-HAV: presence is marker for past exposure or illness to HAV; noninfectious, and denotes immunity to HAV

Table 8–1 Hepatitis

Hepatitis A	070.1
Hepatitis B	070.30
Hepatitis C	070.51

SIGNS AND SYMPTOMS	TRANSMISSION	DIAGNOSTIC	TREATMENT
Hepatitis A (HAV) Anorexia N/V Fever Aversion to smoke Dark, tea-colored urine Clay-colored stools Jaundiced skin Icteric sclerae Pruritus Liver tenderness and enlargement Persons <6yr may not exhibit symptoms	Fecal-oral route All body fluids can be infective during the acute phase Infected food handlers can spread disease to other persons through food *Incubation is 2–6wk* At-risk persons: 　Household or sexual contacts 　Travelers to underdeveloped countries 　IV drug users Elderly persons have more severe symptoms	Hepatitis panel Anti-HAV IgM (acute infection) Anti-HAV IgG (past infection) AST/ALT	High-calorie diet Bed rest Good hand washing Hydroxyzine HCL 25–50 mg tid–qid for pruritus Prochlorperazine 5–10 mg tid–qid for N/V HBIG 0.02–0.06 ml/kg IM given once to all close contacts within 2 wk of exposure and then start HAV vaccine (Havrix, Vaqta, or Twinrix) Disease is self-limiting and usually resolves within 4–8 wk Encourage hepatitis B vaccine Avoid drugs metabolized in the liver
Hepatitis B (HBV) Onset can be rapid or gradual Myalgia, arthralgia General malaise	Transferred through blood and blood products, sexual contact, IV needle users, self-inoculation, perinatally, semen, and wound exudate	Hepatitis panel LFTs PT/PTT, CBC	Symptomatic measures for comfort with treatment of N/V and malaise Follow AST and ALT levels to monitor liver function

Continued

Table 8–1 Hepatitis—cont'd

SIGNS AND SYMPTOMS	TRANSMISSION	DIAGNOSTIC	TREATMENT
Easily fatigued URI and anorexia out of proportion to illness N/V/D Occasionally fever Abdominal pain in RUQ or epigastrium, increased with jarring Liver tenderness Jaundice	*Incubation* 6 wk to 6 mo	HBsAG, HBeAG, HBcAG HBsAB, HBeAB +HBsAG >6 mo	Bed rest for acute phase Avoid drugs metabolized in liver HBIG 0.02–0.06 ml/kg IM given once to close contacts within 7 days of exposure to provide some protection and then start hepatitis B vaccine series at the same time (do not give HBIG and HBV vaccine in same site)
Hepatitis C (HCV) Usually progresses to chronic state Complaints similar to those for other types of hepatitis Occasional jaundice Few symtoms in acute phase	Transmission through parenteral and possibly sexual contact and perinatally 40% of infected persons have no risk factors *Incubation 14–140 days* Patient may be asymptomatic when first exposed and for up to 20 yr (you may never know you have contracted the disease) Disease worse if: Person >40 yr Co-infected with HBV/HIV Alcohol use or abuse African American males	Hepatitis panel LFTs RIBA/EIA (as confirmatory tests) Anti-HCV HCV RNA with genotype and reflux to genotype	Encourage hepatitis A and B vaccines and routine flu and pneumonia immunizations Refer to gastroenterologist who specializes in hepatitis and co-manage treatment

HBV

- HBsAg: first indication of infection; persists throughout the first 6 months, presence of antigen indicates an infectious state
- HBeAg: presence indicates acute infection and active viral replication
- IgM anti-HBc: onset of acute infection
- IgG anti-HBc: indicates chronic hepatitis or superimposed acute hepatitis from another cause
- HBcAg: indicates active disease or "flare-ups"; may be found before anti-HBs
- Anti-HBs: antibody to HBsAg; occurs after successful immunization with hepatitis B series or signals recovery from HBV
- Persistent circulating HBsAg suggests progressive chronic hepatitis B

HCV

- Anti-HCV: positive as early as 10 to 12 weeks or 9 to 12 months depending on exposure, does not correlate with onset of infection or amount of liver damage
- HCV RNA with genotype: there are currently four genotypes identified; the first one is the most virulent and requires treatment; the others may or may not cause liver failure
- HCV RNA quantitative with reflex to genotype by PCR: indicates the viral load present at this time; viral load can be monitored during therapy to assess progress

NOTES

9

Gynecologic Disorders

Guidelines for Screening Papanicolaou (Pap) Smears

Health care reform groups are attempting to manage timelines for Pap smear screening in the early detection of cancer. Cervical cancer is usually a very slow-growing cancer and annual evaluation with Pap testing may not be needed to determine its presence. Annual pelvic exams are still needed, however, and under certain circumstances Pap smears, HPV testing, and STD testing are indicated at the provider's discretion. Mammography has also been scrutinized in 2012 regarding the best timing and age at which to start testing. The only remaining standardized health screen is colorectal testing, which should start at age 50 (if no past history), with annual hemoccult testing. Initial colonoscopy testing should be followed by a 10-year evaluation (if results were normal). Below is a comparison of the U.S. Preventive Services Task Force (USPSTF) and American Congress of Obstetricians and Gynecologists (ACOG) Pap smear screening guidelines.

Pap Smear Screening Guidelines

USPSTF	ACOG
Pap screen at age 21–65 yr every 3 yr *Or* Pap screen and HPV test at age 30–65 yr every 5 yr No Pap screen: • Under age 21 yr • Age >65 yr with no increased risk (last 2 Pap smears negative within last 5–10 yr) • Hysterectomy for non-cancerous reasons No screen for cervical cancer with HPV test alone or in combination with Pap at age <30 yr Annual clinical breast exam and pelvic exam Mammography every 2 yr between ages 50–74 yr Bone density screen for women age 65+ yr at 2-yr intervals Bone density screen for women age 60+ yr at 2-yr intervals if high risk (history of fracture and/or one or more risk factors*)	Pap screen at age 19–20 yr if indicated Pap screen at age 21–29 yr every 3 yr Pap screen and HPV test at age >30–64 yr every 5 yr or Pap screen every 3 yr No Pap screen at age >65 yr if past 3 screens were negative within 10 yr No Pap screen if hysterectomy for non-cancerous reasons GC/Chlamydia screen at age <25 yr and if sexually active Annual clinical breast exam and pelvic exam Mammography every 1–2 yr starting at age 40 yr and annually after age 50 yr Bone density screen at age 65 yr at 2-yr intervals Bone density screen at age 60+ yr at 2-yr intervals if at high risk (low BMI, history of previous fracture, age, etc.)

*Low body weight is the best predictor for increased risk of fracture.
Data from U.S. Preventive Services Task Force and American Congress of Obstetricians and Gynecologists.

CONTRACEPTIVE METHODS
See Table 9–1

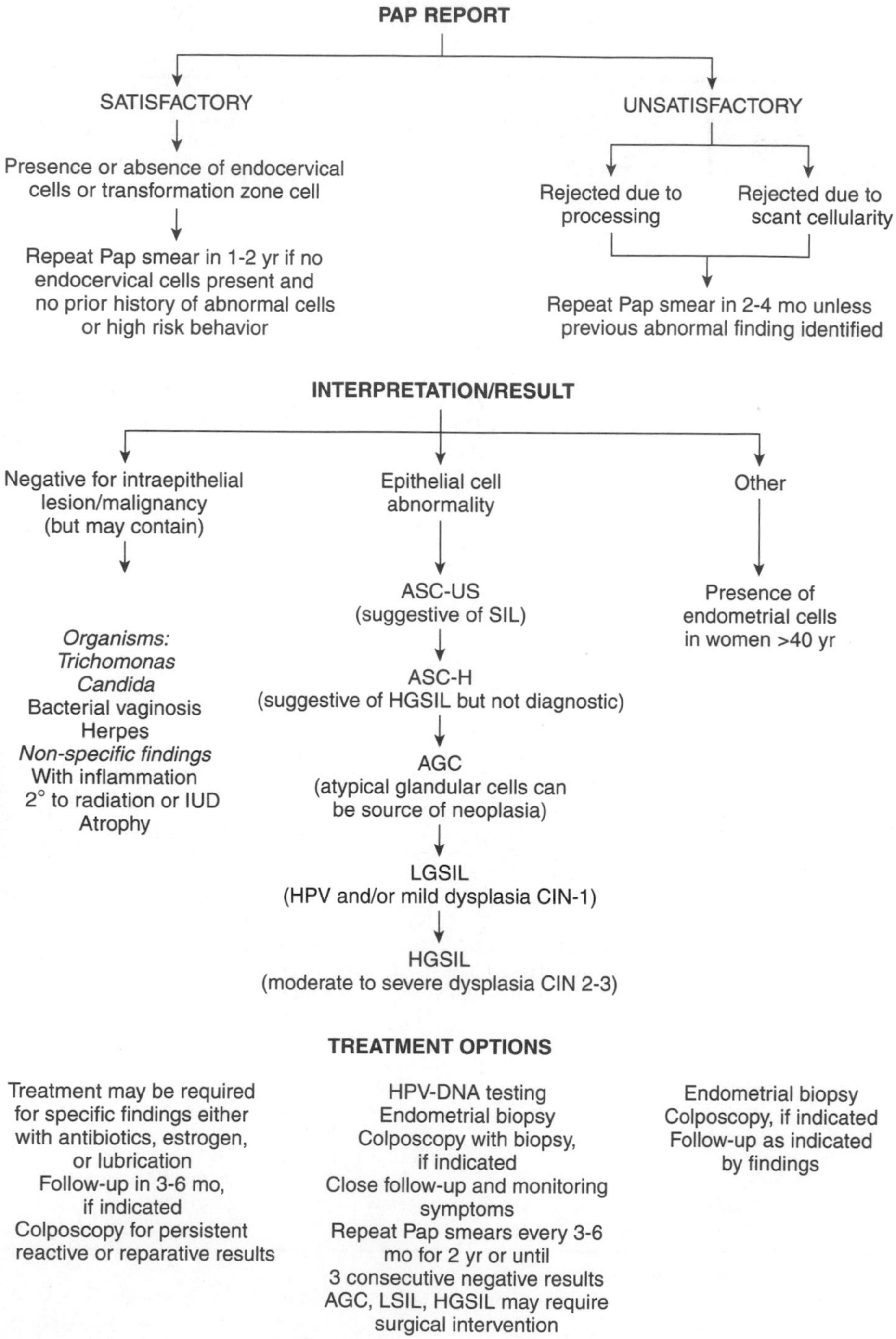

PAP REPORT

SATISFACTORY

Presence or absence of endocervical
cells or transformation zone cell

Repeat Pap smear in 1-2 yr if no
endocervical cells present and
no prior history of abnormal cells
or high risk behavior

UNSATISFACTORY

Rejected due to
processing

Rejected due to
scant cellularity

Repeat Pap smear in 2-4 mo unless
previous abnormal finding identified

INTERPRETATION/RESULT

Negative for intraepithelial
lesion/malignancy
(but may contain)

Organisms:
Trichomonas
Candida
Bacterial vaginosis
Herpes
Non-specific findings
With inflammation
2° to radiation or IUD
Atrophy

Epithelial cell
abnormality

ASC-US
(suggestive of SIL)

ASC-H
(suggestive of HGSIL but not diagnostic)

AGC
(atypical glandular cells can
be source of neoplasia)

LGSIL
(HPV and/or mild dysplasia CIN-1)

HGSIL
(moderate to severe dysplasia CIN 2-3)

Other

Presence of
endometrial cells
in women >40 yr

TREATMENT OPTIONS

Treatment may be required
for specific findings either
with antibiotics, estrogen,
or lubrication
Follow-up in 3-6 mo,
if indicated
Colposcopy for persistent
reactive or reparative results

HPV-DNA testing
Endometrial biopsy
Colposcopy with biopsy,
if indicated
Close follow-up and monitoring
symptoms
Repeat Pap smears every 3-6
mo for 2 yr or until
3 consecutive negative results
AGC, LSIL, HGSIL may require
surgical intervention

Endometrial biopsy
Colposcopy, if indicated
Follow-up as indicated
by findings

FIGURE 9–1 Interpretation of Pap smear report.

Table 9–1   Contraceptive Methods

METHOD	ADVANTAGE	DISADVANTAGE	CONTRAINDICATION	ADDITIONAL POINTS
Male condom	Inexpensive; cost is ~$0.50 per unit Easy to use Reduces risk of STDs 85% effective in preventing pregnancy if used correctly	Skin irritation May interrupt foreplay	Latex allergy	Must be used correctly to prevent semen escaping into vagina Effectiveness against pregnancy increases with use of spermicide Must be accepted by both partners
Female condom	Cost is ~$2.50 per unit Reduces risk of STDs 80%–90% effective in preventing pregnancy if used correctly	Awkward to use More difficult to insert Sexually unappealing	Latex allergy	Must be used correctly Increased effectiveness against pregnancy if used with spermicide
Copper T 380A IUD (nonhormonal)	Cost is ~$350 over 5- to 10-yr period No patient application 95%–99% effective in preventing pregnancy Can be used with history of DVT, CVA, dyslipidemia, migraine	Office visit for insertion Menstrual cramping Spotting Sometimes increased menstrual bleeding No protection against STDs	Pelvic infection Multiple sexual partners Abnormal bleeding Depressed immune system Valvular heart disease (increased risk of subacute bacterial endocarditis [SBE])	Discuss warning signs: Abnormal bleeding Abnormal discharge Fever, rash, and chills Missing string
Levonorgestrel IUD (Mirena)	Same as above *except:* Inserted for 5 years Can be used in smokers Not associated with weight gain Can be used in the obese woman	Requires office visit for insertion Irregular bleeding for the first 3–6 months, then may have greatly lessened bleeding amounts Increased chance for accidental expulsion in first year	Same as above	Cervical mucus is thickened May have increased acne or hair growth Reduced rate of anemia Rapid return to fertility when removed Painful menses, vaginitis,

Continued

9

Table 9–1 Contraceptive Methods—cont'd

METHOD	ADVANTAGE	DISADVANTAGE	CONTRAINDICATION	ADDITIONAL POINTS
	Noticeable reduction in menorrhagia after 6–12 mo	No protection against STDs		and myoma were decreased Can be used in lactating women
Oral contraceptives (OCs)	Cost is ~$15–$35/mo No patient application Easy to take but must be taken on time daily Some protection against PID 99% effective against pregnancy if used correctly Relieves PMS symptoms and decreases cramping with menses	N/V H/A Dizziness Spotting Weight gain Breast pain Depression No protection against STDs Must be taken on time every day	Liver dysfunction Thromboembolic disorders CAD Breast cancer Smoking Hyperlipidemia Third-generation OCs have increased risk of thrombosis	**Discuss warning signs:** Abdomen pain Chest pain Headache Eye problems Severe leg pain Low-dose OCs good for: Lactating women (>4 wk after delivery) Diabetes HTN Women >40 yr
Ortho Evra patch	Cost ~$35/mo Weekly application Easy to use Good adherence of patch 99% effective against pregnancy if used correctly	Skin irritation Patch may inadvertently come off No protection against STDs	Same with OCs	When prescribing, always order one extra patch in case one is lost or comes off; package of three is dispensed Caution if weight >180 lb; may decrease effectiveness
NuvaRing	Cost ~$40/mo Patient-inserted vaginal ring Easy to insert	Patient must insert May accidentally be expelled No protection against	Same as OCs	Discuss warning signs (same as OCs)

Method	Description / Benefits	Side effects / Disadvantages	Contraindications	Notes / Warnings
	Ring inserted for 3 wk/mo 99% effective against pregnancy if used correctly	STDs		Discuss warning signs: Excessive weight gain H/A
Medroxyprogesterone acetate (Depo-Provera)	Cost ~$160–$200/yr 98% effective in preventing pregnancy Requires one shot every 13 wk Decreases anemia Can be used with history of DVT, PE, smoking, CV disease, DM, migraine, seizures Decreases ovulation and endometriosis	Must go to clinic or office for shot Weight gain Depression Bone loss H/A No protection against STDs Irregular bleeding	Obesity Suspected pregnancy Abnormal bleeding Depression	Increase intake of calcium and vitamin D If no bleeding, check estrogen levels annually Bone densitometry q2y If >3 mo since last shot, perform pregnancy test before giving injection
Barrier methods: Diaphragm Caps Sponge	Cost varies with product from $4 per sponge to $50–$100 for diaphragm fitting Easy to use and accessible Reduces risk of STDs 85%–95% effective in preventing pregnancy if used correctly	Pelvic "heaviness" Vaginal discharge	Latex allergy Allergy to spermicide	Protection against pregnancy increases with use of spermicide May irritate cervix Frequent, recurrent vaginal infections Increased chance of toxic shock syndrome if left in for prolonged period of time
Etonogestrel (Implanon) Etonogestrel radiopaque (Nexplanon)	Cost ~$450–$540 99% effective 1 small rod inserted every 3 yr Can be used while breastfeeding May lighten or stop menstrual cycles	Must be removed under local anesthesia and reinserted May be less effective over time with obesity or weight gain Bleeding irregularities	Pregnancy Breast cancer DVT Uncontrolled hypertension Liver disease Undiagnosed genital bleeding	Certain drugs effect efficacy Barbiturates Carbamazepine Phenytoin Topiramate St. John's wort

9

Practice Pearls
- See Figure 9–2 for normal menstrual cycle
- Before prescribing hormonal contraceptives, perform history and physical examination and include Pap smear, pregnancy test, and any necessary cultures
- The new progestins (norgestimate, desogestrel, and drospirenone) have fewer side effects and more benefits than older OCs; benefits include decreased acne occurrence, minimal weight gain, decreased hair growth, decreased LDL levels, and increased HDL levels; the adverse effects that do occur can be serious; the progestin in these newer pills increases the sex hormone-binding globulin (SHBG) and binds more androgens; this allows an increase in circulating estrogen; this can cause an increase in venous thrombosis for some women; do not use these new oral contraceptive progestins if there is any history of venous thrombosis; taking an aspirin every day with the OCs may decrease the risk, but this has not been proved; caution these women against smoking
- If breakthrough bleeding occurs in a patient <35 years who smokes, try increasing progestin potency (e.g., Lo/Ovral, Levlen, Nordette); if the woman is >35 years and smokes, use progestin contraceptive, such as levonorgestrel IUD (Mirena), medroxyprogesterone (Depo-Provera), or the progestin only pills (POPs); encourage woman to stop smoking

Managing Common OC Side Effects

EFFECTS	CHANGE TO
Acne, hair growth	Ovcon-35, Brevicon, Modicon, Demulen-35, Ortho Tri-Cyclen, Yasmin
Weight gain	Alesse, Ortho Tri-Cyclen, Ortho-Cept, Yasmin
Headache, nausea, or breast tenderness	Alesse, Mircette, Loestrin, Ortho-Cept
Breakthrough bleeding:	
Bleeding occurs in first 14 days of cycle	Mircette, Loestrin, Ovcon-35, Ortho-Cyclen, Ortho Tri-Cyclen
Bleeding occurs in last 14 days of cycle (before taking inert pills)	Mircette, Levlen, Ortho-Novum 7/7/7, Estrostep
Bleeding occurs anytime in cycle	Estrostep, Loestrin, Cyclessa, Ortho-Novum 1/35
Skin rash or pruritus	Usually occurs from inactive ingredients; switch to pill with different inactive ingredients
Decreased libido	Yasmin, Ortho Tri-Cyclen Lo, Cyclessa
Amenorrhea	Determine cause and correct; may need to change type of estrogen or progestin

Tips on Taking Oral Contraceptives

In a discussion of OCs the patient should be told how to start the package, that additional contraceptive techniques will be needed for the first month, and what to do if

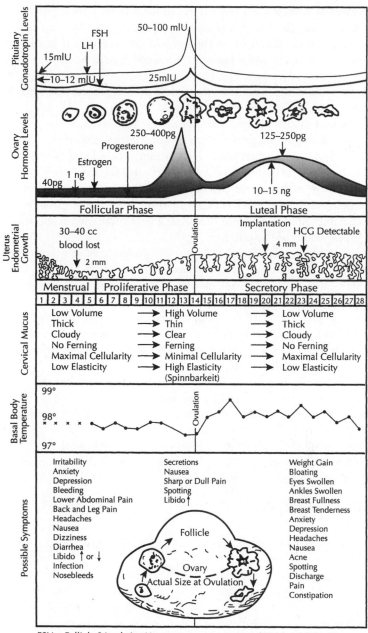

FIGURE 9–2 Occurrences of a normal menstrual cycle. (From *Contraceptive technologies* [16th revised ed.]. [1994]. New York: Irvington Publishers, Inc.)

pills are missed. Following are a few helpful comments on pill usage:

- Start the pill on the first day of menstrual bleeding, on the first Sunday of the week that menses started, or on the day you get your pills if you know for sure you are not pregnant; use a backup contraceptive method for the first cycle or month of your pills
- Take the OCs at the same time every day; if N/V occurs, take with food or at bedtime
- Use a backup method of birth control for the remainder of the pill pack if you miss more than one pill or if you are spotting during any of your cycles
- If a pill is missed, take that pill as soon as remembered and take the next pill as scheduled; use a backup method for birth control for the next 7 days
- If two pills are missed in the first 2 weeks, take two pills for 2 days; if two pills are missed in the last 2 weeks of the monthly cycle, take one pill every day until the active pills are finished and then start a new pack; use backup contraception for the remainder of the pill pack
- If three or more pills are missed, you will probably start a normal menstrual cycle; you can take one pill every day until the active pills are finished and then start a new pack; use a backup method for 7 days after the new pack is started
- Notify the clinician immediately if any of the warning signs occur (see Table 9–1)
- If you miss one period while taking the pill, there is no reason for concern; if you miss two periods while taking the pill, perform a pregnancy test
- Pregnancy is more likely to occur when OCs are missed just before or just after the hormone-free pills are taken
- For patients with seizure conditions, progestin-only birth control or OCs with at least 50 mcg of estrogen will be safe and effective
- Always use condoms; the OCs do not protect against sexually transmitted diseases
- Use backup method of birth control when taking antibiotics
- If you forget two or more pills and forget to use a condom during sex, call your practitioner for emergency contraception

Emergency Contraception

- Criteria
  - Patient is seen within 72 hours of unprotected intercourse
  - Pregnancy test negative
  - Pelvic examination negative
- Options (Table 9–2)

Practice Pearls

- These regimens prevent pregnancy by inhibiting ovulation, not by disrupting the pregnancy
- Relative contraindications are active migraines with neurologic symptoms and preexisting venous thromboembolism
- If no menses in 3 weeks, check a pregnancy test; if no menses in 2 months, come to office

Table 9–2 Oral Contraceptives for Emergency Contraception

FORMULATION	BRAND NAME	FIRST DOSE	SECOND DOSE (12 hr AFTER FIRST DOSE)
Norgestrel 0.50 mg + ethinyl estradiol 0.05 mg	Ovral	2 white pills	2 white pills
Norgestrel 0.03 mg + ethinyl estradiol 0.03 mg	Lo/Ovral	4 white pills	4 white pills
Levonorgestrel 0.15 mg + ethinyl estradiol 0.03 mg	Levlen, Nordette	4 light orange pills	4 light orange pills
Levonorgestrel 0.125 mg + ethinyl estradiol 0.03 mg	Tri-Levlen, Triphasil	4 yellow pills	4 yellow pills
Levonorgestrel 0.1 mg + ethinyl estradiol 0.02 mg	Alesse, Levlite	5 pink pills	5 pink pills
Norgestrel 0.075 mg	Orvette	20 yellow pills	20 yellow pills
Levonorgestrel 0.25 mg + ethinyl estradiol 0.05 mg	Preven	2 blue pills	2 blue pills
Levonorgestrel 0.75 mg	Plan B	1 pill	1 pill

- Copper T IUD may be inserted within 5 to 7 days of exposure; can be left in place for up to 10 years

Gynecologic Conditions Encountered in Primary Care

- Breast conditions (Table 9–3)
- Gynecologic conditions (Table 9–4)

MENOPAUSE

627.2

Condition

- Ovarian failure causing hormonal fluctuation in estrogen and progesterone that eventually leads to deficiency in estrogen and progesterone
- This usually occurs between the ages of 45 and 55 years; the average age of onset can be approximated based on the person's mother's age at menopause (if known)
- Onset can be caused by normal physiologic changes, surgery, or pathologic conditions
- If hormonal replacement is indicated for relief of vasomotor symptoms, short-term use and lowest effective dose to control symptoms should be used
- Because menopause does occur normally in the aging process, monitor the patient for occult medical conditions
- *HRT is not indicated to prevent cardiac or lipemic problems and may not be effective in delaying dementia*

Text continued on p. 260

Table 9–3 Breast Conditions

Breast Discharge 611.29	Premenstrual Syndrome 625.4	
Mastitis 611.0	Dysmenorrhea 625.3	
Breast Mass 611.72	Abnormal Uterine Bleeding 626.0	
Fibrocystic Breast Disease 610.1	Amenorrhea 626.0	
Menstrual Abnormalities 626.4		

CONDITION	SIGNS AND SYMPTOMS	DIAGNOSTICS	TREATMENT
Breast Discharge	Thorough history involving recent	Thorough physical exam of	Consult or refer if abnormal
Physiologic causes include:	pregnancy, lactation history,	breast and nipple	findings/results
Pregnancy and lactation or	amount of personal stimulation	Pap smear of nipple discharge	
recent lactation	LMP and menstrual history	Prolactin level	
OC use	Milky or bloody discharge; can be	TSH, UCG	
Overstimulation of breasts	unilateral or bilateral	Mammogram	
Pharmacologic causes include:	Usually associated with constant	Ultrasound, if indicated	
Herbal products with	or intermittent pain in breast or	MRI of brain, if indicated	
estrogenic effects	nipple but may be painless		
Estrogen products	Nodules present		
Haloperidol	Appearance of nipples: clean or		
Metoclopramide	crusted with exudate		
SSRIs, TCAs			
H$_2$ antagonists			
Pathologic causes include:			
Cancer			
Pituitary lesion			
Severe head trauma			
Mastitis	Red, hot, firm to touch, tender	Breast examination and	Antibiotics (cephalexin is safe)
Inflammation of the breasts	breast; usually unilateral, but	inspection of nipple	Warm, moist packs
	can be bilateral	Discuss infant's nursing habits	Breast-feeding can be continued
	Abscesses may be present	Consider CBC	if patient can tolerate it

Condition / Risk Factors	Signs / Symptoms	Diagnostic	Management
	Often fever >101°F (38.3°C)		Recheck in 3–7 days; Refer to surgeon if condition does not completely resolve
Breast Mass High risk with any of following: Age >50yr; Early menarche; Late menopause; Nulliparity, late first pregnancy; DES exposure in utero; Family history of near-relative with breast cancer; Increased risk if family member has breast cancer before menopause	Mass that does not resolve with normal menstrual cycle; May be associated with pain; Mass firm to hard, nonmobile, poorly defined edges; May see deviation of nipple placement with patient in upright position; May see "orange peel" appearance or dimpling to breast skin; Change in configuration or consistency of breast tissue; Nipple discharge	If not lactating, mammogram and ultrasound; Mammogram; Ultrasound	Refer to surgeon
Fibrocystic Breast Disease (Benign)	Usually multiple, painful bilateral nodules; Nodule is firm, well defined, and mobile; Cyclic symptoms, increasing during premenstrual phase; Rare in postmenopausal women	Mammogram; Ultrasound, if indicated	Teach SBE and encourage monthly examinations; Decrease or stop caffeine, tea, chocolate, and nicotine; Wear support bra; Apply hot or cold compresses to breast; NSAIDs (see Appendix E); Vitamin E 1000IU 1 tab qd; Vitamin B$_6$ 50–100mg 1 tab qd; Evening primrose oil 2 capsules bid; Switch to lowest estrogenic OC or discontinue

9

| Table 9–4 | Gynecologic Conditions |

CONDITION	SIGNS AND SYMPTOMS
Premenstrual Syndrome (PMS)/ **Premenstrual Dysphoric Disorder** (PMDD)	Consistent S/S Occurs on a predictable time frame before menstrual cycles and disrupts life both at home and at work Symptoms reverse when menses starts or within 3 days Breast tenderness Bloating and weight gain (about 2–5 lb [1–2 kg]), edema, oliguria Tiredness, fatigue, and exhaustion H/A Cravings for salt, sugar, and chocolate Joint and muscle pain Decreased libido Acne Greasy or dry hair Nausea, palpitations, sweating Clumsiness, vertigo, tremor Depression, irritability Inability to concentrate, loss of control, and anxiety Feeling tense, sad

DIAGNOSTICS	TREATMENT
CBC, U/A, TSH, FBS, and pelvic examination to R/O pathologic condition	Reassure patient that her complaints are real and that she may have some control over her condition
Have patient complete a symptom diary (Fig. 9–3) for 2–3 mo to plot specific symptoms in relation to phase of menstrual cycle	Teach patient about normal menstrual cycle and effects of hormones (see Fig. 9–2)
May see increase tendency toward OCD behaviors and postpartum depression	Teach patient how to use the symptom diary to prevent or minimize discomfort (see Fig. 9–3)

TREATMENT (continued):

Diet
Eat well-balanced diet that is high in complex carbohydrates and low in sodium, fat, and red meat
Decrease or eliminate caffeine-containing beverages, foods, and medications
Decrease alcohol consumption
Calcium 1200 mg qd
Vitamin B_6 50–100 mg qd
Vitamin E 200–400 IU qd
Zinc 25–50 mg qd
Magnesium 400 mg qd
Manganese 6 mg qd
Can try evening primrose oil capsules qd/bid starting midcycle

Exercise
Aerobic exercise for ~30 min 3–4 times a week; should be activity patient enjoys
Relaxation training to decrease stress or tension, which can aggravate symptoms

Pharmacologic Therapy
Diuretics should be used only for those patients who can document actual weight gain premenstrually; any diuretic will work at the lowest dosage; start dose before weight gain and stop after menses starts
NSAIDs (see Appendix E) should be started 2–3 days before pain is expected; use with caution if the patient has kidney problems, asthma, or ulcers
SSRIs such as fluoxetine 20 mg qd or sertraline 50 mg qd can be used in severe cases to improve mood swings, irritability, anxiety, and depression; dosing can be daily or cyclic—start 10–12 days before next cycle and stop 1–2 days into cycle; can increase dose (if symptoms not controlled) of daily SSRI starting on day 10 before next cycle starts, then decrease when cycle starts

Continued

Table 9-4 Gynecologic Conditions—cont'd	
CONDITION	**SIGNS AND SYMPTOMS**
Dysmenorrhea Primary type defined as a painful menstruation associated with ovulatory cycles Usually induced by release of prostaglandins that stimulate smooth muscle activity	Crampy, spasmodic pelvic pain, back pain, or even leg pain Begins at or several days before menses Usually begins after first year of menses N/V, H/A, and dizziness

Abnormal Uterine Bleeding
Any uterine bleeding that does not result from normal menstruation
Usually painless, irregular vaginal bleeding from the endometrium that is excessive, prolonged, unpatterned, and unrelated to structural or systemic disease
The amount of bleeding exceeds that of normal menstrual bleeding; bleeding is prolonged enough to cause lifestyle changes
 	
Ovulatory Type
Occurs at regular intervals, usually associated with midcycle spotting or with PMS symptoms (breast tenderness, weight gain, mood swings); this usually signals that ovulation has occurred
There is an adequate amount of progesterone for endometrial proliferation but inadequate estrogen for
	History should include:
	    LMP for last two cycles
	    When bleeding occurs
	    Amount of bleeding (pad counts are subjective; ask whether pad is soaked [e.g., "Can you see blood stain through pad backing?"])
	Color of blood passed and any clots noted
	Weight gain or loss
	Breast pain or galactorrhea
	Hirsutism or thinning alopecia
	Presence of petechiae
	Acne
	Pelvic pain either during intercourse or before menses
	Palpated abdominal mass
	Cervical/vaginal discharge
	Amenorrhea that precedes abnormal bleeding cycle (usually caused by pregnancy, OCs, anovulatory cycle)
	Fever (usually STDs, PID, sepsis)

DIAGNOSTICS	TREATMENT
	Anxiolytics can be used at very low doses, started a few days before symptoms, and tapered off after menses
	OCs may stabilize hormonal fluctuations and relieve or eliminate some symptoms; use low-dose estrogen combined, monophasic pills (Yasmin should help control weight gain); can also use progesterone-only contraceptives to stabilize symptoms (e.g., Depo-Provera or POPs)
None needed if history indicates dysmenorrhea	*NSAIDs Commonly Used*
	Mefenamic acid (Ponstel) 250 mg 2 tab initially then 1 tab q6h
	Ibuprofen 400–800 mg q6h
	Naproxen DS (Anaprox DS) 1000 mg qd start 2–3 days before menses is due to start and continue until symptoms subside
	Common Measures
	Warm, moist heat to lower abdomen
	OC therapy
	Exercise
	See also PMS treatment
Tanner's staging (see Table 2–1)	Pregnancy must be R/O first before treatment can be started
Vital signs, including orthostatic readings	Ovulatory menorrhagia can be treated with meclofenamate (Meclomen) 100 mg tid, starting 2–3 days before menses and continuing for 3–4 days during menses; can continue for 3–6 mo, and then stop and monitor bleeding
Height and weight	
CBC, U/A, UCG (if sexually active)	
TSH, FSH	
Liver panel	
Prolactin level (if galactorrhea)	
DHEA (if adrenal tumor suspected)	
PT, PTT	**If no systemic or organic cause can be found for bleeding, then assume bleeding is anovulatory, but if bleeding is not controlled with hormones, look for other causes of abnormal bleeding**
Pelvic examination with Pap smear	
Wet prep	
Pelvic and/or transvaginal U/S (note thickness of endometrium; if >5–6 mm, must do further investigation with biopsy; if woman is not menopausal, get U/S a week after menses; if woman is postmenopausal and taking HRT, U/S may not be reliable)	The woman who has been bleeding for an extended time or who is taking a high-progestational OC or progestin-only contraceptive probably has a thin, fragile endometrial lining; she will need estrogen to slow bleeding on the "raw" endometrial surface and reestablish a normal cycle
Screen for STDs	
Endometrial biopsy recommended for: Women >35 yr old	The woman who has sudden onset of bleeding after having been amenorrhagic probably

Continued

Table 9–4 Gynecologic Conditions—cont'd

CONDITION	SIGNS AND SYMPTOMS
continued proliferation; endometrium becomes friable and heavy bleeding occurs; estrogen replacement should correct problem	Pallor without tachycardia or shock symptoms may indicate chronic, excessive bleeding from anovulatory cause
Common Causes	Headache, visual disturbance, and decreased libido suggest pituitary lesion
Anatomic problems: tumors, infections, lacerations, pregnancy, or complications from pregnancy	Fine, thinning hair with decreased reflexes suggests hypothyroidism
Low platelet count: idiopathic thrombocytopenic purpura (ITP), DIC, leukemia	*Definitions*
Increased bleeding time: von Willebrand's disease	**Menorrhagia:** prolonged or excessive bleeding at regular intervals (>7 days, >80 ml per menses, or more than 6–8 soaked pads qd)
Medications such as warfarin, aspirin, NSAIDs	**Metrorrhagia:** irregular bleeding, variable in amount, usually prolonged
Renal or liver disease	**Menometrorrhagia:** irregular, frequent bleeding that may be excessive and prolonged
Anovulatory Type	**Polymenorrhea:** regular cycles occurring more frequently than every 21 days
Occurs at irregular intervals not associated with PMS	**Oligomenorrhea:** menses occurring at intervals greater than every 35–42 days
Usually at extremes of reproductive life span	
Common Causes	
Puberty: caused by immature HPO axis; usually takes about 20 mo to establish a normal pattern of menses	
Childbearing years (16–40 yr); pregnancy and complications of contraceptives, adenomyosis, endometriosis, fibroids, endometrial hyperplasia, polyps, polycystic ovary syndrome, PID	
With any abnormal bleeding, cancer should be R/O first	
Women who smoke have increased risk for breakthrough bleeding and abnormal bleeding	
As ovarian estrogen production decreases, the pituitary gland secretes more FSH to increase production of estrogen; this means perimenopausal women tend to be hyperestrogenic with lower progestin levels; this increases the risk for endometrial hyperplasia	

DIAGNOSTICS	TREATMENT
All women with risk factors for endometrial cancer (obesity, unopposed estrogen use) Women with heavy, prolonged, or frequent (<21 days) perimenopausal bleeding Women not responding to medical therapy for bleeding CT scan, if warranted by exam	has adequate or thickened endometrium and will benefit from OCs or progestin to reestablish normal cycles Refer for hospitalization if Hgb <7 g/dl with orthostatic signs, patient is in shock, or if pad count is >pad/hr *Treatment of Heavy Bleeding (with Hgb > 7 g/dl but <10 g/dl)* Ovral 3 tabs day 1 2 tabs days 2–9 1 tab qd until pill pack finished Lo/Ovral 1 tab qid × 4 days 1 tab tid × 3 days 1 tab bid for 2 wk then start a new pill pack immediately CEE 1.25 mg or estradiol 2 mg 1 tab q4h × 24 hr 1 tab tid × 7–10 days 1 tab qd for remainder of month and add progesterone 10 mg last 10 days of cycle *Treatment of Mild to Moderate Bleeding* Hgb >10 g/dl, prolonged menses; goal is to stabilize endometrium to stop bleeding Monophasic OCs: 2 tab bid until bleeding slows, 1 tab bid until bleeding stops, then finish pill pack; immediately start new pill pack and take 1 tab qd for 2–3 cycles without stopping or allow withdrawal bleeding and then start new pill pack Once bleeding has been controlled, start OC or HRT for 6 mo as prescribed Start iron replacement therapy (see Table 7–1) Antiemetic treatment for nausea caused by high doses of estrogen: Promethazine 25–50 mg q6h Prochlorperazine 10–25 mg q6h Progesterone therapy alone can be used for anovulatory bleeding: MPA 10 mg/day, 10 days a month Progesterone in oil 100–200 mg IM:

Continued

Table 9–4	Gynecologic Conditions—cont'd

CONDITION	SIGNS AND SYMPTOMS
Amenorrhea	
Primary Amenorrhea	Obvious dysfunctional growth and
Absence of menarche by:	development of secondary sexual
16 yr of age with normal sexual	characteristics
development *or*	May look female but have male
14 yr of age without sexual development	characteristics
Causes of Primary Amenorrhea	History of excess exercise >2 hr/day
Athlete's amenorrhea	Extreme dietary limitations in protein, fat
Anorexia, bulimia	intake, or both
Pituitary lesions	Weight <95 lb
Hereditary conditions	
Secondary Amenorrhea	
Absence of menses for >3 mo in a woman	
who previously had normal cycles or for	
>12 mo in a woman whose cycles have	
been irregular	

DIAGNOSTICS	TREATMENT
	start with 200 mg IM, then repeat q3–4 wk × 6 mo
	IUDs containing progestins
	Compounded progesterones based on individual needs
	Reevaluate anemia in 1 mo
	Refer to gynecologist if bleeding continues or restarts after treatment ceases
	NSAIDs will help reduce cramping, bleeding, or both; caution patients to take with food: Mefenamic acid 500 mg tid Naproxen 550 mg bid Ibuprofen 600 mg tid
	Abnormal bleeding may be a side effect of missing OCs; if scant bleeding is noted during pill-free interval and abnormal bleeding occurs in regular cycle, this may indicate progestin excess
	Try increasing estrogenic effect of contraceptive pill or add supplemental estrogen daily for 7 days of each cycle along with contraceptive dose (do not double up on OCs)
Physical examination to include height, weight, vital signs and Tanner's staging (see Table 2–1) Pelvic exam for normal development TSH, LH, FSH DHEA, testosterone Question regarding drug use (illegal, prescription, and OTC) Consider pelvic ultrasound for pelvic CT if unsure of internal structures	If genetic or physical problem suspected, refer to geneticist or pediatric specialist If amenorrhea caused by too little body fat due to poor nutrition or eating disorder, refer to both nutritionist and pediatric psychiatrist If amenorrhea due to overexercise, counsel person to decrease amount of time spent exercising or change training program to allow more rest; increase daily consumption of calcium, start OCs to prevent bone loss and reestablish hormonal balance
Obtain good, detailed menstrual history, including partners and pregnancy history Pregnancy test (hCG, UCG)	If menses have not started after 3–6 mo, refer to gynecologist See Fig. 9–4 for treatment modalities for secondary amenorrhea Refer to endocrinologist or gynecologist for further evaluation if treatment options fail

Continued

Table 9–4 Gynecologic Conditions—cont'd	
CONDITION	SIGNS AND SYMPTOMS
Causes of Secondary Amenorrhea	

Central Organ Failure
   Athlete's amenorrhea
   Stress
   Severe eating disorders
   Posthormone suppression
   Pituitary lesions
	Central Organ Failure
	   Galactorrhea
	   H/A
	   Visual changes
	   Decreased libido
	   Weight loss, low body mass

Ovarian Failure
   Premature or natural menopause
   Autoimmune disorders
	Ovarian Failure
	   Hot flashes
	   Vaginal dryness
	   Labile moods
	   Weight gain
	   Dry, pale vaginal mucosa

End Organ Failure
   Cervical stenosis
   Uterine surgeries
   Asherman syndrome
	End Organ Failure
	   Cyclic PMS without menses
	   Abdominal bloating
	   Pinpoint cervical os

Anovulation
   Polycystic ovary syndrome
   Nonsynchronous ovulation
	Anovulation
	   Hirsutism
	   Acne
	   Deepening voice

Pregnancy-Related Amenorrhea
   Intrauterine pregnancy
   Extrauterine pregnancy
   Hydatidiform mole
   Missed abortion
	Pregnancy-Related Amenorrhea
	   Enlarged abdomen
	   Enlarged uterus

Drug-Induced Amenorrhea
   Illegal drugs (e.g., "crack," cocaine, heroin)
   Prescription drugs (e.g., haloperidol,
      phenothiazines)
   Herbal medicines (e.g., any herb that
      stimulates estrogen receptor sites, such
      as red clover, black cohosh, DHEA,
      milk thistle, ginseng, etc.)	

- Identification of menopausal conditions caused by loss of estrogen should be initiated early in the perimenopausal period; the potential problems are osteoporosis, vaginal dryness and irritation, emotional lability, increase in the number of UTIs, and yeast infections

Signs and Symptoms

- Gradual or sudden change in menstrual cycle patterns either in amount of bleeding, timing between cycles (either longer or shorter), or sudden cessation of

DIAGNOSTICS	TREATMENT
Prolactin level (if galactorrhea)	
TSH, FSH, LH (if LH >10 mIU/ml and LH/FSH ratio > 2:1, suspect polycystic ovary syndrome)	
DHEA and testosterone level (if androgen excess is suspected)	
Pelvic ultrasound, if indicated	
CT scan of abdomen and pelvis, if indicated	
Endometrial biopsy	

menses; cycles usually lengthen until menses are missed for longer than 12 months; heavy bleeding can occur during this period of time; monitor for developing anemia due to excess blood loss (see p. 204)
- Vasomotor symptoms such as hot flashes/flushes, night sweats are usually noticed first, followed by:
  □ Vaginal atrophy and irritation
  □ Frequent vaginal discharge, bacterial vaginosis, recurrent vaginitis
  □ Frequent UTIs, stress incontinence, dysuria, frequency

Name _____   Month _____

Date	1	2	3	4	5	6	7	8	9	10	11	12	13	14	15	16	17	18	19	20	21	22	23	24	25	26	27	28	29	30	31
Check if menstruating																															
Medication taken																															
Symptoms: 1 = small amount; 2 = moderate; 3 = quite a bit; 4 = extreme																															
Mood swings																															
Irritability																															
Out of control																															
Nervous tension																															
Depression																															
Low interest level																															
Fatigue																															
Energetic																															
Confused																															
Craving for sweets																															
Sleeplessness																															
Headache																															
Breast tenderness																															
Bloated feeling																															
General aches, pains																															
Other																															

FIGURE 9-3 PMS symptom diary.

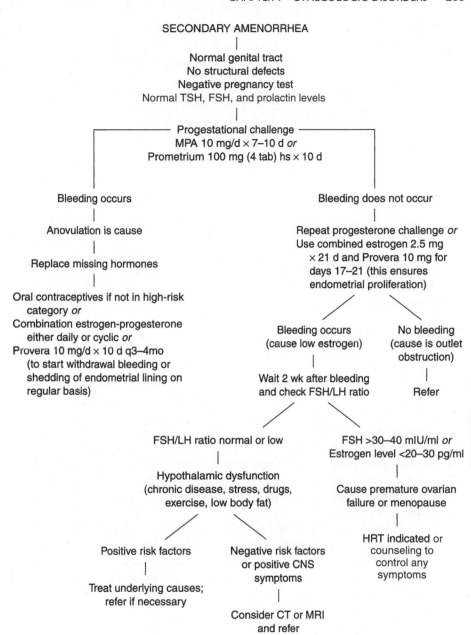

FIGURE 9–4 Secondary amenorrhea chart.

  ▫ Dyspareunia, vulvar itching, vaginal dryness, feeling of pressure in perineum
  ▫ Headaches
  ▫ Labile emotions, crying frequently, anxious without reason
  ▫ Cold hands or feet
  ▫ Forgetfulness or decreased ability to concentrate
  ▫ Weight gain in hips and thighs
  ▫ Altered sleep patterns
  ▫ Decreased skin elasticity
  ▫ Loss of energy, apathy

Diagnostics
  • Complete history and physical
  • FSH/LH; estradiol levels, testosterone/dehydroepiandrosterone (DHEA) levels if indicated
  • TSH/T_4
  • CBC, UCG (if indicated), chemistry profile, lipid profile
  • Pap smear, wet prep, STD testing (if indicated)
  • Mammogram

Perimenopausal Therapies
  • Perimenopausal period is considered the 2- to 6-year transition between reproduction years and menopause
  • During this time, emphasis should be on healthy lifestyles, including weight loss, exercise (aerobic, strength-training, and weight-bearing), smoking cessation, decreased caffeine intake, and multivitamin therapy; healthy behaviors are very beneficial but very difficult to sustain for any length of time
  • If cycles are sporadic, heavy, or both and the woman is not a smoker and has a low-risk profile, use low-dose oral contraceptives for cycle control; at approximately age 50 to 52 years, check FSH on day 5 of pill-free week; if FSH is elevated on two consecutive months, can switch to HRT at low dose (if patient wants to continue hormone therapy)
  • Perimenopausal women taking herbal products for relief of PMS, vasomotor symptoms, fatigue, or irregular cycles should be aware that these products can cause unwanted hormonal side effects (e.g., breast tenderness, irregular or heavy bleeding, bloating) and can increase the risk of endometrial cancer (if unopposed estrogenic product used)

Menopausal Nonhormonal Therapies
  • Osteoporosis prevention or treatment (see p. 356)
  • Vaginal atrophy and irritation
  ▫ OTC lubricants (water-based products [e.g., KY Jelly, Astroglide]) and moisture barriers [e.g., petroleum jelly, Crisco]) should be used 2 to 3 times daily
  • Emotional lability and change in sleep patterns may need a combination of medications to control symptoms

- □ SSRIs help with emotional symptoms
- □ TCA and trazodone may help with sleep disturbances
- Vasomotor symptoms
  - □ Herbal therapies (Table 9–5)
  - □ Venlafaxine (Effexor) 12.5 to 37.5 mg qd to bid
  - □ Fluoxetine (Prozac) 10 to 20 mg qd
  - □ Clonidine 0.1 mg bid to tid
  - □ Bellergal-S/tablet bid

Menopausal Hormonal Therapies

- A woman with an intact uterus must be given both estrogen and progestin product to protect the endometrium; if estrogen is given alone, proliferation of the endometrium will result in higher risk for cancer
- Close monitoring during the annual physical is required for prudent prescribing practices if patient is taking HRT; breast exam, mammogram, and Pap smear should be done annually; perform routine screening for cholesterol level and colorectal cancer
- Testosterone can be added to improve sexual desire (not guaranteed to work); this requires close monitoring for adverse effects: deepening of voice, hirsutism, worsening lipid profiles
- There are many different commercial types of estrogens, progesterones, and combined oral products, along with intravaginal inserts, IUDs, topical creams and transdermal patches; the practitioner can be very creative and individualize therapy to meet the patient's needs; *remember, if the woman has an intact uterus you are obligated to use both estrogen and progesterone* (Table 9–6)
- Compounding of hormone products can help the practitioner to individualize therapy; estrogen, progesterone, and testosterone can be compounded either together or separately in oral capsules, creams, patches, vaginal creams, or troches; listed below are some common equivalent doses for commercially prepared and compounded oral estrogens:
  - □ CEE 0.625 mg = oral estradiol 1 mg = estradiol patch 0.05 mg = TriEstrogen 1.25 to 2.5 mg bid (compounded as 80% estriol, 10% estrone, 10% estradiol)
  - □ CEE 1.25 mg = oral estradiol 2 mg = estradiol patch 0.1 mg = TriE strogen 2.5 to 5.0 mg bid (compounded as 80% estriol, 10% estrone, 10% estradiol)

Practice Pearls

- Exercise is important to every women's overall health; it contributes to stronger bones and prevention of osteoporosis (see p. 356); whenever possible, exercise should consist of weight-bearing activity 30 min/day 4 to 6 times a week; strength training can be beneficial to maintain agility and muscle mass
- Diet is important in maintaining health; for the patient wanting natural products high in phytoestrogens, the diet should be high in soy products (beans, soy milk, flour, tofu), flaxseed (oil, seeds), red clover, alfalfa, celery, parsley, fennel,

Table 9-5 Herbal Products for Relief of Menopausal Symptoms

PRODUCT	DOSE	PRECAUTIONS	VAGINITIS, UTIs	HOT FLASHES	LABILE MOOD	FATIGUE	COLD HANDS OR FEET	FORGETFULNESS
Black Cohosh (Remefemin; Cimicifuga) Can be used for long periods Caution: may stimulate estrogen-positive breast cancers Can be used in women who cannot tolerate HRT	1–2 tab bid	Monitor blood pressure	Yes	Yes	Yes	No	No	Yes
Evening Primrose Oil Can be used for long periods	1–2 caps bid	None known	No	Yes	Yes	No	No	No
Ginkgo Biloba Enhances vascular microcirculation Improves the transmission of nerve signals in brain	40 mg qd	May worsen migraine in some women	No	No	No	Yes	Yes	Yes

6

	Dosage	Contraindications/Cautions						
Vitamin E Improves skin texture and moistness Can be used either orally or topically Also beneficial cardiac protection	800 IU/day po *or* topical oil, cream, or ointment, *or* suppository	None known	Yes	Questionable	No	No	No	No
Promensil Red clover extract	1 tab qd	Not to be used with HRT	Yes	Yes	Yes	Yes	No	No
Wild Yam	¼ tsp bid (on 3 wk, off 1 wk)	Breast or pelvic cancer, uterine fibroid, endometriosis	Yes	Yes	No	No	No	No
Chasteberry	Crude herb extract 20–240 mg bid–tid	Breast or pelvic cancer, uterine fibroid, endometriosis	Questionable	Yes	Yes	Questionable	No	No
Ginseng, Panax	Root extract capsules 100–600 mg qd for 3 wk every month for 3 mo	May worsen migraine in some women	No	Yes	No	Yes	No	No

9

Table 9–6 Hormone Replacement Therapy

ESTROGEN ONLY	PROGESTERONE ONLY	COMBINED ESTROGEN/PROGESTIN
Premarin (CEE) 0.3 mg, 0.45 mg, 0.625 mg, 0.9 mg, 1.25 mg, 2.5 mg	Provera, Cycrin (medroxyprogesterone) 2.5 mg, 5.0 mg, 10 mg	Prempro 0.625 mg/2.5 mg, 0.625 mg/5 mg, 0.45 mg/1.5 mg (oral combined CEE/medroxyprogesterone)
Estrace (estradiol) 0.5 mg, 1 mg, 2 mg	Prometrium (micronized progesterone) 100–200 mg hs	Premphase 0.625 mg/5 mg (days 1–14 estrogen alone; days 15–28 (oral combined CEE/medroxyprogesterone)
Estratab, Menest (esterified estrogen) 0.3 mg, 0.625 mg, 2.5 mg	Aygestin, Nor-QD (norethindrone) 2.5 mg, 5 mg, 10 mg	Activella 1 mg/0.5 mg (oral combined) estradiol/norethindrone)
Ogen (estropipate) 0.625 mg, 1.25 mg, 2.5 mg	Crinone (progesterone vaginal gel) 4%, 8%; use one applicator qod	Femhrt (oral combined ethinyl estradiol/norethindrone)
Cenestin (estrogens conjugated, synthetic) 0.3 mg, 0.625 mg, 0.9 mg, 1.25 mg		Ortho-Prefest (oral combined cyclic estradiol 1 mg/norgestimate 0.9 mg); cycles are in 3-day compliments
Transdermal patches: Vivelle, Alora, Climara, Estraderm (estradiol) Application varies from biweekly to weekly		CombiPatch transdermal system (combined estradiol/norethindrone 0.05/0.14 mg, 0.05/0.25 mg)
Estring (estradiol vaginal ring) inserted every 90 days		Estratest 1.25 mg/2.5 mg and Estratest HS 0.625 mg/1.25 mg (oral combined esterified estrogen/methyltestosterone)
Vaginal creams: Premarin cream (CEE) 0.625 mg/g Estrace vaginal 0.1 mg/g (estradiol) Vaginal tablet (Vagifem) 0.025 mg		

6

apples, nuts, and whole grains; these products must be consumed on a daily basis to get the required amount of natural estrogen and to alleviate vasomotor symptoms

- Many women do not want to take traditional HRT; they wish to try herbal products to relieve symptoms; some herbal products are safe but have not been studied thoroughly (see Table 9–5); some herbal products have been found to cause more harm than help (see Appendix H); educate your patients and guide them; don't shut the door on their health care
- Encourage your patients to dress comfortably in layered clothing; avoid extreme temperature changes and identify foods that may trigger hot flashes
- Postmenopausal women without a uterus can use estrogen products alone or with herbal or nonhormonal therapies; *remember the lowest effective estrogen dose is the safest*
- If you use Estratest or Estratest HS in a woman with an intact uterus, you still have to use a progesterone product to protect the endometrium from unopposed estrogenic effect
- If rash or skin irritation occurs with patch therapy, have the patient use inhaled corticosteroid spray in the area where the patch will be applied, let it dry, and then apply the patch; this should decrease the reaction; the spray dries better than the OTC steroid creams
- Topical estrogen therapy can be used to alleviate vaginal dryness and improve vulvovaginal irritation; these products have minimal systemic uptake and are considered safe for the woman with a uterus (i.e., no progestin needed)
  □ Estrogen cream can be inserted into vagina or applied topically to external genitalia
  □ Estring vaginal ring every 90 days
  □ Vagifem tablets are used qhs × 14 days then twice weekly
- If a person experiences unwanted symptoms with one type of estrogen or progesterone product, switch to another class of drug; dosing is individual; start with the lowest dose and gradually increase dose to control symptom(s)
- Contraindications to HRT
  □ Unexplained vaginal bleeding
  □ Active or chronic liver disease or dysfunction
  □ Recent vascular thrombotic incident or history of varicose veins
  □ Cardiac disease or recent heart attack
  □ Carcinoma of the breast
- HRT is not indicated for prevention of heart disease or improvement of lipids; HRT may cause breast cancer, thromboembolic events, and gall bladder disease; use caution when prescribing HRT to women at high risk for these conditions; HRT is indicated for relief of menopausal and vasomotor related symptoms on a short-term basis; if patient has been undergoing HRT for >10 years, consideration should be given to decrease the dose or stop the dose and evaluate the symptoms; if patient is asymptomatic, can cease the HRT and discuss healthy behaviors and other nonhormonal therapies to prevent bone loss and treat any vasomotor symptoms that recur

- Encourage patient to use vitamin E (synthetic) 1000 IU daily with multivitamin, either initially or when HRT is stopped
- Order bone densitometry to get baseline data and then order every 2 years; encourage daily calcium and vitamin D supplements
- Abrupt cessation of HRT may cause sudden onset of vasomotor symptoms or vaginal bleeding; gradual withdrawal is recommended when patient has been undergoing HRT for more than 6 months
- Concomitant use of gastroesophageal reflux disease (GERD) medications can cause decreased absorption of oral estrogen products; if woman is having increased vasomotor/integumentary symptoms, try holding GERD product and monitor symptoms

POLYCYSTIC OVARY SYNDROME

256.4

Condition

- Polycystic ovary syndrome is a disorder of the ovary and adrenal glands leading to overproduction of androgens and other hormones including insulin, elevated LH, and insulin resistance, which act together to cause ovarian growth, androgen production, and increased ovarian cysts; the increased circulating androgens and increased insulin resistance place the patient at higher risk for DM and CAD because of increased body weight and dyslipidemia
- Polycystic ovary syndrome is also called *functional ovarian hyperandrogenism* and *ovarian androgen excess;* these terms are more descriptive of the disease process; polycystic ovaries (PCOs) are only one component of the disease process; PCOs are a sign of the disease and not diagnostic of the disease
- This common condition usually begins at menarche but may not be identified until later in life; patient usually has a long history of irregular cycles or long periods of amenorrhea, increased hair growth, acne, and central obesity
- Polycystic ovary syndrome does not have a rapid onset; if symptoms have occurred rapidly, think some type of neoplasm
- It may have genetic component
- It is the leading cause of infertility
- It results in increased risk for cardiovascular disease, diabetes and diabetic complications, and endometrial cancer

Signs and Symptoms

- Oligomenorrhea
- Amenorrhea
- Infertility or decreased fertility
- Central obesity (may be normal or underweight)
- Signs of androgen excess
  - Hirsutism
  - Acne
  - Alopecia

- ☐ Acanthosis nigricans
- Insulin resistance
- Increased triglycerides with low HDL on lipid profile
- HTN, weight gain, and obesity

Diagnostics

- TSH (elevated results indicative of thyroid disorder)
- Prolactin level (elevated results indicative of pituitary tumor)
- LH/FSH (usually is seen as a 2:1 ratio, but normal ratio does not exclude diagnosis of polycystic ovary syndrome; elevated FSH level indicative of premature ovarian failure
- 17 OH progesterone level (level >5 ng/ml is abnormal and should be investigated, cause could be congenital adrenal hyperplasia); may need to do ACTH stimulation test
- Total testosterone and DHEA (elevated results indicative of androgen-producing tumor; testosterone levels >200 ng/dl or DHEA levels >800 mcg/dl are not seen with polycystic ovary syndrome and may indicate a virilizing adrenal tumor)
- Complete chemistry panel and 2-hour GTT (elevated results [2-hour GTT >200 mg/dl] indicative of insulin resistance)
- Lipid panel (used to monitor for cardiac disease)
- Endometrial biopsy and pelvic transvaginal ultrasound (prolonged estrogen stimulation in the endometrium without opposing progesterone can increase risk for endometrial cancer; virilizing ovarian tumors are identified earlier)
- UCG

Treatment

- Weight loss (even 5% to 10% weight loss can improve insulin resistance and lipid profile and may decrease circulating androgens enough to restart menses)
- Exercise
- Hair removal techniques such as electrolysis or waxing
- May consider eflornithine (Vaniqua) to remove unwanted hair; apply thick layer of cream to affected areas of face bid
- Metformin for insulin resistance; may also correct anovulation; usual dose is 1500 to 2000 mg qd in three divided doses
- OCs to reestablish normal hormonal levels; progesterone alone can be used to protect the endometrium from unopposed estrogen stimulation; Yasmin is OC of choice because drospirenone component acts like spironolactone and blocks androgens
- Antiandrogens such as spironolactone and finasteride possibly decrease hair growth and improve acne; effects may take as long as 3 to 6 months to be noticed
- Monitor FBS and GTT annually; lipid profile every 3 to 5 years if normal initially
- Infertility specialist if pregnancy is desired

Gynecologic Infections

See Table 9–7

Table 9–7   Gynecologic Infections

Infectious Vaginitis 112.1	Pelvic Inflammatory Disease 614.9
Trichomonas Vaginitis 131.01	Gonorrhea 098.0
Noninfectious Vaginitis 627.3	Chlamydial Infection 079.98
Vulvovaginal Candidiasis 112.1	Syphilis 097.9
Stress Leukorrhea 623.5	Herpes Genitalia 054.10
Vulvitis 616.10	Genital Warts 078.19

CONDITION	SIGNS AND SYMPTOMS
Infectious Vaginitis *Bacterial Vaginosis (BV,* Gardnerella *Vaginitis)* Most common cause of vaginal discharge; may be associated with multiple sex partners (*not* sexually transmitted), tampons and douching	Usually asymptomatic Foul- or fishy-smelling vaginal discharge that frequently increases before menses and after sexual intercourse Increased vaginal discharge that has copious, thin, gray-white ("spilled milk") appearance Itching and burning are rare unless coinfection with another pathogen exists
Trichomonas *Vaginitis (Protozoan)*	Yellow-green, frothy discharge and foul odor Vulval itching Dysuria Symptoms increase during and after menses Dyspareunia

DIAGNOSTICS	TREATMENT

Presence of 3 of 4 of the following signs is diagnostic for bacterial vaginosis:
Thin, homogeneous, gray-white, adherent vaginal discharge
Vaginal pH > 4.5*
Positive KOH "whiff" test result*
Clue cells with microscopic examination (see microscopic findings, Fig. 1–8)

Antibiotic Therapy
Recommended Therapy
Metronidazole: 500 mg PO bid × 7 days; 0.75% intravaginal applicator once daily × 5 days (pregnancy class B) *or*
Clindamycin: 5 g intravaginal applicator once daily × 7 days (pregnancy class B); no condoms for 72 hr after using

Alternate Therapy
Metronidazole 2 g po once
or
Clindamycin 300 mg po bid × 7 days
or
Clindamycin vaginal 1 application qhs × 3–7 days
Tinidazole 1000 mg po qd × 5 days (non-pregnant)

Recurrent Vaginosis
Vaginal acidifiers (lactate gel and acetic acid gel, acidophilus intravaginal suppositories) for symptom relief near menses
Intermittent treatment with intravaginal metronidazole gel once weekly or 2 g po once monthly; if patient is pregnant, refer her to obstetrician
Encourage patients to wear all-cotton underwear, to avoid douching, and to use sanitary napkins instead of tampons
Encourage patients to avoid alcohol while taking metronidazole and for 72 hr after finishing medication
Betadine gel or suppository intravaginally bid × 14–28 days; treat for any concurrent candidal infection with diflucan 150 mg × 1

Trichomonads (see Fig. 1–8)
WBCs >10/HPF with microscopic examination
"Whiff" test may or may not have positive results
pH >4.5

Metronidazole: 2 g po as single dose (recommended); 250–500 mg bid × 7 days
Alternate Therapy
If resistant to metronidazole, try
Betadine or vinegar douche qd × 1 mo; recheck in a month
Tinidazole 2 g × 1

*Highest sensitivity is pH; highest specificity is positive amine odor. If both positive, treat for BV; if one or both are negative, continue testing.

Continued

Table 9–7	Gynecologic Infections—cont'd

CONDITION	SIGNS AND SYMPTOMS
	Strawberry, friable cervix that bleeds easily
	Painful inguinal lymph nodes
	May be dormant for years
Noninfectious Vaginitis *Atrophic Vaginitis*	
	Burning and irritation
	Feeling of dryness
	Pruritus
	Vaginal bleeding (minimal amount)
	Can occur during postpartum, perimenopausal, or postmenopausal period
	Painful sexual intercourse with spotting afterward
	Gray-yellow, nonodorous vaginal discharge
	Pale, smooth vaginal walls
	Sparse, brittle pubic hair
	Punctate hemorrhages on vagina and cervix
Vulvovaginal Candidiasis (VVC)	
	Erythema, pruritus, excoriation, and swelling of external genitalia
	May occur while taking antibiotics or OCs
	External dysuria
	Whitish-yellow, cottage cheese–appearing discharge that is adherent to vaginal walls
	Musty odor
	Candidiasis in men may be demonstrated by urethritis, balanitis, and cutaneous lesions on penis

DIAGNOSTICS	TREATMENT
	Encourage patients to avoid alcohol during and for 24 hr after finishing antibiotic therapy Treat partner(s) Encourage "safe sex" practices Refer pregnant patient
Decreased lactobacilli with microscopic examination Wet prep negative FSH/LH ratio	HRT and/or topical estrogen therapy (see Table 9–6) Water-soluble lubricants Black cohosh Mix equal portions of OTC hydrocortisone cream and petroleum jelly (Vaseline) and apply topically to relieve itch and dryness
KOH positive for hyphae and budding yeast (see microscopic findings, Fig. 1–8) pH < 4.5 Whiff test negative If recurrent or difficult to treat, evaluate fasting glucose level	*OTC Vaginal Preparations* Butoconazole 2% cream 1 applicator hs one time (pregnancy class C) Clotrimazole 100 mg vaginal tablet hs × 7 days (pregnancy class B) Clotrimazole 500 mg vaginal tablet one time *Prescription Preparations* Terconazole cream 1 applicator hs × 3 or 7 days or 1 suppository hs × 3 days (pregnancy class C) Fluconazole 150 mg po once (pregnancy class C) Tell patients to wear sanitary napkins to protect clothing and to change them frequently, to wear all-cotton underwear, and to avoid too-tight clothing, panty hose, and use of harsh soaps and perfumes in vulval area If partner has balanitis, treat him with any imidazole cream followed by nystatin powder; keep foreskin retracted for treatment

Continued

Table 9–7 Gynecologic Infections—cont'd	
CONDITION	SIGNS AND SYMPTOMS

Other Vulval and Vaginal Disorders

Stress Leukorrhea

Breakdown of vaginal cells increases production of lactic acid; the lactic acid produces hydrogen peroxide, which is irritating to the vulval skin, and pruritus begins

Possible causes: decrease in estrogen or increase in progesterone from some type of change in the hormone environment; can be induced by stress

Yeastlike presentation with itching and discharge

Cyclic, usually premenstrual symptoms (not present during rest of cycle)

Discharge is usually white to clear but irritating

Discharge usually doubles during premenstrual period

Vulvitis

Can be caused by *anything:* too-tight clothing; perfumed soaps, sprays, pads, or shampoos; hot tub or pool chemicals, colored undergarments; laundry detergents; birth control methods including MPA (a decrease in estrogen can lead to atrophic vulvitis); oral sex; postpartum period, perimenopause, menopause; overuse of OTC yeast products, latex allergy (condoms); *these are just a few causes*

Consider vulvar cancer with persistent vulvitis

Severe itching and burning to vulval and perineal area

May see diffuse redness without specific lesions (if lesions present, they do not resemble herpes)

Symptoms may be cyclic or daily; person may attribute the symptoms to change in environment

Usually bilateral, but can be unilateral involvement of labia

DIAGNOSTICS	TREATMENT
	Recurrent VVC (>4 episodes/yr)
	Fluconazole 150 mg × 1 tablet now and repeat in 3 days
	or
	Give one of the following for 6 mo:
	Clotrimazole 500 mg vaginal tablet once weekly
	Ketoconazole 100 mg qd (pregnancy class C)
	Fluconazole 100–150 mg once weekly
	Itraconazole 400 mg once monthly (pregnancy class C)
	Boric acid 600 mg capsule intravaginally bid × 2 wk
	Check blood glucose status
	Discourage anal to vaginal intercourse without washing
Wet mount is usually normal without clue cells or hyphae	Discourage use of yeast medications
WBC count may vary but not enough to consider infection	No douching or use of tampons
	Reduce stress before menses
pH usually normal	Increase rest before symptoms occur
Person needs to keep a symptom diary because each episode should be evaluated	Decrease intake of sugar prior to symptoms
	Try OCs such as Ortho Tri-Cyclen; use back to back for 3 mo (no withdrawal bleeding) and then reevaluate symptoms
Diagnosis by exclusion	Remove cause if known
Biopsy if long-standing condition	Treat any known cause
Consider colposcopy if irritation extends into vaginal vault or cervix	Individualized care for symptoms
	Decrease stress if this is a factor
Consider and test for noncyclic causes such as BV, *Trichomonas*, STDs, HPV, herpes, HIV	Have person keep a personal diary for several cycles if possible
	Discourage any type of scrubbing of vulval area; pat dry after urination; use soft, unscented toilet tissue or in the initial period have person use soft cotton cloth wipes after urination; use mild soap after defecation to cleanse perineal and anal areas
	No tight clothing; wear all-cotton, white underwear that is laundered with mild detergent before it is worn

Continued

Table 9–7	Gynecologic Infections—cont'd
CONDITION	**SIGNS AND SYMPTOMS**
Sexually Transmitted Diseases *Pelvic Inflammatory Disease (PID)* Usually sexually transmitted infection, especially *Neisseria gonorrhoeae*, and *Chlamydia trachomatis*; other organisms involved are anaerobes, *Gardnerella vaginalis*, *Haemophilus influenzae*, enteric gram-negative rods Chronic PID can cause infertility Can mimic other lower abdominal problems	*Minimum Criteria for Diagnosis* Lower abdominal tenderness Adnexal tenderness Cervical motion tenderness (CMT) If woman is sexually active, no other cause is identified, and she meets these three criteria, treat *Additional Criteria* Oral temperature >101° F Abnormal cervical or vaginal discharge Elevated ESR Elevated C-reactive protein Laboratory documentation of infection with *N. gonorrhoeae* or *C. trachomatis* These additional criteria may be used to increase specificity; these support a diagnosis of PID *Definitive Criteria* Histopathic evidence of endometritis on biopsy Transvaginal or pelvic U/S showing thickened, fluid-filled tubes or free pelvic fluid Laparoscopic findings consistent with PID
Gonorrhea Caused by *N. gonorrhoeae* After exposure, approximately 60%–90% of women become infected	May be asymptomatic for both men and women Men may have dysuria, urinary frequency, and purulent penile discharge

DIAGNOSTICS	TREATMENT
	If you suspect a hormonal problem, change OC or stop injections
	For initial treatment, try topical steroid cream for short time, such as Zonalon, Diprosone, Vagicort (OTC), or Lotrisone
	Consider topical estrogen cream, if indicated
	May try some type of topical skin protectants such as zinc oxide, Vaseline, A&D creams, OTC topical yeast preparations, or topical anesthetic
Obtain cultures from cervix for *N. gonorrhoeae* and *C. trachomatis* Obtain specimen from vaginal walls for *G. vaginalis* and wet prep for number of WBCs; if vaginal discharge normal, PID is unlikely CBC ESR, CRP UA/UCG If laboratory evidence of *N. gonorrhoeae* or *C. trachomatis,* the partner must be treated	Ceftriaxone 250 mg IM × 1 plus doxycycline 100 mg bid × 14 days with or without metronidazole 500 mg bid × 14 days *or* Cefoxitin 2 g IM with probenicid 1 g plus doxycycline 100 mg bid × 14 days with or without metronidazole 500 mg bid × 14 days *or* 3rd generation cephalosporin IM plus doxycycline 100 mg bid × 14 days with or without metronidazole If allergy to above: levofloxacin 500 mg qd or ofloxacin 400 mg bid × 14 days with or without metronidazole 500 mg bid × 14 days Patients should respond to treatment within 72 hr; if symptoms are resolving, follow-up in 4–6 wk; if symptoms are worsening, refer for hospitalization Refer if patient is pregnant, a potential surgical risk, or does not comply with outpatient therapy and for severe illness, N/V, high fever, tubo-ovarian abscess, immunodeficiency Treat partner empirically; consider HIV testing and counseling
Cervical culture Gonococcal and *Chlamydia* culture Urine NAAT	*Antibiotic Therapy* Ceftriaxone sodium 125 mg IM once (safe during pregnancy) *plus* azithromycin 1 g orally once *or* Doxycycline 100 mg bid × 7 days

Continued

Table 9–7 Gynecologic Infections—cont'd

CONDITION	SIGNS AND SYMPTOMS
If untreated, approximately 15% will have PID with possibility of sterility	Women may have purulent vaginal discharge, abnormal menses, and dysuria Positive cervical motion tenderness (CMT) Purulent discharge from cervix
Chlamydial Infection Caused by *C. trachomatis* Most common nonviral STD Leading cause of infertility, ectopic pregnancy, and PID	May be asymptomatic Mucopurulent cervicitis or vaginal discharge Spotting usually after intercourse Possibly dyspareunia Cervical friability, erosion, and irritation Positive CMT Occasional lymphadenopathy Abdominal or pelvic pain Dysuria
Syphilis Caused by *Treponema pallidum* Incubation period between 10 and 90 days There have been recent outbreaks of syphilis associated with the increase in HIV infection, drug use, and increased poverty conditions	*Primary Syphilis* Chancre, a painless, indurated ulcer, is usually found at the site of inoculation *Secondary Syphilis* Skin rash Enlarged lymph nodes Malaise Alopecia Anorexia Arthralgia

DIAGNOSTICS	TREATMENT
	Other injectable cephalosporin (cefoxitin 2 g with probenicid 1 g or ceftizoxime 500 mg) *plus* azithromycin 1 g or doxycycline 100 mg bid × 7 days; if allergy to cephalosporin, use azithromycin 2 g orally
	Treat also for *Chlamydia*
	Educate on transmission and prevention techniques
	Patient should avoid intercourse until therapy completed and symptoms resolved
	Report to health department
	Treat all contacts if possible
	If uncomplicated infection, no return for test-of-cure; if complicated infection, return in 3 mo
Chlamydia culture	*Antibiotic Therapy (po for 7–10 days)*
May need CBC if PID is suspected	Doxycycline 100 mg bid (pregnancy class D)
Screen all women ≤25 yr of age	*or*
Screen all women >25 yr of age if >2 partners in past 2 mo, or new male partner in past 2 mo, or Hx of STDs	Azithromycin 1 g (one time only) (pregnancy class B) *or*
Urine NAAT	Erythromycin 500 mg qid (safe with pregnancy) *or*
	Ofloxacin 300 mg bid (not during pregnancy or if <18 yr old) or levofloxacin 500 mg qd (not during pregnancy or if <18 yr old)
	Levoquin 500 mg qd × 7 days
	Teach about transmission, prevention
	Patients should avoid intercourse until therapy completed (or for 7 days after single dose therapy)
	Report to health department
	Test-of-cure not advised unless compliance in question, symptoms persist, or reinfection suspected; retest in approximately 3 mo if suspected reinfection without symptoms
	Also treat for gonorrhea
	Treat all known partners
Need to use combination tests to avoid false-positive results: RPR and VDRL	Report to health department
Test for HIV	*Antibiotic Therapy for Primary and Secondary Syphilis*
Gonococcal and chlamydial culture	Benzathine penicillin-G 2.4 million units IM once
Hepatitis B and C screen	Doxycycline 100 mg bid × 14 days if allergic to penicillin
	Reexamine and order serologic tests at 6 and 12 mo; sustained fourfold increase probably indicates treatment failure or

Continued

Table 9–7	Gynecologic Infections—cont'd

CONDITION	SIGNS AND SYMPTOMS
	Late Syphilis Usually asymptomatic *Neurosyphilis* General paresis Tabes dorsalis Dementia May occur at any stage up to 30 yr after exposure

Herpes Genitalias
Caused by a virus that remains in the ganglia after infection
Recurrence is high; recurrent episodes are usually milder and of shorter duration
Possible triggers:
    Stress
    Menstrual changes
    Illness
    Fatigue
    Poor nutrition
    Intercourse
    Fever
    Trauma
Patient is considered infectious at onset of symptoms and until lesions are dried up
	Vesicular lesions initially followed by ulcerated area on erythematous base; vesicles appear "punched out" area on skin
	Usually does not itch
	Severe burning pain at area of eruption
	May last 7–10 days
	May have watery discharge
	May have "flulike" syndrome with first outbreak
	Lymphadenopathy
	Cervicitis
	Prodromal symptoms may include pain or paresthesias of buttocks, thighs, legs ("boxer shorts" area)

Genital Warts (Condylomata Acuminata) Caused by human papillomavirus (HPV) HPV increases risk of vulval and cervical cancers Highly contagious Most common STD HPV is usually a transient infection, but not always	Painless warts noted on genitalia Sometimes pruritic May cause dyspareunia, dysuria, and bleeding Flat, painless, or papular lesions with fleshy appearance; can be multilobular Usually found on or around vulvovaginal or anal area, on penis, or sites of friction

6

DIAGNOSTICS	TREATMENT
	reinfection; treat again after evaluating for HIV
	Refer to infectious disease specialist
Herpes culture	*Primary Episode (po for 7–10 days)*
STD testing	Acyclovir 200 mg 5 times per day or 400 mg
Serologic testing for herpes	tid (pregnancy class B) *or*
	Famciclovir 250 mg tid (pregnancy class B) *or*
	Valacyclovir 1 g bid (pregnancy class B)
	Recurrent Episodes
	Acyclovir 800 mg bid or 400 mg tid × 5 days *or*
	Famciclovir 125 mg bid × 5 days *or*
	Valacyclovir 500 mg bid × 3–5 days
	If >6 episodes per year, consider daily prophylactic treatment with acyclovir 400 mg bid *or* famciclovir 250 mg bid *or* valacyclovir 500 mg–1 g qd
	Reevaluate after 1 yr; provide patient with prescription so treatment can be started within 24 hr of onset
	General Measures
	See patient tips on p. 476
	Wear loosely fitting undergarments
	Avoid sexual intercourse when lesions are present
	Use condoms for all intercourse
	Teach about transmission, prevention
Use bright light for examination	*Provider-Applied Treatment*
STD testing is recommended, including HIV testing	Trichloroacetic acid (TCA) 85%; apply with cotton applicator, being careful not to touch healthy tissue; may repeat application q2wk
Applying acetic acid 5% solution (vinegar) to skin will cause HPV lesions to turn white	Liquid nitrogen; apply with cotton applicator weekly until resolved

Continued

Table 9–7 Gynecologic Infections—cont'd

CONDITION	SIGNS AND SYMPTOMS

DIAGNOSTICS	TREATMENT
Colposcopy is recommended with presence of perineal or vulval lesions even if Pap smear results are normal (20%–25% Pap smear results false-negative); base treatment on biopsy results, not Pap smear results	Podophyllum 10%–25%; apply a petroleum jelly collar around the lesion and then apply podophyllum with cotton applicator; wash off in 3–4 hr; treat once a week × 4 wk; do not use in pregnancy or with oral, cervical, anal, or urethral lesions *Patient-Applied Therapies* Have patient follow package instructions Podofilox 5% solution (Condylox) Imiquimod (Aldara) 5% cream Sinecatechins (Veregen) 15% ointment *General Measures* Reinforce that there is no cure and that lesions may return; the goal is symptomatic relief Referral for laser surgery may be necessary Advise of routes of transmission and means of prevention Advise patients to use condoms for all sexual encounters; however, this will not prevent transfer of lesions on external genitalia Encourage annual Pap smears for early detection of cervical cancer or further growths Recommend HPV (Gardisil) immunization for males and females of appropriate age See patient tips on p. 476

NOTES

NOTES

NOTES

10

Common Urinary Tract Disorders

The urinary tract system can be a very daunting system to evaluate. After the practitioner has performed the history and physical, a urinalysis will be ordered. Many times the practitioner will review the urine by using a multitest stick, using microscope evaluation or sending the urine out to the reference laboratory for complete review. The physical appearance of the urine and the urinalysis results will tell the practitioner information that can be used for the final diagnosis. Listed below are some common findings related to the urinalysis that can aid in the diagnosis.

Practice Pearls
- Nocturia: think polyuria associated with diabetes or CHF, bladder irritability from caffeine or other stimulant drugs, or incomplete emptying caused by obstruction from a tumor, stool, or an enlarged prostate
- Urethral syndrome (spasm): can be treated with prazosin (Minipress) 1 mg bid; can go up to 2 mg bid; monitor blood pressure closely for hypotension
- Avoid ASA, NSAIDs with renal insufficiency
- Gross hematuria:
  - If at beginning of urination, think urethra or prostate dysfunction
  - If at end of urination, think trigone or bladder neck spasm
  - If throughout voiding, think bladder, ureter, or kidney pathology
  - If cyclic with menses, think endometriosis of urinary tract
- Chronic WBCs too numerous to count on repeat UAs, check CBC (if leukocytes >20,000, think leukocytic leukemia)
- 99% of UTIs in men are due to prostatitis; fluoroquinolones work better than TMP-SMZ in men
- Think UTI in an elderly person with acute confusion, lethargy, N/V, or diarrhea
- Treatment of *asymptomatic* bacteriuria in elderly persons leads to antibiotic resistance only treat if symptoms present
- Cystocele grading: first degree, clearly visible; second degree, at introitus; third degree, protruding from vagina
- Preventative measures for acute or chronic UTI:
  - Do not douche; this may disrupt the normal vaginal flora and encourage migration of bacteria to the urethral opening
  - Always urinate after sexual intercourse to flush harmful bacteria out of urethra
  - Do not use bubble baths and perineal sprays; these cause chemical irritation

- Wipe perineum front-to-back to prevent spread of harmful bacteria
- Increase fluid intake to 6 to 8 glasses of water a day
- Eliminate spermicides (especially nonoxynol-9), which cause irritation and decrease normal vaginal flora
- Only use cranberry juice or cranberry pills at bedtime (too much cranberry can cause overacidification of urine and cause irritation to bladder lining)
- Drinking apple cider vinegar (2 to 4 oz) daily may provide a bactericidal environment for the bladder

Text continued on p. 301

Urinalysis Findings

DESCRIPTION	NORMAL	ABNORMAL	SIGNIFICANCE
Color	Clear, yellow straw color	Colorless/pale	Diabetes insipidus, alcohol, increased fluid intake
		Red or brown	Blood, porphyrin Foods: beets, rhubarb, food color Drugs: sulfisoxazole, phenytoin, cascara, chlorpromazine
		Orange	Decreased oral intake, urobilinogen, fever Drugs: phenazopyridine HCl (Pyridium), sulfa, nitrofurantoin Foods: carrots, rhubarb
		Blue or green	*Pseudomonas* Drugs: amitriptyline, methylene blue
		Brown or black	Lysol overdose, melanin, bilirubin, methemoglobin Foods: cascara, iron
		Cloudy	Bacteria, pus, prostate fluid, semen
		Milky	Pyuria, hyperlipidemia
		Foamy	Cirrhosis, bilirubin, bile, hepatitis, obstructive disease of the liver, proteinuria
Odor	Aromatic	Ammonia	Urea breakdown, increased nitrites

Urinalysis Findings—cont'd

DESCRIPTION	NORMAL	ABNORMAL	SIGNIFICANCE
		Foul	Bacteria
		Mousy	Phenylketonuria
		Fruity	Diabetes, starvation states, anorexia, bulimia, or extreme dieting
pH	4.6–8	<4.6	Acidosis, high-protein diets, severe diarrhea, vomiting, severe COPD
		>8	Bacteriuria, UTI, metabolic alkalosis Drugs: neomycin, sulfa, potassium citrate
Specific gravity	1.005–1.030	<1.005	Diabetes insipidus, increased oral intake, severe potassium deficit
		>1.030	Decreased oral intake, fever, excess vomiting or diarrhea, iodine dye, DM
Protein	Negative (trace/1$^+$: think exercise and recheck early morning specimen)	Positive If >2$^+$ get 24-hr urine for protein and creatinine clearance	Pyelonephritis, glomerulonephritis (1$^+$–2$^+$ or 1000–2000 mg/ 24 hr), bladder cancer, UTI, CHF, myeloma, fever, lead poisoning, toxemia, DM, nephrosis (3$^+$–4$^+$ or 3000– 4000 mg/24 hr) Drugs: barbiturates, sulfa, neomycin
Glucose	Negative	Positive	DM, CVA, anesthesia, extreme stress Drugs: ASA, cephalosporin, vitamin C, epinephrine
Ketone	Negative	Positive	High-protein diet, decreased oral intake, heat exhaustion, DKA, fever, hyperthyroidism

Continued

10

Urinalysis Findings—cont'd

DESCRIPTION	NORMAL	ABNORMAL	SIGNIFICANCE
Bilirubin	Negative	Positive	Hepatitis, cirrhosis, obstructive disease of the gall bladder
Urobilinogen	Negative	Positive	Hepatitis, cirrhosis, CHF, hyperthyroidism Drug: neomycin
Leukocyte esterase	Negative	Positive	Infection
Nitrite	Negative	Positive	Infection
Blood	Negative	Positive	Kidney stones, cancer, infection, menses, transfusion reaction, Foley catheterization, polycystic kidneys, trauma Drugs: anticoagulants
Microscopic Findings			
RBCs	<2/HPF	>2/HPF >3/HPF: repeat UA; if 2 abnormal tests: further evaluation	Renal disease, kidney stones, cancer, strenuous exercise, prostatitis, cystitis, trauma to GU tract Drugs: ASA, warfarin sodium
WBCs	<4/HPF	>4/HPF	Lower UTI, fever, renal disease, strenuous exercise, TB, SLE, AGN, interstitial cystitis, analgesic abuse
Hyaline casts	<5/HPF	10–30/HPF	Strenuous exercise, CHF, fever, benign HTN, AGN
RBC cast	0	>2/HPF	AGN, renal cancer, SBE, vasculitis, GABHS, malignant HTN
WBC cast	0	>2/HPF	Pyelonephritis

10

Common Urinary Tract Disorders in Men and Women

Acute Cystitis   595.0
Acute Pyelonephritis   590.10
Acute Glomerulonephritis   580.9
Bladder Cancer   188.9
Kidney Stone (Renal Calculi)   592.0

SIGNS AND SYMPTOMS	DIAGNOSTICS	TREATMENT
Acute Cystitis/Lower Urinary Tract Infection		

Suprapubic discomfort, pain, pressure
Dysuria, frequency
Nocturia
Hematuria
Incontinence
Usually afebrile
Elderly patients may have somnolence, confusion, decreased appetite and urine output, change in normal behavior
	Urinalysis
	Positive for leukocyte esterase
	Positive for nitrites
	May be positive for blood
	pH >7 (usually)
	
	Microscopic Examination
	Positive for bacteria
	WBCs >5–10/HPF
	No RBC or WBC casts
	May see many epithelial cells
		Uncomplicated
		This refers to young, nondiabetic persons, without structural defects, and/or nonpregnant women experiencing their first or second UTI
		May treat with single dose:
		  TMP-SMZ DS 1 tab bid × 3 days
		  Nitrofurantoin 100 mg bid × 5 days
		  Fosfomycin powder 3 g × 1 dose
		  Ciprofloxacin 250 mg bid × 3 days
		Alternate Therapy Due to Allergy
		  Augmentin 500 mg bid × 3 days
		  Cefdinir 100 mg bid × 5 days
		  Cephalexin 500 mg tid × 5 days
		
		Complicated
		This refers to persons who have experienced more than 2–3 UTIs, may have structural or functional defects, are elderly, or have other risk factors
		Antibiotic therapy may be given for 7–10 days depending on need and PMH:
		  TMP-SMZ DS 1 tab bid
		  Ofloxicin 200 mg bid × 10 days
		  Nitrofurantoin 50–100 mg 1 tab qid
		  Levaquin 750 mg qd × 5 days *or* 250 mg qd × 10 days
		  Ciprofloxacin 250–500 mg 1 tab bid
		
		Pain Relief
		For adults, phenazopyridine HCl (Pyridium) 100–200 mg 1 tab tid × 3 days
		For children, try lidocaine HCl (Xylocaine HCl) jelly applied sparingly to urethra for pain
		
		Prophylaxis Therapy
		Used when >2 UTI in 6 mo or >3 UTI in 12 mo
		Medications qd indefinitely:
		  Nitrofurantoin 50–100 mg

Continued

Common Urinary Tract Disorders in Men and Women—cont'd

SIGNS AND SYMPTOMS	DIAGNOSTICS	TREATMENT
		TMP-SMZ DS 1 tab
		Cephalexin 500 mg after intercourse
		Methenamine 500–1000 mg 2–4 × day
		Refer to Urologist:
		Boys with first time UTI
		Girls with second UTI
		All children with gross hematuria
		Adults with gross hematuria not cleared with first round of antibiotics
Acute Pyelonephritis		
Acute onset fever, chills, flank pain (either side), and malaise	*Urinalysis*	Consider hospitalization, especially if pregnant or unable to keep fluids down because of vomiting
	Positive for leukocyte esterase	
N/V	Positive for nitrites	Outpatient antibiotic therapy for mild to moderate cases:
Positive costovertebral angle tenderness (CVAT)	Positive for blood	Ciprofloxacin 250–750 mg 1 tab bid × 14 days
	Microscopic Examination	Levofloxacin 250–500 mg qd × 10 days
Hematuria, dysuria frequency and urgency	Positive for bacteria, protein	Gatifloxacin 400 mg qd × 10 days
	WBCs >5–10/HPF	Ceftriaxone 1 g IM qd × 3 days
May give history of recent UTI or history of long retention of urine for any reason	RBCs >1–2/HPF	TMP-SMZ DS 1 tab bid × 14 days
	WBC or RBC casts	If no improvement in 24 hr, consider referral or hospitalization
	Culture should be obtained and may show the following:	Recheck urine 3 days after antibiotic therapy is completed
	Escherichia coli (most common)	Oral rehydration with 3–4 L/day
	Klebsiella, Proteus, Pseudomonas	Discuss common causes and prevention of UTI with patient
		Refer all pregnant women with symptomatic pyelonephritis
Acute Glomerulonephritis		
Acute onset oliguria, hematuria, facial edema, weight gain, and abdominal pain	*Urinalysis*	Consultation and hospitalization
	Smoky, rust-colored urine	Decrease salt in diet
	Positive for protein	Decreased fluid intake
Increased BP and anemia	Positive for blood	Monitor potassium and calcium levels
	Microscopic Examination	Follow-up UA monthly until clear
Back pain	RBC and WBC casts	Monitor BP at each visit
May have history of recent strep infection	WBC >5–10/HPF	
Fever	RBC >5–10/HPF	

Common Urinary Tract Disorders in Men and Women—cont'd

SIGNS AND SYMPTOMS	DIAGNOSTICS	TREATMENT
	No bacteria *Other Tests* 24-hr urine for protein and creatinine clearance Urinary protein: creatinine ratio	
Bladder Cancer Unintentional weight loss Persistent hematuria, either gross or microscopic Dysuria, frequency Suprapubic mass Usually no fever or infection May see urinary retention or overflow incontinence in patient who was previously continent	*Urinalysis* Cloudy, concentrated urine Positive for blood, protein May see leukocyte esterase *Microscopic Examination* WBCs >2–3/HPF RBC casts; no WBC casts RBCs >5–10/HPF	Refer to urologist Encourage the patient to quit smoking

Kidney Stones (Renal Calculi)
Sudden onset sharp, severe pain
May start in the back and radiate to groin area or may be localized to RLQ or LLQ
Patient frequently states "this is the worst pain I have ever had"
Unable to find a comfortable position, may be pacing the room
	Urinalysis
	May be clear or cloudy
	Positive for blood
	Positive for protein
	May see frank hematuria
	
	Microscopic Examination
	RBCs >5/HPF
		Refer for an IVP or non-contrast CT for stone location
		Push fluids either orally or IV (minimum 3–5 L qd)
		Use strainer for urine to obtain stone if it passes
		Analgesic for pain
		Refer to urologist if unresolved
		Prophylaxis:
		  Oral hydration daily (2–3 L/day)
		  Low sodium, oxalate, and purine diet
		  Increased intake of fruit juices (especially lemonade)

Continued

Common Urinary Tract Disorders in Men and Women—cont'd

SIGNS AND SYMPTOMS	DIAGNOSTICS	TREATMENT

Oliguria
Hematuria, either gross or microscopic
		Calcium stone prevention:
		    Low-dose hydrochlorothiazide
		    12.5–25 mg qd
		Uric acid stone prevention:
		    Low-dose allopurinol 300 mg qd
		    with potassium citrate 10–30 mEq
		    bid (this regimen will alkalinize
		    the urine)
		Oxalate stone prevention:
		    avoid foods high in oxalate:
		    Beets
		    Chocolate
		    Coffee, tea
		    Cola
		    Wheat bran
		    Cranberry
		    Nuts
		    Rhubarb
		    Soy
		    Spinach
		    Strawberries

Chronic Kidney Disease (CKD)

CHARACTERISTIC	DIAGNOSTICS	TREATMENT
Chronic kidney disease (CKD) is a slow, insidious, irreversible disease of the kidney CKD is present when serum creatinine >1.5 mg/dl in women or >2.0 mg/dl in men, but significant renal dysfunction may be present without significant increase in the serum creatinine, especially in the elderly **Risk Factors** DM HTN NSAID use Obesity Hyperlipidemia	BUN/Cre U/A for urinalysis, protein, and creatinine (calculate ratio of protein to creatinine: >3.5 = nephrotic proteinuria; <3.5 = nonnephrotic proteinuria) CBC Electrolytes Calcium, PTH level Phosphorous Magnesium Iron HbA_{1c} Renal ultrasound Protein to creatinine ratio (should be <200 mg/g)	Identify high-risk groups and monitor yearly creatinine level Slow the progression of the disease and monitor comorbid conditions Maintain B/P <130/85; with proteinuria, B/P <125/75 Maintain HbA_{1c} <7.0 Adequate hydration Calcitriol 0.25–1 mcg (Rocaltral) qd ACEI/ARBs for HTN and renal protection (monitor K^+ level) Avoid nephrotoxic or herbal products (e.g., NSAIDs, contrast dyes, aminoglycosides, cimetidine, colchicine, probenecid, metformin, acarbose, glyburide, mineral supplements, chromium 3,

Chronic Kidney Disease (CKD)—cont'd

CHARACTERISTIC	DIAGNOSTICS	TREATMENT
Cigarette smoking High-protein diet Elderly Glomerulonephritis Polycystic kidney disease **Stages (GFR in ml/min)** Normal: GFR >90 Mild: GFR 60–89 Moderate: GFR 30–59 Severe: GFR 15–29 Kidney failure: GFR <15	Albumin to creatinine ratio (should be <30 mg/g/day) Can use Cockroft-Gault formula* to calculate CrCl (equal to GFR), see formula below	guarana, ephedra) Vitamin E 800 IU qd Give erythropoietin 100–150 U/kg weekly for anemia with HCT ≤30% Consider iron supplements IM or IV with iron deficiency, in addition to erythropoietin to raise Hgb/Hct Low-protein, low-sodium, low- potassium, low-phosphorous diet Skin moisturizers and diphenhydramine 12.5–25 mg bid for pruritus Kayexalate 15 g qd–qid oral or 30–50 g per rectum q6h to decrease high potassium levels Refer to nephrologist when GFR <59 ml/min

*Calculation of creatinine clearance *(CrCl)* or glomerular filtration rate *(GFR)* is used to monitor kidney function with suspected kidney disease and when giving medications that are toxic to the kidneys. With diminished kidney function, drugs can build up to a toxic level quickly because of poor excretion. Serum creatinine is excreted through the kidney and is elevated when there is a loss of more than 50% of the kidney nephrons. This is a fairly sensitive test of glomerular function. Serum creatinine is more specific than BUN and less influenced by hydration and medications. Elevated levels are indicative of kidney failure, either acute or chronic.

The following formula can be used to calculate the CrCl in both men and women. This should be calculated on an annual basis for all high risk persons. Normal values are 90 to 120 ml/min.

$$CrCl\,(men) = \frac{(140 - age) \times weight\ in\ kilograms}{72 \times serum\ creatinine}$$

$$CrCl\,(women) = \frac{(140 - age) \times weight\ in\ kilograms \times 0.85}{72 \times serum\ creatinine}$$

Common Genitourinary Tract Disorders in Men

Prostatitis 601.9		Testicular Torsion 608.2	
Prostatic Cancer 185.		Testicular Cancer 186.9	
Epididymitis 604.90		Erectile Dysfunction (Impotence) 302.72	

SIGNS AND SYMPTOMS	DIAGNOSTICS	TREATMENT
Prostatitis Fever, chills Boggy, tender prostate Lower back pain	May need to obtain multiple voidings for accurate specimen;	Analgesics for pain Stool softeners Increase fluids

Continued

SIGNS AND SYMPTOMS	DIAGNOSTICS	TREATMENT
Difficulty initiating urine stream, decrease in force of urine stream, and decrease in amount of urine flow Frequency, dysuria, nocturia Pain may refer to the end of the penis Arthralgias, myalgias	use specimens 2 and 3 WBCs >10–15/HPF Positive for bacteria Urine culture Culture any penile secretions for STDs Use caution when examining prostate to lessen possibility of causing bacteremia	Rest **Antibiotics for 14-30 days:** TMP-SMZ DS 1 tab bid Ciprofloxacin 500 mg 1 tab bid Norfloxacin 400 mg bid Follow-up in 1–2 wk unless symptoms are worsening Caution patient against using decongestants
Benign Prostatic Hypertrophy (BPH)		
Poor initiating of urine stream, hesitancy Difficulty in stopping urine stream Decrease in force of stream Postvoiding dribble Urge or overflow incontinence, frequency Nocturia Distended bladder, hematuria	Increased postvoid residual >100 ml Pyuria pH > 7 PSA may be elevated "Normal" PSA (ng/ml): 40–50 yr ≤2.5 51–60 yr ≤3.5 >61 yr ≤4 Digital rectal exam (enlargement of prostate without nodule) Serum creatinine	Tell patient not to drink large amounts at one time but to take smaller amounts frequently during the day and to decrease fluid intake after evening meal Void frequently during the day Avoid OTC "cold" preparations (containing pseudoephedrine or antihistamines), antidepressants, anticholinergics, and ETOH Consider using: Terazosin HCl 1–10 mg hs and titrate Finasteride 5 mg qd Doxazosin 1 mg hs, titrated for symptom control up to 8 mg Tamsulosin 0.4–0.8 mg 1 qd Saw palmetto 160–320 mg 1–2 × daily (for symptom relief) Refer to urologist if symptoms persist
Prostatic Cancer		
Localized, nodular, painful prostate Unexplained weight loss Urine obstruction, UTI Anemia, bone pain, SOB (with metastasis) Pelvic heaviness Low back pain Usually slow-growing; symptoms may go unnoticed Hematuria	Increased PSA Increased acid phosphatase Increased alkaline phosphatase Digital rectal exam	Refer to a urologist

SIGNS AND SYMPTOMS	DIAGNOSTICS	TREATMENT
Epididymitis		
Tenderness to posterior epididymis with induration, scrotal pain, and swelling	Pyuria and increased WBCs in urine	Ice packs and scrotum elevation
	Leukocytosis	Bed rest for 1–2 days or during acute phases
Urinary frequency, hematuria, and cloudy urine	Culture penile secretions for gonorrhea and *Chlamydia* infection	Increase fluids
Fever and chills		For men <45 yr, consider treating for possible STDs by using the following:
		Doxycycline 100 mg 1 tab bid × 10 days and ceftriaxone 250 mg IM
		If STD not suspected, treat with one of the following:
		Tetracycline 500 mg 1 tab qid × 10 days
		TMP-SMZ DS 1 tab bid × 14 days
		Ciprofloxacin 500 mg 1 tab bid × 14 days
		Levofloxacin 250 mg qd × 14 days
		Pain management with NSAIDs (see Appendix E)
		Follow-up in 48 hr; if no improvement, consult with or refer to a urologist
Testicular Torsion		
Sudden onset of *severe* scrotal pain	UA results may be normal	*Immediately* send to emergency department
Scrotum is enlarged, red, swollen with unilateral testicular pain	May see hematuria	
Testes are high in scrotal sac		
N/V		
Cremasteric reflex absent on affected side		
Testicular Cancer		
Nodule or swelling in scrotum with sensation of fullness or heaviness in scrotum	Increased α-fetoprotein	Refer to urologist or surgeon
	Increased β-HCG	
Firm, nontender mass	Increased placental alkaline phosphatase	
Gynecomastia		
Usually a rapid-growing tumor		
Unexplained weight loss		
Mass does not transilluminate		

Continued

Common Genitourinary Tract Disorders in Men—cont'd

SIGNS AND SYMPTOMS	DIAGNOSTICS	TREATMENT
Erectile Dysfunction (Impotence)		
Sudden or slow onset of symptoms	Obtain a *good* sexual history	Establish a good rapport with patient and significant other and have an open discussion regarding sexual function and problems that can occur before or during intercourse; sexual counseling can be initiated in the office setting; if symptoms do not resolve, further counseling can be started
Inability to obtain an erection	Fasting blood sugar	
Inability to maintain an erection either during masturbation or during sexual intercourse	Morning free-serum testosterone	
	Serum prolactin (may indicate a pituitary adenoma)	
Inability to get or maintain an erection satisfactory for intercourse ¾ of time	TSH	
	Rigiscan (can be rented and used at home)	Review *all* medications that patient is taking, both prescription and OTC
Patient may exhibit:	Postage stamp test* (high accuracy differentiating organic from psychogenic cause)	Discuss amount of alcohol patient is drinking
Decreased or absent femoral and lower extremity pulses	PSA	Smoking cessation
Gait disturbances	Rectal examination	If significant decrease in testosterone and hypogonadism is identified, testosterone can be given either IM, 1% gel, or patch transdermal
Loss of sensation to skin in perineal area		
Loss of bulbocavernosus reflex		
Cause can be organic, psychogenic, or an interaction of both; if man is <40 yr, problem is usually psychogenic; if man is >40 yr, problem may be organic		Yohimbine (an α_2-adrenergic antagonist touted as an aphrodisiac) 15–30 mg qd
		Sildenafil (Viagra) 25–50 mg one dose about 1 hr before sexual activity (discuss side effects with patient); maximum dose is 100 mg qd
Psychosocial Risk Factors		
Drugs, alcohol, tobacco use, poor sexual knowledge or techniques		Tadalafil (Cialis) 10–20 mg ~30 min prior to sexual activity (do not take more often than 72 hr) or 2.5–5 mg daily
Organic Risk Factors		Vardenafil (Levitra) 10 mg 1 hr prior to sexual activity
DM, hypogonadism, HTN, vascular disease, depression, priapism, neurogenic disorders		Refer to urologist if treatment fails

*Place a roll of stamps around the penis at bedtime. If the stamps are broken apart in the morning, erection occurred.

URINARY INCONTINENCE (UI)

788.30

Diagnosis
- Thorough history to exclude common causes of transient incontinence
- Physical examination
- Urinalysis

Use the patient's history and physical exam to determine which type of urinary incontinence is present; UI affects all ages, but primarily affects the postmenopausal woman or the elderly man; if no reversible causes are found and additional evaluation is required, then refer to urologist or urogynecologist

There are many causes of incontinence, and most patients can give a detailed account of symptoms; Resnick's mnemonic device DIAPPERS can be a helpful guide in assessing the elderly patient with transient incontinence

Common Causes of Transient Incontinence*
- *D*elirium or confusional state
- *I*nfection, urinary (only symptomatic)
- *A*trophic urethritis or vaginitis causes inflammation with bladder irritation and uncontrolled bladder contractions
- *P*harmaceuticals
  - □ Sedatives or hypnotics, especially long-acting agents
  - □ Loop diuretics
  - □ Anticholinergic agents (antipsychotic agents, antidepressants, antihistamines, antiparkinsonian agents, antiarrhythmics [disopyramide], antispasmodics, opiates, and antidiarrheal agents)
  - □ Alpha adrenoceptor agonists and antagonists
  - □ Calcium channel blockers
  - □ Vincristine sulfate
  - □ Caffeine
- *P*sychologic, especially depression (rare)
- *E*ndocrine disease causing excess urine output (e.g., CHF, hyperglycemia, SIADH)
- *R*estricted mobility causes urge incontinence due to inability to toilet self
- *S*tool impaction causes excess urine retention by blocking bladder outlet and overflow incontinence

10

---

*Reprinted with permission of Blackwell Publishing Ltd., by Resnick N. M. (1990). Initial evaluation of the incontinent patient, *Journal of the American Geriatrics Society, 38*(3):311–316.

Overview of Urinary Incontinence

Urge Incontinence	788.31
Stress Incontinence	788.32
Overflow Incontinence	788.39
Transient Incontinence	788.30

TYPE	SIGNS AND SYMPTOMS	DIAGNOSTICS	TREATMENT
Urge Incontinence Involuntary urine loss associated with sudden strong desire to void Caused by overactive, unstable detrusor muscle and leads to incontinence from uncontrolled muscle contractions Urge incontinence occurs in the absence of stress maneuvers Urge incontinence can occur while asleep or awake Can become both a social and a health problem	Sudden, uncontrollable urge to void without warning Urinary frequency as often as q1–2h Nocturia and dysuria Suprapubic tenderness Occurs after, but not during, exertional exercise Skin irritation in perineum and upper thighs	Basic history and physical to include pelvic examination (during bimanual exam, evaluate pelvic floor muscles by having patient contract the muscles around your fingers) UA with culture (if indicated) Postvoid residual should be obtained *Questions to Ask:* Can you sit through a 2-hr movie or meeting without voiding? Do you have accidental loss of urine before you make it to the bathroom? Do you void more than 2 times at night?	*Behavioral Modification* Spread out intake of fluids during the day; refrain from any large intake of fluids at one time Avoid or reduce food or beverages that irritate the bladder: Tomatoes Spicy foods Chocolate Aspartame Caffeine Alcohol Citrus juice Carbonated drinks Sun-brewed tea Planned schedule of voiding Use of superabsorbent adult diapers or condom catheters if no control is possible When urge is felt, stop and contract pelvic muscles for 2–10 sec; relax and repeat until urge subsides; then proceed to bathroom

Pharmacologic Treatment

Tolterodine 1–2 mg bid or extended release 4 mg qd

Oxybutynin chloride extended release 5–15 mg qd

Oxybutynin patch (Oxytrol), applied twice a week

Imipramine HCl 10–25 mg tid or 10 mg at hs

If caused by BPH that results in overactive bladder:

Doxazosin 1–8 mg qd

Finasteride 5 mg qd

Tamsulosin 0.4–0.8 mg qd

Anticholinergic drugs may cause confusion, agitation, dry mouth, blurred vision, and constipation; contraindicated in narrow-angle glaucoma

Refer to urologist or urogynecologist if symptoms persist and medicines do not work

History and physical examination, including pelvic examination to determine whether atrophy or prolapse exists, whether there is poor muscle tone or hypermobility of urethra, and whether there can be any fluid

Behavioral Therapy

Pelvic muscle exercises (Kegel's) up to 100–200 times daily; warn the patient to start slow and work up slowly; this may cause pain

Change fluid intake pattern to

Continued

Stress Incontinence

Instantaneous leakage of urine in response to stress maneuvers

Caused by intrinsic urethral sphincter insufficiency or decreased urethral resistance and pelvic muscle relaxation

Loss of urine with any activity that increases intraabdominal pressures, such as sneezing, coughing, running, bouncing, straining, or laughing

Incontinence decreases at night but occurs frequently during

10

Overview of Urinary Incontinence—cont'd

TYPE	SIGNS AND SYMPTOMS	DIAGNOSTICS	TREATMENT

Usual history of multiple pregnancies with incontinence, trauma to urethra, atrophic urethritis or vaginitis
Young women may have hypermobility of urethra and bladder neck; surgery may be successful
Many women may have both stress and urge incontinence
Men may experience this condition after prostate surgery
	the day while the person is active
	Occurs simultaneously with activity
		expressed from urethra
		UA with culture is indicated
		Measurement of postvoiding residual:
		    >200 ml: abnormal
		    50–199 ml: questionable
		    <50 ml: normal
		Stress test for leakage
		Rule out genitourinary prolapse in older persons
			include smaller amounts during the day
			Encourage more frequent voiding during the day and especially before activity that might stimulate incontinence
			Avoid alcohol and caffeine
			Weight loss
			Pharmacology
			Pseudoephedrine HCl 15–30 mg bid or tid
			Estrogen vaginal cream or Estring
			Imipramine HCl 10–25 mg tid or 10 mg at hs
			Combination therapy with alpha agonist and estrogen may be beneficial, especially if neither works alone
			Vitamin C 500 mg tid
			Vitamin E 800–1000 IU qd
			May refer for surgery or nonsurgical interventions (e.g., pessary, urethral occlusion inserts)

Overflow Incontinence Urine loss associated with overdistended urinary bladder Dysfunctional detrusor muscle causes hypotonia and lack of	Periodic or continual dribbling Urinary frequency with small amounts of urine loss Occurs anytime	History and physical examination to determine whether there is a physical cause for obstruction based on possible causes	Determine cause of obstruction and refer appropriately if indicated: Enlarged prostate to urologist

contraction *Possible Causes* Prolonged retention or overstretching of detrusor muscle over long periods of time Fecal impaction that causes obstruction to outflow of urine Benign prostatic hypertrophy Long-term use of tranquilizers Vitamin B_{12} deficiency Herniated disc	Abdominal distention	CBC, electrolytes, BUN, creatinine, and PSA UA with culture if indicated CXR and abdominal series Postvoiding residual tested; will usually see amounts >500 ml	Abdominal mass to surgeon If obstruction due to fecal impaction, remove the impaction If appropriate, teach the patient or family how to perform clean, intermittent catheterization for long-term treatment Use indwelling Foley catheter as a last resort to solving problem *Pharmacology* Bethanechol chloride 10–30 mg tid Alpha-blocking medications such as: Terazosin HCl 1–5 mg hs Prazosin HCl 2–4 mg hs
Transient Incontinence New onset incontinence in a previously continent patient Possible causes see p. 301	Incontinence usually related to the cause May be febrile, have urinary dysuria, frequency, change in stool pattern, elevated blood glucose, or change in mentation	CBC, electrolytes, BUN and creatinine; may need blood cultures UA with culture if indicated CXR and abdominal series	*Treat the Cause* Evaluate current medications Check for fecal impaction and bladder distention; catheterize if necessary Assess GU tract for dysfunction and vaginal atrophy

10

NOTES

11

Neurologic Disorders

For in-depth physical and cognitive assessment, see Chapter 1.

EQUILIBRIUM DISTURBANCES
See Tables 11–1 and 11–2.

Practice Pearls
- Immediately hospitalize a patient with new onset vertigo accompanied by neurologic signs/symptoms such as diplopia, limb numbness, or slurred speech
- Consider cerebellar dysfunction or peripheral neuropathy if patient complains of dizziness plus imbalance, clumsiness, or incoordination
- Vertigo lasting <1 minute and occurring with position changes (e.g., turning over in bed) indicates benign paroxysmal positional vertigo
- Vertigo associated with Meniere's disease may last minutes to hours; if symptoms last >24 hours, rule out CNS cause
- Be aware of syncope and severe light-headedness as common accompaniments of pregnancy; faintness or light-headedness can be side effects of many antihypertensive medications

Referral Guidelines
Emergency department
- Symptoms suggestive of aortic aneurysm or dissection or MI
- Syncope with unstable VS

Neurologist
- CNS signs and symptoms
- Progressive, disabling Meniere's disease
- Patient with benign paroxysmal positional vertigo who has neurologic signs or who does not respond to therapy

Cardiologist
- Any cardiovascular related cause of dizziness not responsive to standard therapy
- New-onset murmur

Psychiatrist
- Co-morbid psychiatric disorder (e.g., panic disorder or depression) that does not respond to simple reassurance and standard drug management

Table 11–1 Equilibrium Disturbances

Equilibrium Disturbances	780.4
Dizziness	780.4
Vertigo	780.4

DISTURBANCE	SYMPTOMS	DIFFERENTIAL DIAGNOSIS
Dizziness	Weakness	Labyrinthitis
	Light-headedness	Vestibular neuronitis
	Unsteadiness	Tumor
		Head trauma
		Drug toxicity
Vertigo	Feeling of objects in environment spinning	Labyrinthitis
	Dysequilibrium	Meniere's disease
	May be accompanied by N/V and ataxia	Vestibular neuronitis
	Often associated with nystagmus	Positional vertigo
	Recurrent	Multiple sclerosis
		Drug toxicity

Table 11–2 Potential Causes of Syncope

Potential Causes of Syncope	780.2
Cardiac	780.2
Carotid Sinus Hypersensitivity	337.0
Postural (Orthostatic Hypotension)	458.0
Vasovagal	780.2

CHARACTERISTICS	POSSIBLE DIAGNOSTICS
Cardiac	
Sudden onset and resolution; feels fine afterwards	Listen for bruits in the neck and abdomen
	Orthostatic VS*
Evidence of CHF	CXR
Evidence of aortic aneurysm or dissection	ECG, Holter monitor
History of heart disease (angina, MI, HTN)	Echocardiogram
Murmur of aortic stenosis or mitral valve prolapse	Cardiac enzymes, complete metabolic profile
Arrhythmias, often associated with or after palpitations	Carotid Doppler
Myocardial infarction (MI)	Medication levels, as appropriate
Use of medications such as digitalis, quinidine, beta blockers, calcium channel blockers	
Carotid Sinus Hypersensitivity	
Often occurs during shaving or when wearing constrictive collars	Can be reproduced by carotid sinus massage

*Orthostatic hypotension: at least 20 mm Hg drop in systolic BP or 10 mm Hg in diastolic BP.

Table 11-2   Potential Causes of Syncope—cont'd

CHARACTERISTICS	POSSIBLE DIAGNOSTICS
Metabolic	
Onset and resolution usually gradual	Complete metabolic profile
Often associated with light-headedness and paresthesias	TSH, possibly T_4
	2- or 3-h GTT
Associated with infrequent eating (low blood sugar)	CT/MRI of brain
	Reproducible during examination (hyperventilation)
Postural (Orthostatic)	
Often occurs when sitting upright from supine position	Orthostatic VS*
Occurs as an adverse effect of many medications	Complete metabolic profile, CBC
	Stools for OB
Often preceded by light-headedness or dizziness; lying down relieves the symptoms	ECG
Postural changes* in BP are reproducible	Romberg test
History of vomiting, often with diarrhea (dehydration)	
Diabetes (associated with autonomic failure)	
History of anemia and/or fecal occult blood (hemorrhage)	
Vasovagal	
Onset and resolution gradual; feels horrible afterwards for up to 1–2 days	Diagnosed primarily by patient's history
Precipitated by physical or emotional stimuli	
Usually preceded by "vagal" symptoms: nausea, weakness, yawning, sweating, blurred vision	
Usually occurs when upright, but can occur when sitting and straining (as with defecation)	
Seizure Related	
Usually abrupt onset and gradual resolution	EEG, if new onset or changing pattern
Occurs during postictal state	CT/MRI of brain
May have jerking, convulsions, incontinence, or tongue-biting during syncopal period	Medication levels, as appropriate

*Orthostatic hypotension: at least 20 mm Hg drop in systolic BP or 10 mm Hg in diastolic BP.

SEIZURES

| 780.39 |

Definition

- Paroxysmal and disorderly discharge of neuronal impulses and the spread of the impulses throughout brain tissue

Incidence or Prevalence

- Five to 8 per 1000 persons

Causes

- Intracranial lesions
- Congenital abnormalities
- Trauma
- Vascular disorders
- Toxic-metabolic disorders
- Anoxia
- Environmental exposures
- Infections

Classification

See Figure 11–1 and Table 11–3.

Diagnosis

- Electrolytes, CBC, lead levels, alcohol, and toxicology screen
- CT or MRI scan to rule out space-occupying lesion or hemorrhage
- EEG, sleep studies
- Closed-circuit TV with EEG monitoring

Treatment

- Consult with a physician if seizures are different or new onset
- Treatment is based on the seizure type
- Never stop anticonvulsants abruptly; wean over weeks to months
- If patient is taking more than one drug, withdraw sequentially, not simultaneously
- Monotherapy is the treatment of choice when possible
- Refractory seizures (i.e., do not respond to therapy) should be referred for further workup
- Educate the patient on the importance of medication adherence; many treatment failures are due to poor compliance

TREMORS

| 781.0 |

New onset tremor often warrants consult or referral to neurologist; the most important diagnostic distinction is between parkinsonian and essential tremors; for classification see Table 11–4.

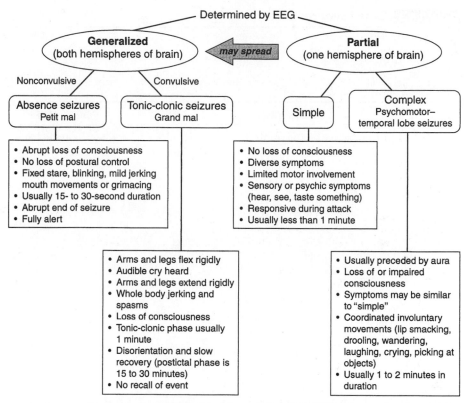

FIGURE 11–1 Types of seizures. (Modified from Agins, A. P. [1999]. *Parent & educators' drug reference*. Providence, RI: PRN Press.)

HEADACHES

784.0

History (Pertinent to H/As)

- Onset, age at onset, and chronic or acute onset; if the patient is >50 years and with new onset or change, check for giant cell (temporal) arteritis (i.e., obtain an ESR)
- Similar H/A before, frequency, and patterns of recurrence
- Duration of pain
- Pain intensity (mild, moderate, or severe), crescendo or plateau pain
- Location, localized or radiating
- Triggers of pain
- Type of pain: throbbing, burning, aching, pressing
- Associated symptoms (e.g., fever, sinus pain, N/V, lacrimation)
- Neurologic symptoms (e.g., diplopia, photophobia, ataxia, ptosis, paresis)
- Treatments used to relieve pain

Table 11-3 Other Seizures

Atonic   345.0
Febrile   780.31
Infantile Spasms   345.6
Myoclonic   333.2
Pseudoseizures   780.39

SEIZURE TYPE	CLINICAL FINDINGS	DURATION	POSTICTAL PHASE
Atonic	Abrupt loss of posture and muscle tone Loss of consciousness Prone to serious injury Incontinence Indicates underlying structural abnormality	Seconds to minutes	Flaccid muscle tone Confusion
Febrile	Usually occurs within first 3 yr of life Usually due to infectious illness Generally occurs with fever >102.5° F (39.2° C), but rapid rise of fever also important Loss of consciousness Generalized muscle contractions	Brief	Variable
Infantile spasms	Usually occur between 4 and 18 mo of age Primarily generalized spasm of head, neck, and trunk Not necessarily accompanied by fever or illness May indicate severe underlying brain pathologic condition	Varies	None
Myoclonic	Loss of consciousness Abrupt, shocklike muscle contractions Contractions may be isolated or repetitive; symmetric or asymmetric	Seconds to minutes	None
Pseudoseizures	Rhythmic movements Unpredictable No aura Chewing or swimming movements No autonomic signs	Variable	No postictal phase No amnesia of event

Table 11–4   Tremors

Physiologic	306.0
Essential	333.1
Cerebellar	781.0
Parkinsonian	332.0

TYPE	CHARACTERISTICS	MANAGEMENT
Action: typically increased with muscle activity and reduced or absent at rest		
Physiologic	Most evident in hands and fingers Low amplitude, fast Little functional impairment	Reassure patient that no disease is present Avoid caffeine and other stimulants Propranolol 10–20 mg tid is sometimes helpful Anxiolytics for *occasional* use in stressful situations
Essential	Most evident during use of affective muscles; may involve extremities or head and neck Low to moderate amplitude, fast May cause significant functional impairment	Avoid caffeine and other stimulants Propranolol 20 mg tid; increase as needed and tolerated *or* Primidone 50 mg hs; gradually increase to 250–300 mg qd in divided doses
Cerebellar	Classic "intention" tremor Moderate or high amplitude, relatively slow Often causes severe functional impairment	Usually very difficult to treat unless underlying disease can be treated Refer to neurologist
Resting: typically most noticeable when the involved extremities are at rest and is relieved or absent during voluntary activity		
Parkinsonian	May be a result of Parkinson's disease or other causes May be asymmetric, involving the extremities but sparing the head and neck The typical movement is the forearm alternating pronation and supination or "pill-rolling" movement of the fingers	Stop or reduce any drugs that might exacerbate parkinsonism Refer to neurologist if Parkinson's disease is suspected

- Recent or past exposure to environmental toxins, recent infection
- Recent or longer personal stressors, change in personal life
- Family history of H/A

Physical Examination (Suggested Steps to R/O Organic Cause of H/A)

- Craniocervical examination: patient supine, examiner at head

□ Ears: press fingers in ears; pain worsens with ear-related cause
□ TMJ: press against TMJ
□ Teeth: look at teeth and percuss with a tongue depressor
□ Sinus: ask the patient to close his or her mouth and exhale; then press nares closed and have the patient try to deeply inhale; increased pain usually indicates sinusitis; this maneuver may relieve the pain of a migraine
□ Eyes: gently press on closed eyes; increased pain may indicate glaucoma, but other symptoms would be present
□ Scalp: inspect and palpate for point tenderness
□ Arteries

Tenderness over temporal arteries: if the patient is >40 years, think temporal arteritis; <40 years, think migraine if present for more than 24 hours

Carotidynia: tenderness associated with episodic, unilateral H/A
□ Meninges: have the patient touch the chin to the chest (flexes low cervical spine) and the chin to the Adam's apple (flexes high cervical spine); if the patient is unable to do these maneuvers, *refer*
□ Veins and venous sinus: gently occlude jugular veins bilaterally; if pain increases, consider venous sinus thrombosis
□ Cervical vertebrae: press on spinous processes; head pain is not associated with a lesion below C4; cervical spondylosis is usually C5 or lower
□ Cervical muscles: palpate for muscle pain and tenderness
• Mental status: at the end of the history, repeat some questions to better evaluate the patient's mental status
• Also observe the patient walking.
• Are the results of the rest of the physical examination normal?
• Are the neurologic examination results normal (including cranial nerves)?

Red Flag H/A
• First or new type or worst-ever H/A (possible intracranial bleed)
• New H/A in patient >50 years (possible temporal arteritis, tumor, or intracranial bleed)
• A change in pattern to usual H/A (possible tumor)
• Signs/symptoms of systemic illness (e.g., fever, vomiting, nuchal rigidity [possible CNS infection])
• H/A with exertion (e.g., cough, sneeze, intercourse [possible increased intracranial pressure])
• Focal neurologic signs (possible CVA, intracranial aneurysm)
• Patient taking anticoagulants (possible intracranial bleed)

H/A in Children
• Listen for a bruit over the carotid arteries; if asymmetric or continuous, *refer immediately*
• If the child has a stiff neck during a severe H/A, *refer immediately* for workup for subarachnoid hemorrhage or meningitis

- Always visualize the fundi
- Measure head circumference if hydrocephalus suspected
- Rule out hypertension

Diagnostic studies
- Electrolytes, CBC, thyroid function tests, UA, ESR, toxicology screen
- CT or MRI scan

Treatment

- Inform patient to treat H/A in mild stages so that it won't become disabling
- A H/A diary can be invaluable to determine triggers and also to evaluate the H/A treatment
- If the complaint is H/A, think migraine first

Refer to H/A specialist

- Patient with complex medical or psychiatric conditions (e.g., cardiovascular disease, DM, renal disease, bipolar D/O)
- If treatment options have not helped

Classification of Common Headaches

See Table 11–5.

Potential Migraine Triggers

See Table 11–6.

IDIOPATHIC PARKINSON'S DISEASE

| 332.0 |

Incidence and Prevalence

- Affects approximately 1 in 1000 persons
- Equal distribution of men and women
- Usually diagnosed at or after the fifth decade of life

Etiology

- Exact cause is unknown
- Theories include atherosclerotic vascular disease, environmental toxins, viral infections, and genetic predisposition

Clinical Features (Early Stages)

- Tremor: observed best with the extremity relaxed; usually begins in the finger and thumb, unilaterally ("pill rolling"); stops during voluntary movement
- Rigidity: detected earliest in neck muscles; cogwheel rigidity on passive motion; have the patient stand with his or her arms at sides, and examiner twists the

Text continued on p. 320

Table 11–5	Classification of Headaches

Cluster **346.2**
Migraine **346.9**
Temporal Arteritis **446.5**

CHARACTERISTICS	ASSOCIATED SYMPTOMS	TREATMENT
Cluster		
In, around, or behind eye	Ipsilateral lacrimation	Oxygen at least 7 L by mask
Exquisitely severe,	Nasal congestion	for 15 min
nonthrobbing	Rhinorrhea	Sumatriptan injection
May worsen when	Agitation (may pace or rock)	Dihydroergotamine
lying still	Facial flushes, sweating	(Migranal) 1 mg IM; may
Occurs up to 10 times		repeat ×2, 1 hr apart *or*
a day; often cyclical,		nasal spray 1 spray each
occurring at the same		nostril; may repeat in
time of day		15 min one time
Lasts 10 min–3 hr		Steroids with a slow taper
Triggers: ETOH, tobacco,		Cyproheptadine 4 mg
histamines, vasodilators		
Migraine		
Unilateral or	Anorexia, N/V	***Abortive Treatment***
predominately	Drowsiness	*"Mild" Migraine*
unilateral	Irritability	NSAIDs, especially
Moderate to severe	Photophobia	naproxen 500 mg initially,
intensity (inhibits or	Phonophobia	then 250 mg q6h prn
prohibits daily	May have nasal symptoms	Excedrin Migraine 2 tabs
activities)	and sinus pressure	
Throbbing	(not tender to	*"Mod-Severe" Migraine*
Lasts 4–72 hr (untreated)	palpation, though)	Triptans (may repeat dose
Often aggravated by	Neck pain	once in 2 hr if needed):
postural changes or	Pallor and vomiting	Sumatriptan (Imitrex)
cough or sneeze	in children	6 mg SQ or 50–100 mg
May be preceded by an		PO or nasal spray *or*
aura (flashing lights or		Zolmitriptan (Zomig)
colors, certain smell or		2.5–5 mg PO or 2.5 mg
sound); the aura is		dissolving wafer *or*
completely reversible		Naratriptan (Amerge)
and lasts >60 min;		2.5 mg PO *or*
headache follows aura		Rizatriptan (Maxalt)
within 1 hr (untreated		10 mg
or unsuccessfully		PO or orally dissolving
treated)		tablet *or*
Many patients may		Almotriptan (Axert)
experience a prodrome		6.25–12.5 mg PO *or*
hours to days before the		Eletriptan hydrobromide
H/A (e.g., mood		(Relpax) 20–40 mg PO
		Dihydroergotamine

*Try one medication for at least three H/A before deciding it will not help.

Table II–5 Classification of Headaches—cont'd

CHARACTERISTICS	ASSOCIATED SYMPTOMS	TREATMENT
changes, stiff neck, restlessness, cold feeling, difficulty concentrating) Most patients have a family history positive for H/A; rarely starts after 50 yr of age Triggers (see Table 11–6)		(Migranal) 1 mg IM or 1 spray each nostril *Prevention (consider with >8 H/A monthly or H/A refractory to abortive treatment)* Propranolol LA 80 mg qd; titrate up to 160–240 mg qd Divalproex sodium (Depakote ER) 500 mg 1–2 tabs qd Amitriptyline 10 mg hs; increase by 10 mg q2wk; usual dose 30–50 mg qd For <12 yr of age, may try NSAIDs, propranolol 0.6–1.5 mg/kg qd (given in 2 doses) or cyproheptadine 2–4 mg Magnesium 350–1000 mg qd Riboflavin 400 mg qd *Patient Education* Must stop daily use of analgesics to prevent rebound H/A Avoid known triggers (see Table 11–6) Biofeedback, stress management, stretching exercises, relaxation techniques, or hypnosis may help H/A diary is useful to monitor triggers and treatment effectiveness *Menstrual Migraines* If taking OCs: Continuous cycling (fixed dose) for 4 mo, then have a period Estradiol gel 1.5 mg qd or patch 50–100 mg qd for the 7 days of inactive pills

Continued

Table 11-5   Classification of Headaches—cont'd

CHARACTERISTICS	ASSOCIATED SYMPTOMS	TREATMENT
		Naratriptan 1 mg bid × 5 days Nortriptyline 25 mg qd Midrin 2 caps at start; may repeat 1 cap q1h, up to 5 caps in 12 hr (C-IV)
Temporal Arteritis Temporal area, unilateral Exquisitely tender; burning, throbbing Constantly present Trigger: chewing	Jaw pain on chewing Increased ESR Tenderness over temporal artery	Urgent referral for possible biopsy and steroids Analgesics (usually opiates)
Tension "Tight band" around head Mild to moderate intensity (nondisabling) Dull, diffuse pressure Can last from 30 min to 7 days Often related to stressful situations or cold temperatures; *not* aggravated by physical exertion	Irritability No N/V	NSAIDs (see Appendix E) or OTC pain reliever with or without caffeine Butalbital-acetaminophen-caffeine compound (Esgic Plus, Fioricet) 1q4h prn (has potential for addiction) Stress reduction Biofeedback, stretching exercises may help Muscle relaxants may help Triptans may help

Table 11-6   Potential Migraine Triggers

TRIGGERS	AVOID OR LIMIT	ALLOWED
Beverages	*Red wine, beer* *Coffee, tea, caffeinated colas* *Chocolate or cocoa*	Whiskey, Scotch, vodka, fruit juices, and sauterne and Riesling wines No more than 1 cup coffee, 2 cups tea, 2 soft drinks Noncola soft drinks, flavored waters, decaffeinated drinks
Dairy products	Milk, buttermilk, cream *Sour cream, yogurt* *Hard (aged) cheeses: cheddar* *Brie, processed cheeses*	Low-fat or skim milk No more than ½ cup yogurt Cottage cheese, cream cheese Butter, margarine, cooking oils

Italicized foods are the most common triggers.

11

Table 11-6 Potential Migraine Triggers—cont'd

TRIGGERS	AVOID OR LIMIT	ALLOWED
Meats/poultry	*Processed meats: hot dogs, bologna* *Aged, cured, smoked, marinated meats* Organ meats: liver	Fresh or frozen meats Limit eggs to ≤3 a wk
Fish	Dried, smoked fish, *pickled herring*	Fresh or frozen fish, canned tuna or salmon
Vegetables	Most beans and peas Onions Pickles, olives, sauerkraut	String beans Asparagus, beets, carrots, spinach, tomatoes, squash, corn, zucchini, broccoli, lettuce, potatoes
Grains, breads, cereals	Yeast breads (white), sourdough breads	Rice, pasta Whole wheat and rye breads English muffins, Melba toast, bagels Most cereals
Soups	Soups containing MSG or yeast Soups from bouillon cubes	Homemade soups
Fruits	*Citrus fruits, bananas,* figs, raisins, papaya, kiwi, plums, pineapples, avocados	Limit citrus and bananas to ½ to 1 qd Apples, prunes, cherries, grapes, apricots, peaches, pears
Desserts, snack foods	*Chocolates* Ice cream Cookies or cakes made with yeast Potato chip products Nuts, seeds Peanut butter	Sugar candies Sherbet, ices, sorbets Cookies or cakes made without yeast Pretzels Jam, jelly, honey
Additives	*MSG (may be in Chinese foods)* Seasonings and spices *Soy sauce*	Salad dressings (in small amounts) White vinegar
Miscellaneous nonfood triggers	Oral contraceptives Air travel Stress Weather (low pressure system)	

Italicized foods are the most common triggers.
MSG, Monosodium glutamate.

patient's shoulders side to side; the patient's arms will not swing freely; DTRs are usually normal
- Bradykinesia: slow, fluid movements; gait disturbances; difficulty initiating voluntary movements

Clinical Features (Later Stages)
- Impaired righting reflex
- Akinesia, rigidity, ataxia, festinating gait, and stooped posture
- Excessive salivation, dysphagia, and constipation
- Low volume, pitch monotony, and dysarthric speech
- Expressionless face and decreased blinking
- Increased cogwheel rigidity and tremor
- Positive Romberg's test and inability to walk backward
- Confusion, hallucinations, and dementia

Diagnosis
- Can only be confirmed on autopsy
- CT or MRI scan to R/O treatable disorders
- Electrolytes, thyroid function tests, lead levels; R/O exposure to environmental toxins
- R/O depression

Treatment
- Refer to a physician for an initial diagnosis, then co-manage with the physician
- Inform the family of state and community resources and support groups

NEUROMUSCULAR DISORDERS
See Table 11–7.

COMMON CNS INFECTIONS
See Table 11–8.

COMPARISON OF CVA AND TIA
See Table 11–9.

Table 11-7 Neuromuscular Disorders

Multiple Sclerosis	340.
Guillain-Barré Syndrome	357.0
Myasthenia Gravis	358.0

DISORDER	COURSE	SYMPTOMS	DIAGNOSIS	TREATMENT
Multiple sclerosis	Remitting and relapsing or chronic progressive Age: 20–40yr	Visual changes Fatigue, weakness Gait instability Intention tremor Clumsiness Tingling, numbness, and bandagelike tightness	CSF: increased cell count, protein, and gamma globulin EMG: abnormal evoked potentials CT or MRI scan: plaques EEG: may have slow wave abnormality	Referral to neurologist May co-manage care
Guillain-Barré syndrome	Acute, rapidly progressive Preceded by viral infection May occur after immunizations Any age group	Acute onset of hyperalgia or myalgia Paraplegia, quadriplegia, paresthesia Ataxia, weakness Papilledema May cause respiratory insufficiency	CSF: increased protein during acute phase EMG: delayed conduction times CT or MRI scan: to R/O other disease	Immediate referral for aggressive respiratory assessment and intervention
Myasthenia gravis	Slow, gradual onset with possible remissions May have acute onset with rapid progression Age: 20–70yr	Ptosis, fatigue Muscle weakness Dysphagia Myasthenic crisis: abrupt worsening of symptoms (hypertension, tachycardia, respiratory distress, dysphagia, incontinence, generalized weakness)	Tension test EMG: evoked potentials CXR or chest CT scan PFTs	Immediate referral for myasthenic crisis Co-manage after crisis

11

Table 11–8 CNS Infections

Viral Meningitis   047.9
Bacterial Meningitis   320.9
Neurosyphilis   094.9
Tick-Borne Disease   088.81

SYMPTOMS	DIAGNOSIS	TREATMENT
Viral Meningitis		
Acute onset	CT or MRI scan	Consult or refer
Fever, H/A, nuchal rigidity, drowsiness	LP: no organisms	Treat symptomatically
	History of exposure	
Fatigue, photophobia	to viral infection or	
May have negative Brudzinski's*	insect bites	
and Kernig's† signs	Serology	
	Cultures	
	CXR	
Bacterial Meningitis		
Fever, H/A, fatigue, nuchal rigidity, seizure, drowsiness	CT or MRI scan	Immediate referral
	LP: organisms seen	Broad-spectrum antibiotics
Positive Brudzinski's* and Kernig's† signs	Cultures	until sensitivities
	Serology	identified
With meningococcal: purpura, red papules; maybe faint pink macules	CXR	
	Skull and sinus x-ray examination	
Neurosyphilis		
May mimic meningitis	CT or MRI scan	Aqueous penicillin
H/A, nuchal rigidity, papilledema, N/V, mental status changes	LP: increased protein and lymph	
	RPR or VDRL (blood tests for syphilis)	
Tick-Borne Diseases (see p. 115)		

*Brudzinski's sign: flex chin on chest; resistance and pain is a positive (abnormal) response.
†Kernig's sign: raise leg straight or flex thigh on abdomen and extend knee; resistance to straightening, pain down posterior thigh is a positive (abnormal) response.

11

Table 11-9 Comparison of CVA and TIA

SYMPTOMS	POSSIBLE CAUSES	TREATMENT
Cerebrovascular Accident: Sudden Onset of a Focal Neurologic Deficit		
Carotid circulation:	Ischemic: carotid	Refer immediately for inpatient
Hemiplegia	atherosclerotic disease	evaluation and treatment
Hemianesthesia	Cardiac: embolism resulting from:	Post-CVA with atrial fibrillation:
Neglect	Mitral valve disease	warfarin (see p. 199 for dosing)
Aphasia	Decreased ventricular wall	Post-CVA without atrial fibrillation: low-
Visual field defects	movement (usually related to AMI	dose ASA or clopidogrel 75 mg qd
May have H/A, seizures,	or CHF) with mural thrombus	
amnesia, facial paresis	Arrhythmia, such as atrial fibrillation	
Vertebrobasilar circulation:	Hypercoagulable states, including	
Diplopia	those due to OCs	
Vertigo	Miscellaneous	
Ataxia	Spontaneous	
Facial paresis	Posttraumatic	
Horner's syndrome*	Artery dissection	
Dysphagia	Vasculitis	
Dysarthria	Drugs (e.g., cocaine, amphetamines)	
Impaired LOC	Hemorrhagic	
Cerebellar lesion in patients with	HTN	
H/A, N/V, and ataxia	Vascular malformations	

Continued

11

Table 11–9 Comparison of CVA and TIA—cont'd

SYMPTOMS	POSSIBLE CAUSES	TREATMENT
Transient Ischemic Attack: Sudden Onset of a Focal Neurologic Deficit Lasting <24hr		
Carotid circulation:	Carotid atherosclerotic lesion	Consult or refer for further studies
Hemiplegia	Small, deep vessel disease	(e.g., ECG, carotid Doppler U/S,
Hemianesthesia	associated with HTN	coagulation studies)
Neglect	Cardiac: embolism related to:	Counsel to stop smoking
Aphasia	Mitral valve disease	Strict control of risk factors (e.g., HTN,
Visual field defects	Decreased ventricular	diabetes, hyperlipidemia)
May have H/A, seizures, amnesia, confusion	wall movement (usually related to	Encourage ASA 81–325 mg qd and
Vertebrobasilar circulation:	AMI or CHF) with mural	vitamin E 400–800 IU qd
Diplopia	thrombus	May take clopidogrel 75 mg qd
Vertigo	Arrhythmia, such as atrial	
Ataxia	fibrillation	
Facial paresis	Hypercoagulable states, including those	
Horner's syndrome*	due to OCs	
Dysphagia	Miscellaneous:	
Dysarthria	Spontaneous	
Cerebellar or brainstem lesion with H/A, N/V,	Posttraumatic	
and ataxia	Arterial dissection	

*Horner's syndrome: sympathetic paralysis of the eye with ptosis and miosis.

NOTES

NOTES

12

Musculoskeletal Disorders

History

A chief complaint ascribed by the patient to a joint may not originate there. Bones and joints can be affected by systemic diseases as well as by local problems. One of the most important points is to determine whether the symptoms are due to structural damage or inflammatory joint disease (see the following lists). Elicit all factors of the chief complaint and associated symptoms and obtain a careful review of systems.

Structural Lesion	Inflammatory Joint Disease
Pain occurs on use, improves with rest	Morning stiffness, especially for more than 30 min
Usually involves weight-bearing joints	Involves also non-weight-bearing joints
No acute exacerbations	Often has flare-ups
No systemic symptoms	Systemic symptoms common

COMMON CHIEF COMPLAINTS

Pain with or after injury: try to mentally "plot" the axis of stress

Pain without injury: think arthritis, bursitis, or infection (Table 12–1), or metastatic cancer (primarily in spine and/or ribs)

Absence of pain in presence of obvious joint disease: think neuropathy

Limp with pain: think neuromuscular involvement

Limp without pain: think muscle disease

Asymptomatic lump

Joint swelling

Joint dysfunction

Fatigue and malaise (Table 12–2)

Table 12-1 Painful Joint Disorders

Rheumatoid Arthritis 714.0
Osteoarthritis 715.90
Gout 274.9

	RHEUMATOID ARTHRITIS	OSTEOARTHRITIS	GOUT	"ITIS"**
Age	Any age	Usually middle age and older	Usually older than 40 yr	Any age
Sex	Mainly female	Either	Mainly male	Either
Cause	Autoimmune disease	Trauma, degenerative changes	Increase in serum uric acid	Overuse of a joint
Inflammatory condition	Yes	No	Yes	Yes†
Joints involved	At least three, including small joints of hands and feet; typically symmetric	Weight bearing (e.g., hip, knee, spine) and DIP/PIP joints and base of thumb	Several but only one at a time; often affects the big toe (MTP joint)	Usually just one
Joints spared	DIP joint and thoracic and lumbar spine	Wrist	Spine	
Joint stiffness	On rising, lasting >1 hr; often improves with activity	On rising, lasts <30 min More at the end of the day		Pain with movement of affected joint
Associated symptoms	Fever with acute stage Affected joints red, warm, swollen Painless SQ nodules over ulna and olecranon Ulnar drift or deformities of fingers (swan neck, boutonniere) Often with malaise May have many extraarticular manifestations (e.g., pleural effusion, pericarditis, anemia, vasculitis)	No fever Affected joints swollen but *not* red or warm; pain is dull, aching; it worsens with activity and is relieved with rest Nontender Heberden's (DIP) and Bouchard's (PIP) nodes Irregular bony margins; may have crepitus No extraarticular manifestations	With acute stage, joint effusion: joint is red, warm, and tender Large, painless nodules (tophi) especially over MTP joint of big toe with chronic gout	No fever May have localized swelling; skin may be warm and red

Treatment	Refer to rheumatologist Monitor patients taking tumor necrosis factor (TNF) inhibitors (e.g., Remicade, Enbrel) for signs of heart failure	Analgesics: acetaminophen is as effective as NSAIDs Physiotherapy Glucosamine‡ 2000–4000 mg qd, with or without chondroitin Joints improve with rest	Acute therapy: Indomethacin 25 mg qid or Naproxen 750 mg stat then 250 mg q8h; taper over 48 hr as attack resolves May also use Kenalog 60 mg IM; may repeat the next day Review risk factors for hyperuricemia (ETOH use, medications, obesity) After second or third attack, consider prophylactic therapy; check serum uric acid level (treatment goal is <6.5 mg/dl) The most commonly used medicine is allopurinol 100–300 mg qd	"RICE" (see p. 357) NSAIDs (see Appendix E) Possible joint injection with steroids Joint rest until pain lessens, then begin gentle ROM to prevent joint stiffness

*For example, bursitis, epicondylitis, or tendinitis.

†Erythema and warmth should also raise the suspicion of an infectious cause.

‡No glucosamine if patient has shellfish allergy; it is made from oyster and crab shells.

12

Table 12–2 Possible Causes of Fatigue and Malaise

ASSOCIATED SYMPTOMS	POSSIBLE DIAGNOSIS	DIAGNOSTIC TESTS
Fever, lymphadenopathy, weight loss	Malignancy	CBC, ESR Possibly chest x-ray, CT, or MRI
Increasing fatigue over time	Malignancy or anemia	CBC, ESR, chemistry profile Probably chest x-ray Possibly CT or MRI
Daytime somnolence, snoring (especially if increased), obesity	Sleep apnea	Sleep studies
Flat affect, appetite or sleep changes, maybe sexual dysfunction	Depression	None if no other history findings suggest a physical cause
Change in skin or hair texture, heat or cold intolerance, weight changes	Thyroid disorder	T_4 and TSH
Fever, cough; sometimes sore throat and lymphadenopathy	Infection	Treat empirically or obtain lab work and x-rays as indicated (e.g., CBC, strep screen, Monospot, chest x-ray)
Weight loss but no fever or signs or symptoms of infection	Malignancy, poor nutrition, malabsorption syndromes	CBC, chemistry panel Possibly x-rays
Pallor	Anemia	CBC; possibly serum folate and B_{12} Stools for occult blood if indicated
Weight loss, polydipsia, polyuria	Diabetes mellitus	FBS (usually also electrolytes, BUN, and creatinine)

Physical Examination

- Knowledge of surface anatomy is critical to the musculoskeletal examination; dermatomes are illustrated in Figure 12–1
- Paired joints usually provide a comparison, and both should be examined; also look above and below the complaint site
- Range-of-motion testing provides quantitative results about joint function; in active ROM the patient performs the movements; in passive ROM the examiner moves the patient's limbs
- Inspection and palpation are the primary techniques; percussion is occasionally used to elicit point tenderness, which may indicate a fracture
- Remember that joint pain may be referred or may be radicular (resulting from nerve compression or injury)

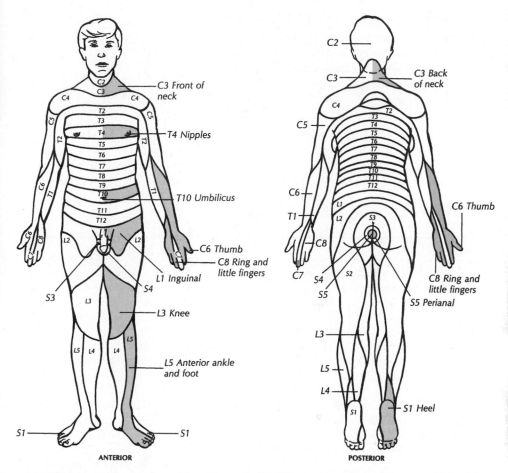

FIGURE 12–1 Dermatomes. (From Bates, B. [1991]. *A guide to physical assessment* [5th ed.]. Philadelphia: J. B. Lippincott Co.)

The rest of the chapter is divided into the major joints. Each section is written in a concise format; the quick examination steps are meant to be helpful in the order written. For more in-depth information, refer to the bibliography.

FIBROMYALGIA SYNDROME AND CHRONIC FATIGUE SYNDROME

Fibromyalgia Syndrome	729.1
Chronic Fatigue Syndrome	780.71

FBS and CFS are common conditions affecting more women than men. Fibromyalgia commonly occurs between 20 and 55 years of age; its incidence increases with age. CFS often starts in the late 30s. Neither condition has physical changes, and they are not life threatening, but both are usually chronic and often disabling from a functional viewpoint.

Fibromyalgia is currently considered to be a disorder of pain regulation. It is believed that any muscle pathology is due to pain and inactivity and not actual muscle damage or disease. Fibromyalgia is often associated with the following:

- A lack of Stage 4 (deep) sleep
- Depression, panic disorder
- Osteoarthritis
- Migraine
- Irritable bowel syndrome, bruxism
- An increased incidence of SLE and rheumatoid arthritis

Currently, the cause of CFS is also unknown, but possibilities include viral (e.g., Epstein-Barr virus, enterovirus), immune dysfunction, or neurochemical disturbances.

Diagnosis

FIBROMYALGIA	CHRONIC FATIGUE SYNDROME
Characterized by widespread aching above and below the waist and both the right and left sides of the body for at least 3 mo *plus* Multiple tender points (Fig. 12–2); they often come and go. Check for tender points using the same amount of pressure used to blanch the thumbnail; in clinical practice, a specific number of tender points is not required to make the diagnosis Spinal or anterior pain must be elicited with palpation	Severe, unexplained fatigue for longer than 6 mo with: New or definite onset Not resulting from ongoing or continued exertion Not resolved or alleviated by rest Functional impairment in occupational, social, educational, and personal activities *and* At least four of the following new symptoms must be present: Impaired memory or concentration Sore throat Tender or enlarged lymph nodes, especially in cervical or axillary areas Arthralgias of multiple joints without joint edema or inflammation Exertional malaise lasting >24 hr New pattern H/A Sleep disturbances or unrefreshing sleep

- Fibromyalgia also has associated symptoms; the more that are present, the more secure the diagnosis:
  - □ Fatigue* (especially when arising from sleep but also mid-afternoon)
  - □ Morning stiffness*
  - □ Sleep disturbances* (not insomnia, but not restful)
  - □ Paresthesias* (often migratory and may last for hours)

*Major associated symptoms.

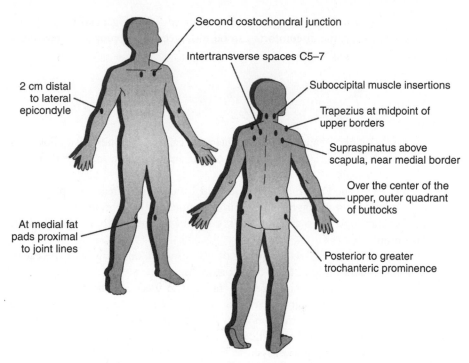

FIGURE 12–2 Tender points for fibromyalgia syndrome.

- □ H/A (includes migraine and muscle tension headaches)
- □ Anxiety and depression (includes problems with attention and concentration)
- □ Subjective swelling
- □ Irritable bowel syndrome
- □ Breathlessness, palpitations
- □ Dizziness
- Fibromyalgia is often made worse with:
  - □ Anxiety and stress
  - □ Temperature changes
  - □ Humidity and weather changes (barometric pressure)
  - □ Fatigue, poor sleep
- Diagnostic studies are of little benefit except to rule out other causes:
  - □ Hypothyroidism (TSH, T_4)
  - □ Muscle disease or polymyalgia rheumatica (ESR, liver enzymes)
  - □ Chronic infection (CBC)
  - □ Sleep apnea and restless leg syndrome (overnight polysomnogram)
- A detailed history and examination are the most helpful; x-rays, CT and MRI scans, and EMG studies are unnecessary unless some other diagnosis is suspected
- Differences between fibromyalgia and chronic fatigue syndrome:
  - □ Muscle aches and pains are worse with FMS

12

□ CFS is likely to improve with time; patients with FMS generally do not get better, although the discomforts can be managed with appropriate treatment, support, and education

Treatment

- A multidisciplinary team works best: primary care practitioner, psychologic, or psychiatric support, physical therapist, occupational therapist, massage therapist, and rheumatologist
- Because there is no known cure, an individualized, holistic treatment plan offers the best chance for management and improvement of the symptoms
- Nonpharmacologic care (some patients respond to these without the need for medication):
  □ Education: diagnosis and treatment of fibromyalgia, uncertainty of the cause, and the patient's role in their own treatment
  □ Gentle, low-impact aerobic exercise, tailored to meet specific needs; suggestions include walking slowly and consistently (e.g., 5 minutes) on alternate weekdays and increase 5 minutes every 2 weeks, with a goal of 20 to 30 minutes 3 to 5 times weekly by the end of the first year, or water therapy
  □ Physical therapy modalities, such as heat and gentle massage
  □ Biofeedback, hypnosis, and acupuncture may be of benefit
  ⊔ Smoking cessation
  □ Adequate sleep and nutrition; consider sleep studies if sleep apnea is suspected
- Pharmacologic therapy (symptomatic; no treatments are curative):
  □ NSAIDs, opiates, and corticosteroids are ineffective
  □ Amitriptyline (Elavil) 10 mg hs; may increase by 5 mg every 2 weeks to maximum relief of symptoms without unacceptable side effects (usually 35 to 50 mg qd)
  □ Cyclobenzaprine (Flexeril) 5–10 mg hs
  □ Tramadol (Ultram) or tramadol with acetaminophen (Ultracet) 1 to 2 tabs every 4 to 6 hours, up to 8 tabs in 24-hour period can help pain (try amitriptyline or cyclobenzaprine first)
  □ If not responding to amitriptyline or having intolerable side effects, try duloxetine (Cymbalta) 20 mg qd, up to 60 mg qd, or pregabalin (Lyrica) 25–50 mg hs, increasing up to 300–450 mg qd
  □ Gabapentin (Neurontin) 100 to 300 mg hs for peripheral pain

Practice Pearls

- Inform patient there is no cure, but teamwork between patient and providers can be beneficial
- If "resistance" develops to amitriptyline or cyclobenzaprine, stop the medicines

for 4 weeks and avoid all medicines that inhibit serotonin uptake receptors; consider

- ▫ Alprazolam 0.5 to 1 mg *or* clonazepam 1 mg hs
- ▫ Carisoprodol 350 mg hs (patient can also take 1 to 2 tablets tid)
- Encourage patient to prioritize time and activities (e.g., work, leisure, ADL)

NECK

| Neck Pain   723.1 |

Inspection

Observe for deformities and abnormal posture

Palpation

Assess for tenderness
- Cervical spine processes (Figure 12–3)
- Trapezius muscles
- Sternocleidomastoid muscles
- Muscles between scapulae

ROM

Ask the patient to do the following (Figure 12–4):
- Touch the chin to the chest (flexion)
- Touch the chin to each shoulder (rotation)
- Touch each ear to respective shoulder without raising the shoulder (lateral bending)
- Tip the head back (hyperextension)
- Axial compression—patient seated: examiner presses down on top of head and turns head side-to-side; positive test with radicular symptoms
- Spurling's maneuver—patient seated with head flexed to one side and rotated: examiner presses down on head; positive test with radicular symptoms: ipsilateral side, think compression; contralateral side, think stretch (traction)

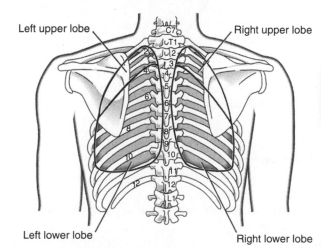

Left upper lobe

Right upper lobe

Left lower lobe

Right lower lobe

FIGURE 12–3 Upper spine and landmarks.

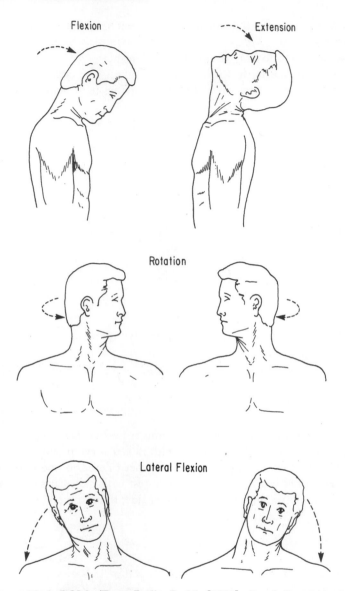

Flexion

Extension

Rotation

Lateral Flexion

FIGURE 12–4 Neck ROM. (From Reilly, B. M. [1991]. *Practical strategies in outpatient medicine* [2nd ed.]. Philadelphia: W.B. Saunders.)

Practice Pearls
- A general physical examination should be done with any suggestion of an unusual source of neck pain
- Pain that is not caused by injury and not relieved by rest or is progressive, think cancer or infection

- No treatment has been shown to change the natural course of mechanical neck pain; management is toward patient comfort until it resolves
- Possible causes of referred neck pain (i.e., no neck tenderness, loss of motion, or pain with motion) include:
  □ Shoulder (bursitis, tendinitis, arthritis)
  □ Reflex sympathetic dystrophy
  □ Thoracic outlet syndrome
  □ Bronchogenic cancer
  □ CAD
  □ Aortic dissection
  □ Peptic ulcer disease
  □ Pancreatitis
  □ Cholecystitis

Neck Pain Diagnosis
See Table 12–3.

SHOULDER PAIN

719.41

With shoulder pain, attempt to answer the following questions:
- Is ROM normal or abnormal?
- Are any structures tender (Figure 12–5), and does the palpation reproduce the patient's pain?
- Are the results of the neurologic examination of the arm and shoulder normal?

Inspection
For swelling, deformity, inequality, and muscle atrophy:
- Anteriorly: shoulders and shoulder girdle
- Posteriorly: scapula and related structures

Palpation
For tenderness and crepitus:
- Site where the patient locates pain
- Sternoclavicular joint
- Acromioclavicular joint: think AC joint strain or osteoarthritis
- Subacromial area (between the humeral greater tubercle and the acromion process)
- Bicipital groove

ROM (DESIGNATE BY DEGREES)
Examine the patient from behind and ask the patient to:
- Raise arms forward and then overhead with palms touching (elevation, flexion)
- Keep elbows at sides, swing forearms out: perform with and without resistance
- Place each thumb between scapulae: "back scratcher" (adduction, extension, internal rotation)

12

Table 12-3 Neck Pain

DESCRIPTION	DERMATOME RADIATION	MUSCLE TENDERNESS	MUSCLE SPASM	LIMITED ROM	PAIN WITH MOVEMENT	EXTREMITY WEAKNESS	ADDITIONAL POINTS
			POSSIBLE SIGNS				
Stiff neck: acute pain, localized and episodic; often present when waking and lasts 1–4 days		X			X		Pain relief with relative rest, NSAIDs, or acetaminophen, muscle relaxers, and hot and/or cold
Neck ache: dull, persistent ache in the back of the neck, often radiating to the occipital area		X			X		If neck tenderness associated with other tender areas in the body, consider fibromyalgia (see p. 333)
Torticollis: involuntary rotation or lateral bending of the head		X	X	X	X		May be acute or chronic
Cervical strain: acute or recurrent pain, more severe and lasts longer than a stiff neck; may be associated with whiplash injury or sudden movement; symptoms increase with ipsilateral rotation and contralateral bending of the neck		X	X	Maybe	X		Neurologic examination of upper extremities is normal; if related to trauma or an accident, refer to or consult with a physician and obtain cervical spine x-ray with oblique view
Neck pain with radiation: pain similar to cervical strain but with sharp, burning, or tingling pain to the shoulder, back, or arm(s)	X	X	X	X	X	Possible	Refer; could be herniated cervical disc or degenerative joint disease with a bone spur

12

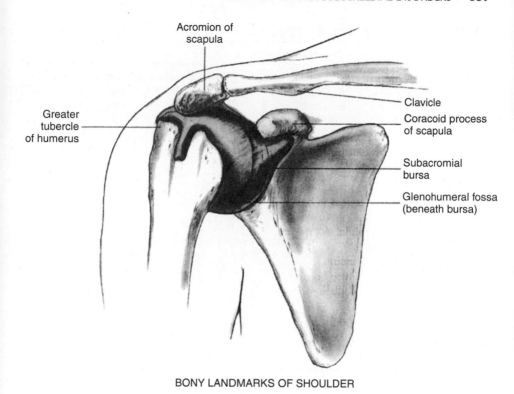

BONY LANDMARKS OF SHOULDER

FIGURE 12–5 Anatomy of shoulder. (From Jarvis, C. [2002]. *Physical examination and health assessment* [3rd ed.]. Philadelphia: W.B. Saunders.)

- Raise arms straight out to side (abduction, extension) with thumbs up and then rotate thumbs down (evaluates rotator cuff): perform with and without resistance
- Flex arm at elbow against resistance (evaluates biceps tendon)

ROM Testing Results

- ROM full, symmetric, and painless: check for referred pain (Table 12–4)
- Active ROM is painful or impaired: perform passive ROM
  - □ If passive ROM is normal with abnormal active ROM, it is probably musculotendon weakness or neurogenic weakness; the most common causes are rotator cuff tear and cervical spine disorders causing deltoid weakness
- Active and passive ROM are both limited: try to localize the restriction; restrict scapula movement by placing the heel of your hand over the upper scapula and your fingers over the shoulder; feel the shoulder as active or passive abduction of the arm is attempted
  - □ Restriction seems inflexible: bony (e.g., degenerative joint disease)
  - □ Restriction "gives" with pressure and is due more to pain and muscle spasm: periarticular (e.g., tendinitis, bursitis, muscle spasm or strain)

12

Table 12–4 Referred Shoulder Pain

SITE	POSSIBLE CAUSE(S)	ADDITIONAL POINTS
Trapezius ridge	Diaphragmatic Pleuritis Pericarditis Subdiaphragmatic disease Ruptured organ (e.g., ulcer) Ectopic pregnancy Splenic rupture	Perform cardiorespiratory and abdominal examinations Check for postural hypotension
Acromioclavicular area	Diaphragmatic or subdiaphragmatic disease (e.g., cholecystitis)	
Lower scapula	Gallbladder disease	
Back of neck, interscapular area, and posterior shoulder	Cervical spine disease (most common site for referred pain)	Perform neck examination
Deltoid area	Articular and periarticular disorders of the shoulder (e.g., arthritis, bursitis)	
Mid-humerus (brachial insertion site)	Rotator cuff problem	

- Determine what part of the shoulder motion causes pain or limitation (Figure 12–6)
  □ All directions of movement: glenohumeral joint itself (e.g., arthritis of the joint)
  □ Initial 30 degrees of abduction impaired: rotator cuff muscles
  □ Initial 90 degrees of abduction impaired, but 90 to 180 degrees normal: rotator cuff muscles, tendons, or bursae
  □ Initial 90 degrees of abduction normal, but 90 to 180 degrees impaired: disorders of the AC joint
  □ Internal and external rotation impaired: rotator cuff muscles, other muscle spasm, impingement syndrome (most common cause of shoulder pain)

Screening Neurologic Examination
- ROM of neck (see Figure 12–4)
- Muscle testing
  □ Shoulder shrug against resistance (cranial nerve XI or cervical [C] nerve 3–5)
  □ Scapular retraction: "stand at attention" against resistance (C5)
  □ Motor strength of biceps, triceps, and wrist extensors and flexors
- Deep tendon reflexes
  □ Biceps (C5)
  □ Brachioradialis (C6)
  □ Triceps (C7)

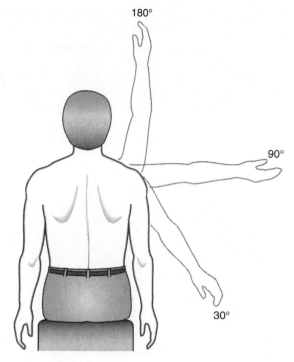

FIGURE 12–6 Shoulder ROM.

- Sensory examination using light touch along dermatome and peripheral nerves (see Figure 12–1 for dermatome distribution)

Adson's Test for Thoracic Outlet Syndrome

Thoracic Outlet Syndrome	353.0

- The patient sits with arms at sides; the examiner palpates radial pulse and auscultates subclavian artery
- The examiner abducts and externally rotates the patient's arm as the patient turns head toward arm and inhales deeply
- Positive (abnormal) results reproduce the patient's symptoms along with bruit over artery and decrease or loss of radial pulse
- Test both sides

Practice Pearls

- Night pain is often worse with bursitis and rotator cuff inflammation
- With burning, constant pain, think neurogenic cause
- If considering an MRI or CT, refer to orthopedic surgeon
- Bilateral shoulder pain after 50 years of age, think polymyalgia rheumatica

Treatment of Common Shoulder Problems

- Rotator cuff tendinitis

726.10

□ Treat with rest and ice for acute pain; may take NSAIDs in full strength (see Appendix E) for 3 to 4 weeks
□ Restrict overhead reaching, any movement with elbow away from body, and sleeping on involved side
□ Weighted pendulum stretch exercises with 5 to 10 lb (2.5 to 4.5 kg) for 5 minutes 1 to 2 times a day after first week
□ Discourage sling, which may hasten development of frozen shoulder
□ Refer if no improvement after 3 weeks
• Rotator cuff tear: refer to orthopedic surgeon

Rotator Cuff Tear	840.4

• Bursitis or tendinitis: see Table 12–1

Bursitis	727.3
Tendinitis	726.90

• AC strain

840.9

□ Goal is to allow ligaments to reattach
□ Activity limited for 30 days

Avoid sleeping on either side

Do not reach overhead or across chest

Do not lift more than 20 lb (9 kg) and lift close to body

□ Apply ice (see RICE mnemonic, p. 357)
□ Shoulder immobilizer, probably for 3 to 4 weeks
□ If no improvement in 2 weeks, consult with or refer to a physician
□ Patient education: if ligament not allowed to reattach, symptoms will recur
• Thoracic outlet syndrome: refer to a physician

ELBOW

Elbow Pain	719.42

Support the patient's forearm so the elbow is flexed at about 70 degrees

Inspect and Palpate

For nodules, swelling, or tenderness:
• Extensor surface of ulna
• Olecranon process (including groove on each side)
• Lateral and medial epicondyles

Perform

Tinel's test at cubital tunnel (where the ulnar nerve crosses the elbow)

ROM

Ask the patient to:
• Bend and straighten elbows; if checking ROM against resistance, examiner resists at wrist, not hand
• Rest arms at sides with elbows flexed, then pronate and supinate hands (Figure 12–7)

FIGURE 12–7 Elbow ROM test.

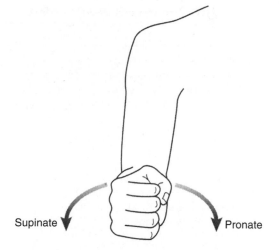

Supinate ▼   Pronate ▼

If pain history sounds as if source was radicular (e.g., tingling, numbness), examine cervical spine (see Figure 12–4 for neck examination)

Practice Pearls
- A patient with an elbow overuse injury frequently also has rotator cuff tendinitis
- Referred pain can be from:
  - Angina
  - Cervical radiculopathy
  - Carpal tunnel syndrome

Common Elbow Disorders
See Table 12–5

WRIST AND HAND

Wrist Pain	719.43
Hand Pain	719.44

Inspection
Inspect for swelling, redness, nodules, deformity, or muscle atrophy. Also, have patient make a fist and look at knuckle (MCP) profile for symmetry.

Palpation
Palpate the following for swelling, bogginess, or tenderness:
- Medial and lateral aspects of each DIP and PIP joint (Figure 12–8)
- MCP joints, just distal to and on each side of the knuckle (use your thumbs for examination)
- Wrist joint (your thumbs on the dorsal side and your fingers beneath it)
- Capillary refill and radial and ulnar artery pulses

Table 12–5 Common Elbow Disorders

FINDING	POSSIBLE CAUSE(S)	ADDITIONAL POINTS
Swelling over olecranon (can move without difficulty and is not painful)	Olecranon bursitis	Pull-on elbow brace may help See Table 12–1 Consult with or refer to a physician for possible aspiration of bursa for specific diagnosis Often recurs
Swelling over grooves along olecranon	Arthritis	See Table 12–1
Pain or tenderness over lateral epicondyle, aggravated by resisting wrist extension	Epicondylitis ("tennis elbow")	Caused and aggravated by hand and wrist movements; splint the wrist A tennis elbow band may prevent recurrence
Pain or tenderness over medial epicondyle	Epicondylitis ("golfer's elbow")	See Table 12–1
Pain in elbow and limited ROM	Nurse maid's elbow	Refer

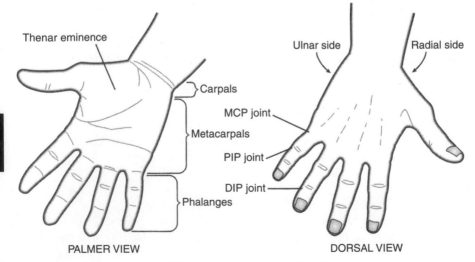

PALMER VIEW   DORSAL VIEW

FIGURE 12–8 Anatomy of hand.

ROM

Ask the patient to
- Make a fist, with the thumb across the knuckles
- Extend and spread fingers
- Touch each finger with the thumb of the same hand (thumb-finger opposition)
- With palms down, move the fingers laterally (ulnar deviation) and medially (radial deviation)
- Flex and extend wrists, with and without resistance

Additional Tests

- For carpal tunnel syndrome
  - Phalen's maneuver: have the patient press backs of hands together (flexes wrists at 90 degrees) for 60 seconds; positive (abnormal) results are numbness and tingling in thumb and first two fingers
  - Tinel's sign: percuss lightly over the median nerve on the palmar side approximately 1 cm proximal to the wrist; positive (abnormal) results are tingling or shocklike sensations across the palm, thumb, and first two fingers
- Finkelstein's test for de Quervain's tenosynovitis: thumb is held in palm with closed grip; wrist is passively, ulnarly deviated; positive (abnormal) result is pain from radial styloid to "snuff box"

Practice Pearls

- Remember that hand or wrist pain may be referred from cervical nerve roots, brachial plexus, or peripheral nerves; "radicular," or nerve pain, is often described as tingling, burning, or numbness and follows dermatomes (see Figure 12–1) or peripheral nerve distributions; if such pain is present, check DTRs and sensory status; the following sensory areas are to be tested:
  - Tip of the index finger (median nerve)
  - Tip of the little finger (ulnar nerve)
  - Dorsal first web of fingers (radial nerve)
  - Dorsal-ulnar surface of the hand (dorsal branch of ulnar nerve)
- If pain persists, repeat x-rays in 2 to 8 weeks to check for carpal fracture or osteonecrosis, which may not be evident on initial films
- Refer all patients with fractures early to an orthopedic surgeon; splint until seen
- For carpal tunnel syndrome, medical suggestions that can help:
  - Have patient hold elbow next to body and, using other hand, forcefully extend the wrist for 10 seconds, 10 times tid or qid; this stretches the carpal tunnel
  - Wear a wrist splint at night
  - Vitamin B$_6$ 100 mg bid may help with paresthesias; NSAIDs prn for pain

Common Wrist and Hand Conditions

See Table 12–6

HIP AND LOWER BACK PAIN

Hip Pain	719.45
Lower Back Pain	724.2

Table 12-6 Common Hand and Wrist Disorders

FINDING	POSSIBLE CAUSE(S)	ADDITIONAL POINTS
Hand or finger swelling, pain, or deformities	Osteoarthritis Gout Rheumatoid arthritis	See Table 12-1
Thenar atrophy	Carpal tunnel syndrome	Refer to an orthopedic surgeon
Painless swelling (cyst) on dorsum of hand or wrist	Ganglion	No treatment necessary unless painful
Pale fingers and slow capillary refill	Raynaud's phenomenon Ulnar or radial artery lesion	See p. 197 Consult or refer immediately if problem is acute
Loss of resistance against extension or flexion	Cervical nerve root lesion	Refer
Passive ROM normal with absent active ROM; may or may not have pain	Peripheral nerve lesion (i.e., radial, median, ulnar) Brachial plexus lesion	Refer
Unable to flex DIP or PIP joint		Refer to an orthopedic surgeon
Asymmetric knuckle profile	Metacarpal fracture Degenerative joint disease	X-ray, refer if fracture present

History

- In addition to the usual questions, ask every patient about the following signs and symptoms, which are *red flags* warranting immediate referral:
  - Bowel or bladder incontinence: think lower disc disease or cauda equina syndrome
  - Numbness in the "saddle area"; if present, think cauda equina syndrome
  - Pain suggestive of dissecting aortic aneurysm (severe "tearing" pain) or cancer (back pain, especially worse supine, and history of cancer)
  - Fever and/or weight loss (particularly in a patient with immunosuppression, DM, or history of substance abuse or recent spinal surgery)
  - Is the patient younger than 20 years or older than 55 years with no prior history of back pain (think ankylosing spondylosis or osteoporosis)

Physical Examination

- Watch the patient walk (abnormal gait often indicates hip disease); have the patient walk on heels (L5) and then on toes (S1); if the patient is able to do this, cauda equina syndrome is ruled out
- Patient standing:
  - Look at the patient's back for deformities (e.g., kyphosis, scoliosis) or lateral curves

12

- □ Look for height differences of shoulders, iliac crests, and skin crease below buttocks
- □ Palpate for levelness of iliac crests (not level—probably pelvic tilt)
- □ Check ROM: forward, backward, and to both sides

  Forward flexion decreases pain in spinal stenosis and increases pain in sciatica

  Look for flattening of lumbar curve

- □ Twist the patient's shoulders both ways
- Patient sitting:
  - □ Palpate for point tenderness; may percuss vertebrae for pain
  - □ Palpate paravertebral muscles for tightness or bulge
  - □ Check DTRs
  - □ Examiner straightens the patient's legs, one at a time (passive straight leg raise)
- Patient supine:
  - □ Check motor and sensory status (e.g., flexion of the great toe against resistance, sensation along dermatomes [see Figure 12–1 for dermatomes], capillary refill)
  - □ Passive SLR bilaterally; note the degree of elevation causing pain and any radiation of pain down the leg (15 to 30 degrees with severe, 30 to 60 degrees with milder cases); pain *must* go down the leg to be a positive test
  - □ Flex the patient's knee and hip and check internal and external rotation in relation to pain
  - □ Abduct and adduct straight leg (testing hip ROM)
  - □ Have the patient bend each knee (individually) up to the chest and pull firmly against the abdomen; opposite thigh should remain on the table, fully extended
- Patient prone:
  - □ Check sacroiliac joints and sacral spines for levelness
  - □ Check leg length for equality

Practice Pearls

- A patient with an acute herniated disk (herniated nucleus pulposus [HNP] prefers to stand
- Disk disease and myofascial pain are most common in adults <50 years of age
- Spinal stenosis, cancer (CA), Paget's disease usually occurs in adults >50 years of age
- Bilateral hip pain that starts with walking and is relieved with rest, think vascular or neurogenic claudication
- Spinal stenosis: also has numbness and/or weakness in legs with standing; improves or resolves with sitting or bending forward
- Plain x-rays showing osteoarthritis do not necessarily rule out other causes of hip pain
- Referred pain to the hip may be from:
  - □ Testicular torsion
  - □ Lumbar spinal problem

□ Disorder of the pelvic cavity
□ Vascular or neurogenic claudication
- A phrase to help remember which type of CA metastasizes to the bone: "BLT with mayo and a Kosher Pickle" (Breast, Lung/lymphoma, Thyroid, Multiple myeloma, Kidney, Prostate)
- Refer all patients with positive neurologic findings for consultation and x-rays
- Treatment for mechanical low back pain
  □ Advise patient to avoid bed rest (including sitting in bed) and to simply limit activities that increase pain
  □ Encourage cold packs; patient may alternate cold and hot
  □ NSAIDs are given for pain (see Appendix E); opioids may be needed short term to enable the patient to begin exercise (see below)
  □ Exercise is key to treatment (e.g., walking, swimming, bicycling)

  Start walking as soon as possible

  Start with 5 to 10 minutes and work up to 20 to 30 minutes a day

  Abdominal and back strengthening exercises may help prevent future problems

  □ Instruct in lifting and carrying techniques
  □ Recheck if not improved in 1 week
  □ Additional therapy modalities for cervical, thoracic, and lumbosacral strains

  Spinal manipulation (e.g., osteopathic, chiropractic)

  Myofascial release, deep massage

  Muscle relaxants (to help with sleep)

  Physical therapy for commonly used modalities

  Trigger point injections with saline, Marcaine, or Xylocaine

- Hip and lower back pain diagnosis (Tables 12–7 to 12–9)

Table 12-7 Common Lower Back Pain Disorders

FINDING	POSSIBLE NERVE COMPRESSION	MUSCLE SPASM
"Radicular" pain	X	
Pain radiates below knees	X	
Asymmetry on inspection or palpation		X
Limited ROM	X	X
Paravertebral muscle bulge		X
Positive SLR	X (usually at 40–60 degrees)	Possible
Asymmetric DTRs	X	
Asymmetric motor or sensory findings	X	
Unequal sacroiliac joints, sacral spines, or leg length		X

Table 12-8   Common Hip Disorders

FINDING	POSSIBLE CAUSE(S)	ADDITIONAL POINTS
Unequal leg length	Fracture or dislocation	Internal or external rotation also seen Refer after examination
Limited ROM	Arthritis Fracture Dislocation	With arthritis, rotation is lost early
Active hip and knee flexion of one leg results in passive flexion of other leg	Flexion deformity of passive hip	Consult with physician
Pain radiates to lateral knee	Iliotibial band syndrome	Often found in joggers Treat with NSAIDs (see Appendix E) and hip adduction stretching exercises
Tender to palpation along lateral hip/greater trochanter	Trochanteric bursitis	Treat with NSAIDs (see Appendix E)

Table 12-9   Comparison of Lumbar Nerve Roots

FINDING	L4	L5	S1
Pain	Lateral hip and anterior leg	Midbuttock to lateral buttock, lateral leg	Midbuttock, posterior leg, lateral foot
Numbness	Distal anterior thigh and knee	Lateral calf	Posterior calf and lateral foot
Motor weakness	Evaluation of quadriceps extension	Evaluation of dorsiflexion of great toe	Evaluation of plantar flexion of foot
Reflexes	Diminished patellar reflex	—	Diminished Achilles reflex
Screening examination (unable to perform)	Squat and stand	Walk on heels	Walk on toes

RESTLESS LEG SYNDROME

333.99

Restless leg syndrome is a syndrome characterized by unpleasant sensations in the legs that occur at rest and are relieved by movement. Because this usually occurs at night, interference with sleep is a common complaint. There is no particular age of onset. Although long remissions are possible, the condition is generally chronic.

Diagnostic Criteria

- The desire to move legs usually associated with paresthesias
- Motor restlessness
- Symptoms are worse or present only at rest and at least partially or temporarily are relieved during activity
- Symptoms are worse in the evening or at night

Additional Findings That May Be Present

- Sleep disturbances (e.g., difficulty falling and remaining asleep, exhaustion)
- Involuntary movements (e.g., periodic jerking)
- Normal neurologic examination
- Positive family history

Treatment

- Levodopa/carbidopa (Sinemet) 25/100 mg sustained-release ½ tab hs; may titrate up as needed and tolerated
- If Sinemet is unsuccessful, opioids (e.g., hydrocodone 1 to 2 tabs hs) or tramadol (with or without acetaminophen) may be used
- Cyclobenzaprine 10 mg hs may help
- Some patients respond to anticonvulsants (e.g., gabapentin 100 mg hs) or benzodiazepines (e.g., clonazepam 0.5 mg hs [unlabeled use])
- Iron supplement to get ferritin level to 50 to 60 mcg/L (check serum iron and ferritin levels)

KNEE

Knee Pain	719.46

History

- Pain related to mechanical use (e.g., brought on by walking, climbing, bending)
- Pain atypical of mechanical use may be referred from a lower back, hip, or circulatory disorder; a quick check of these areas may be warranted
- "Locking" of knee
  - □ Acute: usually related to trauma
  - □ Recurrent: usually due to a torn meniscus but may be degenerative arthritis
- "Clicking": common and does not imply disease; may be associated with a torn meniscus, arthritis, or chondromalacia
- Buckling (knee "gives away")
  - □ True: the patient *cannot* bear weight; associated with anterior cruciate tear, torn meniscus, patellar dislocation
  - □ Pseudo: transient; usually related to a disorder of the extensor mechanism (e.g., patellofemoral disorder or weak quadriceps muscles, especially in elderly or sedentary individuals)
- Pain
  - □ Worse with repetitive flex-extend with weight bearing (e.g., going up or down stairs or squatting and standing): stress on extensor mechanism

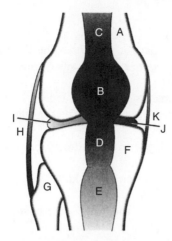

A = Femur
B = Patella
C = Quadriceps tendon
D = Patellar tendon
E = Tibial tuberosity
F = Tibia
G = Fibula
H = Lateral collateral ligament
I = Lateral meniscus
J = Medial meniscus
K = Medial collateral ligament

FIGURE 12–9 Right knee. (Adapted from Reilly, B. M. [1991]. *Practical strategies in outpatient medicine* [2nd ed.]. Philadelphia: W.B. Saunders.)

- □ Worse with pivoting: meniscus or patella
- □ Increases during the day: degenerative arthritis
- □ Decreases during the day: inflammatory conditions (e.g., arthritis, tendinitis)

Examination

With the patient undressed below the waist, compare both knees during the examination (Figure 12–9)

Inspection

Patient in the supine position with legs extended and relaxed:
- Atrophy of quadriceps muscles
- Effusion (loss of normal knee hollow on sides of patella)

ROM

- Limited ROM may be due to joint effusion, pain, or a mechanical problem of the joint, menisci, or ligaments
- Incomplete extension is the most subtle limitation

Palpation

With the patient's legs extended and relaxed:
- For thickening or swelling above and to the sides of the patella; to identify a large effusion, perform ballottement
  - □ Firmly grasp the thigh just above the patella (forces fluid into the space between the patella and femur)
  - □ Using two fingers of the other hand, push the patella sharply back against the femur
  - □ Positive (abnormal) result is a palpable click

- Patellofemoral compartment
  - □ Move the patella side to side
  - □ Push the patella distally and ask the patient to tighten the knee against the table (contracts quadriceps muscles); note pain ("patellar grind") or crepitus (crepitus alone has little significance)
- Test the integrity of the collateral ligaments
  - □ Medial: with the patient's leg extended, exert pressure on the lateral side of the knee and medial side of the ankle
  - □ Lateral: with the patient's leg extended, exert pressure on the medial side of the knee and lateral side of the ankle
  - □ Positive (abnormal) result is pain and movement of knee
- Perform McMurray's test
  - □ Flex the patient's knee, holding the heel of the foot in your hand, with the ball of the foot resting on your wrist
  - □ Place your other hand on the joint line of the knee
  - □ Rotate the foot laterally and extend the leg: checks the medial meniscus; rotate the foot medially and extend the leg: checks the lateral meniscus
  - □ Positive (abnormal) result is a palpable click
- Tibiofemoral joint: flex the patient's knee to 90 degrees with the foot on the examination table
  - □ With your thumbs, press into the joint space on either side of the patellotibial tendon and let your fingers surround the sides of the leg (resting on top of the collateral ligaments and menisci); palpate for tenderness or irregular bony ridges along the joint space
  - □ Palpate the extensor mechanism for tenderness: quadriceps tendon on superior patella and patellotibial tendon on inferior patella
  - □ Palpate medial and lateral areas of the knee for tenderness
  - □ Palpate the posterior surface of the knee for hamstring muscles (knee flexors)
  - □ In an adolescent with knee pain, press on the tibial tuberosity and note swelling or tenderness
- Test the integrity of the cruciate ligaments (drawer tests)
  - □ Knee flexed with the foot on the table; sit on the foot and grasp both sides of the tibia at the knee
  - □ Pull the tibia forward: tests the anterior cruciate ligament
  - □ Push the tibia back: tests the posterior cruciate ligament
  - □ Positive (abnormal) result is movement of the tibia away from the joint

Practice Pearls

- Sharp, stabbing pain—think mechanical problem
- Dull, aching pain—probably degenerative and overuse problems
- With vastus medialis oblique (VMO) exercises, it takes 3 to 6 weeks to start seeing results; to perform, have patient sit with legs extended, either on the floor or sitting in a chair with legs supported on another chair or footstool; fully dorsiflex the foot, press the knee down (i.e., against the floor), and hold for 10 seconds; he/she needs to do this 10 times bid

- Referred knee pain may be from:
  - Adults:
    Herniated disk
    Muscle strain
    Hip injury
  - Pediatrics: hip pathology

Common Knee Disorders
See Table 12–10

| Table 12–10 Common Knee Disorders |||
FINDING	POSSIBLE CAUSE(S)	ADDITIONAL POINTS
Loss of knee "hollows"	Effusion Synovial thickening	Warm and tender: may be synovitis Nontender: osteoarthritis Positive bulge sign or fluid wave with effusion
Positive patellar ballottement	Large effusion	See above Consult or refer
Crepitus or pain with quadriceps tightening	Osteoarthritis patellofemoral syndrome (PFS)	PFS is the most common knee problem—treat with NSAIDs and decreased knee stress until improvement seen with VMO exercises (see p. 352)
Pain and abnormal movement when testing collateral ligaments	Tear of medial or lateral collateral ligament	Refer
Positive results from McMurray's test	Torn meniscus	Refer
Pain with palpation of tibiofemoral joint	Damaged menisci or collateral ligament(s)	Positive results from McMurray's test or weakness of medial or lateral collateral ligament
	Bursitis	Pain more over tibial tubercle
Bony ridges along tibiofemoral joint	Osteoarthritis	See Table 12–1
Swelling or pain over tibial tuberosity	Osgood-Schlatter disease	See p. 454 Normal quadriceps strength and ROM of knee
Positive result from drawer tests	Cruciate ligament tear	Refer

FOOT AND ANKLE

Foot and Ankle Pain   719.47

The foot is not often a site of referred pain; most significant structures are either palpable or easily tested during a physical examination; try to localize the problem to either the forefoot, the midfoot, or the hindfoot (Figures 12–10 to 12–12)

Inspection and Palpation

Inspect and palpate all surfaces for swelling (unilateral [i.e., localized] or bilateral [i.e., systemic]), deformities or nodules, calluses or corns, or point tenderness; begin away from the area of maximal pain

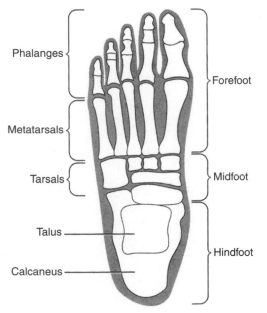

FIGURE 12–10 Areas of foot. (Adapted from Reilly, B. M. [1991]. *Practical strategies in outpatient medicine* [2nd ed.]. Philadelphia: W.B. Saunders.)

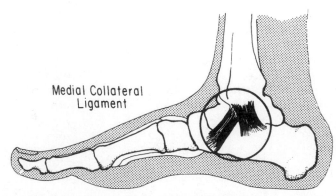

FIGURE 12–11 Medial ligaments. (From Reilly, B. M. [1991]. *Practical strategies in outpatient medicine* [2nd ed.]. Philadelphia: W.B. Saunders.)

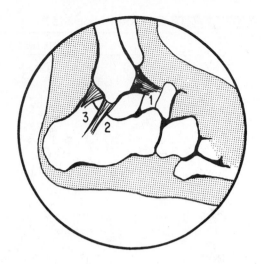

FIGURE 12–12 Lateral ligaments. *1,* Anterior talofibular ligament. *2,* Calcaneofibular ligament. *3,* Posterior talofibular ligament. (From Reilly, B. M. [1991]. *Practical strategies in outpatient medicine* [2nd ed.]. Philadelphia: W.B. Saunders.)

- Ankle joint: over the anterior aspect, the lateral and medial malleoli, and the ligaments
- Achilles tendon
- MTP joints
  - By "squeezing" the forefoot with your thumb and fingers just proximal to the distal ends of the first and fifth metatarsals
  - Palpate the distal end of each metatarsal individually, using your thumb and index finger
- The area between the proximal end of the fifth metatarsal and the lateral malleolus
- With ankle injuries, squeeze the sides of the lower leg just distal to the knee (tibia-fibula "squeeze test")

ROM

Perform ROM actively or passively or both
- Dorsiflexion (point foot toward the patient)
- Plantar flexion (point foot away from the patient)
- Inversion (twist the sole of the foot inward)
- Eversion (twist the sole of the foot outward)
- Flexion of toes

Practice Pearls

- Distinguish warts from calluses by interruption of skin lines, blood vessels in the core, and tenderness with squeezing
- Stress fractures of the foot are common and often don't show up on x-rays; maintain a high degree of suspicion; a bone scan is the "gold standard" for diagnosis

Common Foot and Ankle Disorders

See Table 12–11

Table 12-11 Common Foot and Ankle Disorders

FINDING	POSSIBLE CAUSE(S)	ADDITIONAL POINTS
Heel pain	Plantar fasciitis Bone spur Tendinitis	Treat with rest, NSAIDs (see Appendix E), heel pad, or orthotics Local steroid injection may help Roll arch of foot over frozen juice can Refer if no improvement
Pain with palpation	Sprain or fracture	Consider consultation
Ankle pain with tibia-fibula "squeeze test"	Fracture	Refer to an orthopedic surgeon
Unable to bear weight immediately after accident	Severe sprain or fracture	Refer to an orthopedic surgeon
Unable to plantar flex foot or walk on toes	Rupture of Achilles tendon	Refer to an orthopedic surgeon
Unable to dorsiflex foot	Injury to tibiotalar joint	Refer to an orthopedic surgeon
Pain at base of toes increases with squeezing forefoot	Morton's neuroma	Good support shoes or extra padding NSAIDs (see Appendix E) Refer if no improvement

Severe Ankle Injury

959.7

The following findings suggest a severe ankle injury, and the patient should be referred to an orthopedic specialist soon:
- Eversion injury (more serious because medial support is stronger)
- Immediate diffuse swelling (often indicates bleeding)
- Unable to bear weight immediately
- Tender "squeeze test" of tibia and fibula
- Positive drawer test
- X-ray examination shows avulsion fracture or fracture of the foot

Strains and Sprains

STRAIN   Excessive stretch of the ligament without disruption of its fibers or avulsion fracture

SPRAIN   Excessive stretch of the ligament with disruption of its fibers

GRADE OF SPRAIN	CLINICAL FINDINGS	SUGGESTED TREATMENT
I	Minor tearing of ligament Lateral pain and tenderness with little or no swelling; no joint instability	RICE* NSAIDs round-the-clock, not prn, for 48 hr Non-weight-bearing crutches for 24–72 hr, then according to pain When pain is gone, begin active or passive ROM 3–4 times qid
II	Significant but incomplete tearing of ligament Moderate pain, swelling, and ecchymosis with slight to moderate instability "Pop" felt and often heard; defect palpable	RICE* NSAIDs round-the-clock, not prn for 48 hr Non-weight-bearing crutches for 24–72 hr and posterior splint, air cast, or soft brace When pain free, begin ROM 3–4 times qid May need opiates for pain
III	Complete ligament tear Marked pain, swelling, and ecchymosis with significant instability	Posterior splints and crutches NSAIDs round-the-clock, for 48 hr and opiates for prn use Refer to orthopedic surgeon

RICE is an acronym for the treatment of many joint injuries:

R Rest: avoidance of activities that cause pain; the length of time varies with the injury.

I Ice: 20 minutes qid, usually for 2 to 3 days; a convenient ice pack is to use a bag of frozen peas or corn, which can "mold" around an injury and be refrozen as often as necessary (caution the patient to somehow mark the bag so the vegetables are not accidentally eaten after being thawed and refrozen).

C Compression: use of ACE bandage to provide support and limit swelling.

E Elevation: keep elevated as much as possible for 24 to 48 hours.

OSTEOPOROSIS

733.00

Definition

A skeletal disease characterized by bone loss severe enough to predispose to atraumatic fractures.

Types

- Primary
  - □ Type I: postmenopausal estrogen deficiency (most common in Caucasian and Asian women)
  - □ Type II:

    Occurs in men and women older than age 75 years

    Due to subtle, prolonged imbalance between bone resorption and formation or reduction in vitamin D synthesis

- Secondary: due to extrinsic factors such as chronic corticosteroid use, alcoholism, chronic liver or kidney disease, malabsorption syndromes, hyperthyroidism, hyperparathyroidism, chronic PPI use

Signs and Symptoms
- Backache or pain, acute and chronic
- Kyphosis or scoliosis
- Atraumatic fractures
- Loss of height
- No peripheral bone deformities

Risk Factors
- Dietary
  - Inadequate calcium
  - Excessive phosphate
  - Inadequate vitamin D intake in the elderly
- Physical
  - Immobilization
  - Sedentary lifestyle
- Social
  - Alcohol abuse
  - Cigarettes
  - Caffeine (more than 2 cups of coffee a day)
- Medical
  - Chronic diseases (e.g., liver or renal problems, ulcerative colitis, history of Mason shunt)
  - Corticosteroids (e.g., patient with COPD, Addison's disease)
  - Excess thyroid hormone replacement
  - Chemotherapy
  - Loop diuretics or anticonvulsants

Diagnostic Tests
- Bone mineral density (BMD) x-ray examination (to determine bone mass); dual-energy x-ray absorptiometry (DEXA) is most thorough
  - Osteopenia: 1 to 2.5 standard deviations (SD) below expected bone mass
  - Osteoporosis: >2.5 SD below expected bone mass
- X-ray of vertebrae not necessary unless vertebral fractures are suspected
- Consider labs with significant decline in BMD while on therapy: CBC, ESR, possibly protein electrophoresis (to rule out multiple myeloma and leukemia), thyroid and parathyroid function tests, and FBS (to rule out endocrine disease)

Treatment
- Activity
  - Maintain weight-bearing exercise (e.g., walking 45 minutes 4 times weekly)
  - Avoid aerobic exercises (too much stress on bones)
  - Consider physical therapy measures for back muscle spasm

Table 12-12 Comparison of Calcium Supplements

SUPPLEMENT	CALCIUM (mg/pill)	ADVANTAGES
Calcium carbonate Caltrate Os-Cal Spring Valley Tums Calcium oyster shell	250, 500, or 600	Least expensive and most available
Calcium citrate Citracal	200 or 500	Easily absorbed
Calcium phosphate Posture	600	Least likely to cause constipation

- Diet
  - Calcium intake of 1200 mg qd total (food and supplement)
    Food sources (see Appendix B)
    Calcium supplements (Table 12–12) 500–600 mg bid with meals
  - Avoid excess phosphate (e.g., beverages containing phosphoric acid)
  - Encourage vitamin D 800–1200 IU qd
    Sunlight for 15 minutes daily
    Supplements (as with calcium or in a multivitamin)
    Food sources: seafood, eggs, organ meats, fish liver oils, vitamin D–fortified dairy products
- Medications
  - Biphosphonate therapy: given first thing in the morning with 8 oz (240 ml) of water only; nothing else orally for 30 minutes
    Alendronate (Fosamax): 10 mg qd or 70 mg weekly
    Risedronate (Actonel): 5 mg qd or 35 mg weekly or 150 mg monthly
    Ibandronate (Boniva): 150 mg PO monthly or 3 mg IV q 3 months
  - Raloxifene (Evista): 60 mg qd; if hot flashes occur, stop medication until symptoms stop and then "wean up" (e.g., 1 day week 1, 2 days week 2, 3 days week 4, etc., until taking qd)
- Prevention of falls
- Smoking cessation

Follow-up
- Annual chemistry screening (as indicated), Pap test, and breast examination and mammography

- Repeat BMD in 2 years after initiating therapy; if stable or improving, repeat less frequently. If worsening, verify medication compliance and repeat in 1–2 years
- Patient education
  - ▫ Fall prevention, balance
  - ▫ Body mechanics
  - ▫ Alert patient taking biphosphonates to report any vision loss or eye pain
- Biphosphonates may be stopped after 5 years of use for most patients (no previous vertebral fractures and the BMD is stable); recheck BMD in 2–3 years

NOTES

NOTES

13

Endocrine Disorders

Thyroid Disorders

SCREENING TESTS

Serum thyroid-stimulating hormone (TSH) is the primary test

Serum thyroxine (T_4): many factors may alter serum T_4 measurements because of changes in TBG, including acute illness, high estrogen states and hormone replacement therapy, acute psychiatric problems, kidney and liver disorders, and certain drugs

CONDITION	Free T_4	TSH
Primary hypothyroidism (thyroid disease)	↓	↑
Secondary hypothyroidism (pituitary/hypothalamus disease)	↓	↓ or normal
Hyperthyroidism	↑	↓

DISORDERS OF THE THYROID GLAND

Thyroid Gland	246.9

See Table 13–1

Practice Pearls

- If thyroid dysfunction is suspected, also check serum cholesterol, blood sugar, and CBC levels and obtain an ECG
- If a patient has unexplainable urticaria, check for thyroid dysfunction
- Screen asymptomatic patients, beginning at 60 years of age
- With elevated TSH but normal free T_4, consider subclinical hypothyroidism; if antithyroid antibodies are negative, follow up q6mo; if antibodies are positive or if symptoms develop, treat as for hypothyroidism
- Radioactive iodine scanning determines "warm" vs. "cold" areas; cold is the more serious finding
- Biopsy is preferable with thyroid nodules
- If there is difficulty correcting hypothyroidism using only levothyroxine, consider adding liothyronine (Cytomel), which is T_3

Table 13–1 Disorders of the Thyroid Gland

Endemic Goiter	240.9
Hypothyroidism	244.9
Hyperthyroidism	242.9
Thyroid Cancer	193.

CLINICAL FINDINGS	DIAGNOSIS	TREATMENT
Endemic Goiter Thyroid may be multinodular May be very large and compress trachea Related to low iodine diets	Thyroid U/S TSH and free T$_4$ normal Consider thyroid radioactive iodine scan	Iodine supplementation (goiter usually does not shrink with treatment)
Hypothyroidism *General* Weakness, fatigue Cold intolerance Mild weight gain Depression; confusion (in the elderly, this may be the only sign) *Integumentary* Dry, cold, puffy, sallow skin Hair loss, including the lateral third of eyebrows Brittle nails *Genitourinary* Menorrhagia or menstrual irregularities *Gastrointestinal* Constipation	Signs and symptoms *and* Low free T$_4$ Elevated TSH If patient has signs and symptoms but normal lab results, think depression	Levothyroxine is the drug of choice: Start with 50–100 mcg qd and increase by 25 mcg qd every 2 mo until TSH normalizes; recheck yearly and prn With the patient with heart disease or myxedema or the elderly: 25–50 mcg qd for 2 mo, then titrate as above Some patients may be taking thyroid USP; adjust doses by 15 mg qd; 60 mg thyroid USP = 50–60 mcg levothyroxine in potency; thyroid USP metabolism may be erratic

13

Neurologic
Slow DTRs

Hyperthyroidism	Signs and symptoms	If lab results are abnormal, obtain thyroid radioactive iodine uptake scan and refer for further medical therapy or surgery
Thyroid	*and*	Atenolol 50–100 mg qd can help control symptoms
Firm, smooth, or nodular goiter	TSH <0.1 uIU/ml	Management of hyperthyroidism should involve endocrinologist
	Increased free T$_4$	

General
Hyperactive, nervousness
Anxiety, fatigue
Weight loss
Warm, moist skin
Heat intolerance

Eyes
Stare and lid lag
May have exophthalmos

Cardiac
Tachycardia or atrial
 fibrillation
CHF
Angina

Neurologic
Fine tremor of hands, tongue or closed lids
Hyperreflexia
Proximal muscle weakness

Thyroid Cancer	Normal thyroid function tests	Refer to surgeon
Enlarged thyroid or painless, hard nodule	Thyroid scan shows "cold" areas	
Palpable lymph nodes		

Adrenal Disorders

Adrenal Gland	255.9

See Table 13–2

Diabetes Mellitus

250.00

CATEGORIES

Type 1 (formerly called insulin-dependent diabetes [IDDM]): the pancreas produces no insulin (see Table 13–3)

Type 2 (formerly called non-insulin-dependent diabetes [NIDDM]): the cells are resistant to the insulin produced (see Table 13–3)

DM may develop as a result of pancreatic disease (e.g., cystic fibrosis or chronic pancreatitis), endocrinopathies (e.g., Cushing's syndrome, acromegaly, or pheochromocytoma), or drugs and chemical agents (e.g., thiazide diuretics, glucocorticoids, and phenytoin)

Gestational DM (GDM): develops during pregnancy, due to increased amount of glucocorticoids and other hormones released from the placenta, usually between 24 to 28 weeks' gestation, and usually disappears when the pregnancy ends

Prediabetes: blood glucose higher than normal, but not high enough to meet the criteria for DM

SCREENING

All adults older than 45 years; if normal, repeat testing every 3 years

Adults younger than 45 years if:
- First-degree relative with DM: parent, sibling, child
- Obese: body mass index >25 kg/m² (see Appendix A)
- Member of a high-risk ethnic population: African American, Hispanic, Native American, Asian American, or Pacific Islander
- Has delivered a baby weighing >9 lb or has been diagnosed with GDM
- Previously documented pre-DM
- Hypertensive: BP >140/90 mm Hg
- HDL level <35 mg/dl or triglyceride level >250 mg/dl or both
- Has other clinical conditions associated with insulin resistance (e.g., acanthosis nigricans)

Screening every 2 years for type 2 DM in children (starting at 10 years old) if overweight: body mass index >85th percentile for age and sex (see Appendix A) or weight is >120% of ideal for height PLUS any two of the following risk factors:
- First-degree relative with DM: parent, sibling
- Member of a high-risk ethnic population: African American, Hispanic, Native American, Asian American, or Pacific Islander

Table 13–2 Disorders of the Adrenal Gland

Acute Adrenal Insufficiency (Adrenal Crisis) 255.4		
Chronic Adrenal Insufficiency (Addison's Disease) 255.4		
Cushing's Syndrome 255.0		
Hirsutism 704.1		
Virilization 255.2		
Pheochromocytoma 194.0		

TYPE/DESCRIPTION	CLINICAL FINDINGS	DIAGNOSIS	TREATMENT
Acute Adrenal Insufficiency (Adrenal Crisis)			
Results from lack of cortisol as caused by:	H/A and lassitude	Elevated eosinophil levels	Refer immediately for emergency treatment:
Stress, trauma, infection, surgery or prolonged fasting in patient with Addison's disease	N/V	Hyponatremia	Hydrocortisone sodium succinate (Solu-Cortef) 100–300 mg IV plus normal saline IV stat
	Abdominal pain	Hyperkalemia	
	Diarrhea	Hypoglycemia	
	Impaired LOC	Hypercalcemia	
	Fever	Low serum cortisol levels	
Cessation or insufficiency of steroid therapy in patients receiving glucocorticoids	Hypotension		After acute crisis, maintenance doses of corticosteroids (co-manage with the physician)
	Cyanosis		
May occur as a result of pituitary destruction, after bilateral adrenalectomy or trauma to adrenal glands	Dehydration		
	Skin hyperpigmentation		
Chronic Adrenal Insufficiency (Addison's Disease)			
Autoimmune destruction of adrenal cortices results in chronic cortisol, aldosterone, and adrenal androgen deficiency	Hallmark signs are hypotension and hyperkalemia	WBC: moderate neutropenia, lymphocytosis, elevated eosinophil levels	Refer to endocrinologist
	Other signs are:	Elevated potassium, BUN, calcium levels	Replacement glucocorticoids and mineralocorticoids for life
	Increased skin pigmentation and diffuse tanning (especially over flexor surfaces, palm creases, and areolae)	Low sodium, FBS levels	Hydrocortisone 15–25 mg qd in 2 divided doses, $2/3$ in morning and $1/3$ in late afternoon or early evening

Continued

Table 13-2 Disorders of the Adrenal Gland—cont'd

TYPE/DESCRIPTION	CLINICAL FINDINGS	DIAGNOSIS	TREATMENT
	Volume and sodium depletion Weakness, fatigue Anorexia, N/V, diarrhea Arthralgia, myalgia, muscle stiffness Scant pubic and axillary hair Lymphoid hyperplasia	Low plasma cortisol at 8 AM accompanied by elevation of plasma ACTH Obtain CXR to R/O cancer, TB, fungal infection CT scan of abdomen	Fludrocortisone acetate (Florinef) 0.05–0.5 mgqd or qod
Cushing's Syndrome Cushing's syndrome is caused by adrenal hyperplasia or tumors or extraadrenal malignancies Cushing's disease is generally caused by ACTH hypersecretion secondary to pituitary adenoma	Central (truncal) obesity Moon face, buffalo hump, supraclavicular at pads Protuberant abdomen with purple striae, thin extremities Oligomenorrhea or amenorrhea, impotence Weakness Backache and H/A Acne Easy bruising and poor wound healing Labile mood to psychosis	Pre-DM (see Table 13-4) with adrenal or extraadrenal tumors Dexamethasone suppression test (if <5 mcg/dl, Cushing's syndrome is excluded) 24-hr urine for cortisol and creatinine CT scan of adrenal glands MRI scan of pituitary gland	Refer to endocrinologist
Pheochromocytoma Caused by tumor in adrenal glands or in sympathetic chain	Attacks of H/A, sweating, palpitations HTN Nausea, thoracic or abdominal pain Weakness SOB Visual changes Anxiety, tremor Weight loss Heat intolerance	24-hr urine for catecholamines, metanephrines, vanillylmandelic acid, and creatinine (all elevated) Elevated serum epinephrine and norepinephrine	Refer to surgeon

13

Table 13–3 Overview of Type 1 and Type 2 Diabetes

Diabetes Type 1   250.01
Diabetes Type 2   250.02
Gestational Diabetes   648.8

CHARACTERISTIC	TYPE 1	TYPE 2
Usual age at onset	Younger than 30 yr	Older than 30 yr*
Obesity-associated	Not usually	Frequently
Classic signs and symptoms	Polyuria, polyphagia, polydipsia Weight loss Fatigue, weakness Feeling edgy, moody	Relatively few classic symptoms Repeated or hard-to-heal vaginal yeast or bladder infections May have blurred vision, tingling in extremities, poor wound healing
Etiology	Beta cell destruction due to autoimmune disease Genetic and environmental triggers	Genetic and environmental factors appear to be important Usually arises because of insulin resistance combined with relative insulin deficiency
Ketosis prone	Yes	No, except in periods of acute stress
Dependent on insulin to sustain life	Yes	No, may require insulin therapy to correct hyperglycemia

*More children, even as young as 10 years, are being diagnosed with type 2 DM; this is probably related to increased fast foods and decreased activity in their lifestyles.

- Signs of or conditions associated with insulin resistance (e.g., acanthosis nigricans, HTN, dyslipidemia)

Screening in pregnancy
- Screen between 24 and 28 weeks' gestation; give 50-g oral glucose load and obtain plasma glucose 1 hour later (fasting not necessary); a value >140 mg/dl indicates the need for a diagnostic, fasting 3-hour GTT
- Screen as soon as possible women with a high risk for GDM (e.g., marked obesity, personal history of GDM, glycosuria, or strong FH of DM); if this screening has negative results, repeat it between 24 and 28 weeks' gestation

DIAGNOSIS

The diagnosis is based on criteria set by the Expert Committee of the American Diabetes Association; there are specific criteria for diagnosis (Table 13–4)

Diagnosis of DM and pre-DM should be based on blood glucose values by laboratory determination and not by capillary blood glucose monitors or glycosylated hemoglobin (HbA$_{1c}$) values; laboratory methods are much more accurate and precise, and the levels established for diagnosis are based on blood glucose levels rather than capillary blood

Table 13-4	Criteria for Diabetes, Prediabetes, and Gestational Diabetes	
DM	PRE-DM	GESTATIONAL DM
FBS level >126 mg/dl on at least two occasions* (preferred test) Random plasma glucose >200 mg/dl The 2-hr value during the GTT >200 mg/dl HbA$_{1c}$ >6.5%	FBS level 110–125 mg/dl on at least two occasions* (preferred test) The 2-hr value during the GTT is 140–199 mg/dl	After receiving a 100-g glucose load: positive test result if two values meet or exceed the following: FBS level \ 105 mg/dl 1-hr GTT: 190 mg/dl 2-hr GTT: 165 mg/dl 3-hr GTT: 145 mg/dl

*An oral GTT is not necessary if the fasting glucose level is elevated on two occasions.

Differentiating type 1 and type 2 DM
- Most patients with type 1 DM tend to be lean; most with type 2 DM are generally (but not always) obese
- Most patients with type 2 DM have a family history of DM
- Most patients with type 1 DM have experienced symptoms such as polyuria, polydipsia, and weight loss before diagnosis; most patients with type 2 DM have only mild symptoms, if any at all (fatigue is common)
- Many patients with type 2 DM also have acanthosis nigricans, which is a brownish hyperpigmentation with a velvety appearance, usually most visible on the back of the neck and axilla

INITIAL OFFICE EVALUATION
History
- Symptoms
- Prior HbA$_{1c}$ results
- Eating patterns, nutritional status, weight history; growth and development in children and adolescents
- Previous diabetes treatment, including nutrition and self-management education
- Current treatment: medications, meal plan, self-monitoring of blood glucose (SMBG), and the patient's use of data
- Exercise history
- Frequency, severity, and causes of acute complications (e.g., DKA, hypoglycemia)
- Prior or current infections (especially genitourinary, skin, foot, and dental)
- Symptoms and treatment of chronic complications of diabetes (see Table 13–14)
- Other medications that may affect blood glucose levels
- Risk factors for atherosclerosis (e.g., smoking, HTN, hyperlipidemia)
- History and treatment of other conditions, including eating and endocrine disorders
- Family history of diabetes and other endocrine disorders
- Gestational history and contraception
- Tobacco, ETOH, and/or controlled substance use

• Lifestyle, cultural, psychosocial, educational, and economic factors that may influence diabetes management

Physical Examination

See p. 381 for a flow sheet
- Height and weight (growth chart for children and adolescents)
- Sexual maturation (in peripubertal period) (see Tanner's staging, Table 2–1)
- BP (including orthostatic measurements as appropriate)
- Funduscopic evaluation, preferably with dilation
- Oral examination
- Thyroid palpation
- Cardiovascular examination, including auscultation for bruits and palpation of pulses; ECG in adults
- Abdominal examination
- Hand, finger, and foot examination (for neuropathy)
- Skin examination (for acanthosis nigricans)
- Neurologic examination, including sharp and dull sensations

Diagnostic Evaluation

- Fasting chemistry panel to include glucose, BUN, and creatinine
- HbA_{1c}
- Fasting lipid profile, including total cholesterol, HDL and LDL cholesterol levels, and triglycerides
- UA for glucose, ketones, protein, and evidence of microalbuminuria or infection
- TSH in all patients with type 1 and in patients with type 2, if indicated
- ECG (adults)

Referrals (Possible)

- Diabetes Education Program (this is a standard of care for DM, recommended by the American Diabetes Association and American College of Endocrinologists)
- Annual dilated eye exam
- Dietitian consultation (especially if patient is newly diagnosed); if someone else in the home does the meal planning and cooking, encourage that person also to attend the appointment; this is recommended if it is not part of the Diabetes Education Program or as a follow-up visit for further teaching or clarification
- Podiatrist for orthotics or evaluation/treatment of abnormal exam findings

GOALS

The overall goals for management of DM are:
- Type 1
  □ Avoid excessive hypoglycemia and hyperglycemia, especially when accompanied by ketoacidosis
  □ Balance food intake with insulin and exercise
  □ Maintain an appropriate weight and provide optimal nutrition

- Type 2
  - Eliminate symptoms
  - Improve quality of life
  - Prevent or delay microvascular and macrovascular complications through tight glycemic control

Individualize, taking into account patient's ability to understand and carry out the treatment regimen and understand the risk for hypoglycemia

Emphasize that diabetes is a chronic disease and management of diabetes involves five equal tools: meal plan, exercise, monitoring, medications (if needed), and education
- Meal plan
  - Managing the "diet" is of utmost importance; poor eating habits will lessen or negate efforts to achieve lower blood glucose levels
  - Weight reduction when indicated
- Lifestyle changes
  - Exercise
  - Quit smoking
- Monitoring
  - Blood glucose goals: 80 to 120 mg/dl (before meals), 100 to 140 mg/dl (hs or 2 hr postprandial)
  - HbA_{1c} <6.5%
  - Maintain BP <120/80 mmHg
  - Control hyperlipidemia if necessary; suggested priority is

    LDL <100 mg/dl

    HDL >40 mg/dl

    Triglycerides <150 mg/dl
- Medications (if needed) (Figure 13–1)

For patients with pre-DM
- Emphasize the risk of developing actual DM unless lifestyle changes are made
- The best results are with changes in eating, similar to a person with diabetes; it is a good idea to have the patient meet with a dietitian knowledgeable in DM
- Encourage patient to work up to walking 30 minutes, 5 times a week; it can be split into two 15-minute walks, if this is more feasible; "walking" means faster than a casual stroll, but the patient should still be able to carry on a conversation without difficulty

CURRENT DIETARY RECOMMENDATIONS

If a dietitian is unavailable, the nurse practitioner must be able to do the following:
- Calculate the desired body weight
- Calculate the appropriate caloric level
- Distribute the calories throughout the day while providing the appropriate proportion of carbohydrates, fats, and protein
- Teach the patient how to make adjustments for hyperglycemia, hypoglycemia, illness, and exercise

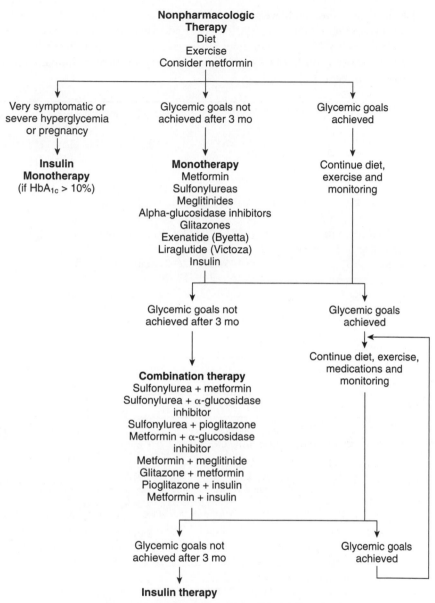

FIGURE 13–1 Suggested therapy for type 2 DM.

Calories

- Goals are to attain or maintain (1) desired body weight (dbw) for adults, (2) normal growth and development for children and adolescents, and (3) adequate nutrition for a mother and fetus during pregnancy and lactation

- To calculate desired body weight (plus/minus 10%, depending on frame size):
  □ WOMEN: 5 feet (150 cm) = 100 lb (45 kg); add 5 lb (2.25 kg) for each additional inch (2.5 cm) of height and subtract 5 lb for each inch less than 5 feet tall
  □ MEN: 5 feet = 106 lb (47.7 kg); add 6 lb (2.7 kg) for each additional inch
- Fiber: 20 to 35 g qd

Birth to 12 years	1000 kcal for first year and 100 kcal/yr older than 1 yr
12–15 yr	
Female	1500–2000 kcal and 100 kcal/yr older than 12 yr
Male	2000–2500 kcal and 200 kcal/yr older than 12 yr
15–20 yr	
Female	13–15 kcal/lb (29–33 kcal/kg) dbw
Male	15–18 kcal/lb (33–40 kcal/kg) dbw
Adults	
Physically active (athletes or strenuous physical activity)	14–16 kcal/lb (31–35 kcal/kg) dbw
Moderately active	12–14 kcal/lb (26–31 kcal/kg) dbw
Sedentary (most Americans)	10–12 kcal/lb (22–26 kcal/kg) dbw
Sedentary, older than 55 yr, obese, or inactive	10 kcal/lb (22 kcal/kg) dbw

Macronutrients

There is no evidence that supports eliminating any one food from the diet, including sugar.

NUTRIENT	SPECIFICS	SERVINGS
Protein	10%–20% of total calories 10% of calories with nephropathy	Meat, poultry, fish, eggs, peanut butter, cheese—2 to 3 qd
Carbohydrate	45%–50% of total calories Try to be consistent throughout the day to prevent blood glucose swings	Grains, beans and starchy vegetables—six or more qd Vegetables (other than above)—at least three qd Fruits—at least three qd
Fat	Total fat varies with treatment goals; usually: 30%–35% of total calories Saturated fat <10% of calories (<7% with elevated LDL) Polyunsaturated fat up to 10% of calories Remainder of fat mainly monosaturated Cholesterol <300 mg qd	Butter, margarine, salad dressing, oils—use sparingly

Sweeteners

- Sucrose (sugar) does not affect blood glucose control in type 1 or 2 DM; it is considered part of the carbohydrate servings

- Sugar alcohols (e.g., sorbitol) have low glycemic effect but may cause diarrhea
- Noncaloric sweeteners approved by the FDA are acceptable

Alcohol

- Avoid in persons with poor metabolic control, those attempting weight loss, those with elevated triglycerides, those with nephropathy, and in pregnant women
- Moderate intake (one to two servings per day for men; one per day for women) is acceptable
- Can contribute to hypoglycemia in patients taking insulin or sulfonylureas; for this reason, recommend that the patient eat protein when drinking alcohol

Micronutrients

- Sodium
  - □ Less than 3000 mg qd
  - □ Less than 2400 mg qd for patients with HTN and nephropathy
- Potassium
  - □ Increase intake in patients taking certain diuretics
  - □ Restrict in patients with renal insufficiency and those taking ACE inhibitors and ARBs
- Vitamins and minerals generally are not needed if patient has adequate dietary intake

Meal Planning Strategies

- Plan should be appropriate for the patient's lifestyle and should provide day-to-day consistency in caloric and carbohydrate intake and mealtimes; update as needed for changes in growth or lifestyle; encourage these guidelines:
  - □ Eat three balanced meals each day, 4 to 5 hours apart
  - □ Eat at the same times each day, whenever possible
  - □ Include a bedtime snack, especially if taking insulin
  - □ Avoid high sugar foods and drinks
- Plan should integrate insulin therapy when appropriate
- SMBG data should be used to make adjustments in food intake or insulin dosage
- Meal planning tools are available from the American Diabetes Association: *Exchange Lists for Meal Planning, Healthy Food Choices, Eating Healthy with Diabetes*, cookbooks and menu planning guides
- The exchange list is only one method of meal planning; the point system, carbohydrate counting, the Plate Method (Figure 13–2), and others may also be used

EXERCISE AND DIABETES

Weight loss and exercise work together to decrease insulin resistance, which is a primary problem in type 2 DM

Exercise Prescription

Individualize based on patient's level of fitness, lifestyle, and motivation

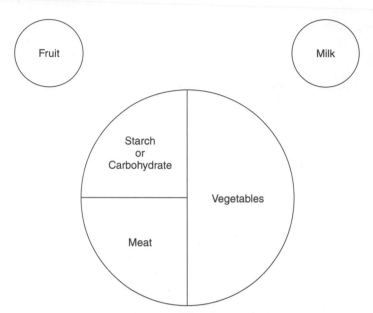

FIGURE 13–2 The plate method.

Important Elements

Important elements for both types DM are listed in Table 13–5
- Warm-up and cool-down for 5 to 10 minutes (walk at comfortable pace; gentle stretching)
- Keep moving (i.e., aerobic activity) for 20 to 30 minutes; patient may have to work up to this
- No matter what activity is chosen, patient should be able to talk without being short of breath
- Wear proper shoes; check feet before and after exercise
- Drink plenty of water to avoid dehydration
  - Two cups 2 hours before exercise
  - One to two cups 30 minutes before exercise
  - One-half cup every 15 minutes during exercise
- Patients may need extra food for up to 24 hours after exercise, depending on duration and intensity of workout

Exercise Restrictions

- Avoid exercise in extreme heat or cold and during periods of poor glycemic control
- Active proliferative retinopathy: avoid weight lifting and head-down positions
- Peripheral neuropathy: avoid weight-bearing activities
- HTN: avoid activities that involve straining

Points for Patients Using Insulin

See Table 13–6

Table 13–5 Exercise and Diabetes

TYPE 1 DM	TYPE 2 DM
Potential Benefits	
Cardiovascular	Cardiovascular
Decreased VLDL and triglycerides	Decreased VLDL and triglycerides
Increased HDL	Increased HDL
Decreased BP	Decreased BP
Increased cardiac work capacity	Increased cardiac work capacity
Weight control	Assist in weight loss and maintenance
Decreased stress	Improved blood glucose control by
Improved sense of well-being	increasing insulin sensitivity
Increased insulin sensitivity	Reduced need for insulin or OHAs
	Improved quality of life
	Decreased stress
	Improved sense of well-being
Potential Risks and Precautions	
Hypoglycemia can be delayed or prolonged	Cardiovascular, ophthalmologic, and
after prolonged or intense exercise	neurovascular complications are
Arrhythmias or MI can be precipitated in	relative contraindications or
patients with cardiovascular disease	precautions to exercise
Some types of exercise may worsen	
retinopathy and may lead to problems	
in patients with neuropathy	
Medical Evaluation Before Institution of an Exercise Program	
Assess glycemic control (e.g., HbA$_{1c}$)	Assess glycemic control (e.g., HbA$_{1c}$)
Cardiovascular examination	Cardiovascular examination (BP,
Neurologic and musculoskeletal examinations,	pulses, bruits, blood lipids, ECG
including examination of the feet	if the patient is older than 35
Ophthalmoscopic examination	years or has history of cardiovascular
	disease)
	Graded exercise treadmill
	Neurologic examination
	Ophthalmoscopic examination

- Do not exercise if blood glucose level is <60 mg/dl or >250 mg/dl
- Always begin exercise at least 1 hour after last insulin injection and avoid exercise during the time of peak insulin action
- If hypoglycemic symptoms occur during exercise, *stop immediately* and check blood glucose level

MONITORING
SMBG

- Safe and effective management of patients with type 1 DM requires SMBG; a standard regimen is before meals and at bedtime (minimum of 4 times a day); frequency is determined by level of glycemic control desired

Table 13-6 Food and Insulin Adjustments for Exercise (Type 1 Diabetes Mellitus)

Blood glucose level <100 mg/dl	Add snack and recheck glucose in 15–30 min
Blood glucose level >250 mg/dl	Adjust insulin
	Delay exercise until glucose decreases
Moderate exercise <30 min	No snack unless blood glucose level <80 mg/dl
Exercise longer than 30 min	Snack every 30–60 min
	Snack should be ~10–15 g of carbohydrate for every 30 min of exercise (see p. 390)
	Snack size may vary from patient to patient and with duration and intensity of exercise
Strenuous activity >45 to 60 min	May require ~20% decrease in corresponding insulin component
	Do not inject insulin into exercising extremity
Prolonged rigorous exercise	May require large decrease in insulin ($\frac{1}{3}$ to $\frac{1}{2}$ usual dose)

- Monitoring may vary
  □ Diabetes regimen variations
  □ Propensity for hypoglycemia
  □ Illness
- Initial monitoring of patients with type 2 DM who are taking insulin or sulfonylureas may be 4 times a day as well; in addition, 1- or 2-hour postprandial testing may be helpful 2 to 3 times per week (allows the patient to see the effects of a particular type of food on blood glucose levels); stable patients may monitor themselves 2 to 4 times a day, 2 to 4 times a week
- Patients with nocturnal hypoglycemia should test $1\frac{1}{2}$ to 2 hours after the evening snack or between 1 AM and 3 AM once or twice each week
- Tips for effective SMBG
  □ Patients should be taught the technique by trained individuals
  □ More frequent testing is necessary when the usual daily schedule is changed (e.g., travel, surgery, hospitalization) or during periods of illness or stress
  □ Patient should record all test results

  Manufacturers of insulin, sulfonylureas, and SMBG devices often provide log books for patient SMBG results

  Teach the patient to record results in a method that allows quick comparison of day-to-day results so that patterns are easily appreciated

  Recording insulin doses along with the blood glucose results is also helpful; be sure the patient knows that he or she must separately enter baseline doses and compensatory doses (e.g., according to a "sliding scale")

  □ Patients should know how to respond appropriately to SMBG results by making adjustments in diet or insulin regimen; the goal is to achieve and maintain blood glucose levels within the desired range, individualized for each patient (Table 13-7)

13

Table 13-7   Suggestions for Adjustments with Blood Glucose Excursions

BLOOD GLUCOSE VALUE	DIET ADJUSTMENTS	INSULIN ADJUSTMENTS	ADDITIONAL POINTS
<50 mg/dl	Include at least 10 g of quick carbohydrate during the meal	Give injection right before meal	Recheck blood glucose level 30–60 min after meal to ensure it is in normal range
50–70 mg/dl	None	Decrease short-acting* by 2–3 units Gives injection right before meal Decrease short-acting* by 1–2 units	Recheck blood glucose 30–60 min after meal to ensure it is in normal range
70–130 mg/dl	None	None	
130–150 mg/dl	None	Increase short-acting* by 1 unit	
150–200 mg/dl	None	Increase short-acting* by 2 units	Recheck blood glucose level 1–2 hr after meal to ensure it is in normal range
200–250 mg/dl	Delay meal ~45 min after injection	Increase short-acting* by 3 units	If pregnant, check urine for ketones with blood glucose level >200 mg/dl
250–300 mg/dl	Delay meal ~45–60 min after injection	Increase short-acting* by 4 units	Recheck blood glucose level 1–2 hr after meal to ensure it is in normal range
300–350 mg/dl	Delay meal ~45–60 min after injection Increase fluid intake if urine ketones are moderate to large	Increase short-acting* by 5 units	Recheck blood glucose level in 2–3 hr
350–400 mg/dl	Delay meal ~45–60 min after injection Increase fluid intake if urine ketones are moderate to large	Increase short-acting* by 6 units	Recheck blood glucose level in 2–3 hr
>400 mg/dl	Delay meal ~50–60 min after injection Increase fluid intake if urine ketones are moderate to large	Increase short-acting* by 7 units	Recheck blood glucose level in 2–3 hr
Any blood glucose value	Planned meal is larger than usual Planned meal is smaller than usual Unusually increased activity after meal: eat extra carbohydrates Unusually decreased activity after meal	Increase short-acting* by 1–2 units Decrease short-acting* by 1–2 units Decrease short-acting* by 1–2 units Consider increasing short-acting* by 1–2 units	Recheck blood glucose level in 2–3 hr Recheck blood glucose level in 2–3 hr Recheck blood glucose level in 2–3 hr If insulin is adjusted, recheck blood glucose level in 2–3 hr

*Regular or Humalog.

Glycosylated Hemoglobin (HbA$_{1c}$)

- Best method for assessing long-term glucose control because it reflects mean blood glucose concentration over the preceding 8 to 12 weeks
- Not affected by blood glucose at the time the blood specimen is drawn
- Several methods for assay are available, and all differ in normal range; *cannot compare results from different laboratories*
- Discrepancies between SMBG and HbA$_{1c}$
  - Inaccurate testing technique
  - Fabricated SMBG results
  - Inappropriate timing or frequency of SMBG
  - Hemoglobinopathies (e.g., sickle cell anemia lowers results; hemoglobin F may elevate results)
  - Represents an average blood glucose concentration, so fluctuations in blood glucose levels may result in near-normal HbA$_{1c}$ levels

Follow-up Office Evaluations

See also p. 381 for a flowsheet

- Frequency
  - Every 3 months in type 1 DM or uncontrolled type 2 DM
  - Every 4 to 6 months in controlled type 2 DM
  - Every 6 months with pre-DM
- History
  - Frequency and cause(s) of hypoglycemia and hyperglycemia episodes
  - Results of SMBG
  - Any changes patient has made in the treatment plan; problems with adherence
  - Symptoms suggesting development of complications of DM
  - Current medications
  - Psychosocial issues (e.g., quality of life issues, depression, ability to pay for medications or tests)
- Physical examination
  - Height and weight
  - BP
  - Cardiovascular examination including bruits and pulses
  - Oral examination for periodontal disease
  - Foot examination
- Laboratory and other testing
  - Fasting blood sugar (FBS)
  - HbA$_{1c}$: every 3 months in type 1 DM or type 2 with poor glycemic control; every 6 months if patient has stable glycemic control or in patient with pre-DM if FBS level remains above normal
  - Annual fasting lipid profile, urinalysis for protein and microalbuminuria, TSH (as indicated)
  - Annual ECG in adults, if indicated
  - Annual dilated-eye examination by ophthalmologist or optometrist
- Counseling
  - Discuss treatment goals and plan

□ Review food plan
□ Discuss exercise, weight reduction plan (if indicated)
□ Review medications

DIABETIC MAINTENANCE FLOWSHEET

Name _____   DOB _____

Referral Dates: Known cardiac risk factors:

Eye _____   Smoker   Yes   No

Foot _____   Hypertension   Yes   No

Education _____   Hyperlipidemia Yes   No

Date															
Weight															
BP															
Glucose															
Microalbumin															
Foot exam															
HbA$_{1c}$															
Creat. clearance*															
Cholesterol															
HDL															
LDL															
Triglycerides															

*For men:
$$\frac{(140 - \text{age}) \times \text{Weight in kilograms}}{72 \times \text{Serum creatinine}}$$

For women:
$$\frac{(140 - \text{age}) \times \text{Weight in kilograms}}{72 \times \text{Serum creatinine}} \times 0.85$$

Referral (to Endocrinologist)

- Concurrent illness (e.g., infection or dehydration requiring hospitalization)
- Diabetic ketoacidosis
- Recurrent hypoglycemia
- Unable to obtain glycemic control

ORAL HYPOGLYCEMIC AGENTS (OHAs)
Practice Pearls
- OHAs are ineffective unless a diabetes food plan, weight loss (as appropriate), and exercise are part of the management plan; in reality, these are more effective than OHAs in decreasing insulin resistance
- Taking an "extra" dose of OHAs to cover excess food intake is ineffective and may be harmful; this should be emphasized to patients
- Reinforce the teaching that OHAs are *not* oral insulin and do not work like insulin
- When one OHA is being changed for another, a delay between regimens is not necessary (unless changing from chlorpropamide)
- Possible causes for OHA failures:
  - Overeating and weight gain
  - Poor compliance
  - Lack of physical activity
  - Stress or concurrent illness (e.g., surgery, trauma, infection)
  - Decreasing beta cell function
  - Increasing insulin resistance
  - Inadequate drug dosage
  - Concomitant therapy with diabetogenic drugs (e.g., corticosteroids)
- Management of OHA failures:
  - Address possible causes before altering therapy
  - Combination therapy may be more successful than monotherapy
  - Insulin may "tune up" insulin receptor initially, after which use of an OHA may be effective
  - Most patients require insulin after 10 to 15 years of OHA therapy because of declining beta cell function
- Consider OHAs when diet and exercise do not achieve glycemic goals after 6 to 12 weeks

Choice of Agent
See also Tables 13–8 and 13–9

INSULIN THERAPY
Practice Pearls
- Patients should see instructor in diabetes care to learn how, when, and where to inject themselves
- As a rule, normalize the fasting blood glucose before normalizing the levels throughout the remainder of the day ("fix the fasting first")
- Teach patient signs and symptoms of hypoglycemia and how to treat them and what to do on sick days (see pp. 390 and 391)
- Intensive glucose control is contraindicated when
  - The patient cannot comply with the regimen
  - The patient is insensitive to signs of hypoglycemia

13

Table 13–8 Suggested Oral Hypoglycemic Agents

PATIENT PROFILE	SUGGESTED AGENT	AGENTS TO AVOID
Elderly	Glipizide or glimepiride	Chlorpropamide
	Glitazones	Glyburide (or use at lower dose)
Hepatic insufficiency		Metformin
		α-Glucosidase inhibitors
		Meglitinides
		Chlorpropamide
		Glipizide (or use at lower dose)
		Glyburide
		Glitazones
Renal insufficiency	Meglitinides	Metformin
	Glitazones	α-Glucosidase inhibitors
		Chlorpropamide
		Glyburide
Obese	Metformin	Sulfonylureas
Patient <18 yr	Metformin	Meglitinides
Irregular schedule or eating habits	α-Glucosidase inhibitors	Sulfonylureas (hypoglycemia is more likely)
	Glitazones	
Hyperlipidemia	Metformin	
	Glitazones	
Also taking insulin	Glitazones (cautiously)	
	Metformin	
CHF		Metformin
		Glitazones
Postprandial hyperglycemia	Meglitinides	

- ▫ The patient has seizures or compromised mental status
- ▫ Comorbid conditions, such as stroke or cerebrovascular disease, are present

Indications

- Type 1 DM: provide insulin to cover basal insulin secretion and to cover postprandial glucose excursions
- Type 2 DM
  - ▫ Hyperglycemia despite adequate trial of OHAs
  - ▫ Pregnancy
  - ▫ Periods of stress, illness, or injury
  - ▫ Renal disease
  - ▫ Uncontrolled weight loss and hyperglycemia
  - ▫ Newly diagnosed with $HbA_{1c} > 10\%$

Pharmacokinetics of Insulin

See Tables 13–10 and 13–11

Text continued on p. 387

Table 13–9 Oral Hypoglycemic Agents

MEDICATION	ACTION	ADMINISTRATION	CAUTIONS
Secretagogues *Sulfonylureas—First Generation* Tolbutamide (Orinase) Tolazamide (Tolinase) Chlorpropamide (Diabinese) *Sulfonylureas—Second Generation* Glyburide (DiaBeta, Glynase, Micronase) Glipizide (Glucotrol, Glucotrol XL) Glimepiride (Amaryl)	Effective only with endogenous insulin secretion Increase beta cell insulin production and secretion Effective for 7–10yr in most patients	Monotherapy or in combination with insulin or any of the other oral hypoglycemic agents Give 30min before breakfast (qd dosing) or 30min before breakfast and the evening meal (bid dosing)	Do not use two sulfonylureas simultaneously First-generation drugs can cause SIADH and disulfram effect May cause severe hypoglycemia and weight gain ***Contraindications*** Type 1 DM Pregnancy or lactation Major surgery Severe infection, illness, trauma History of severe reaction to sulfa
Meglitinides Nateglinide (Starlix) Repaglinide (Prandin)	Stimulates insulin release from pancreas (glucose dependent)	Monotherapy or in combination with metformin Take within 30min of starting the meal; do not take if skipping the meal	Use cautiously in patients with impaired hepatic function May cause hypoglycemia (less risk with nateglinide) ***Contraindications*** Ketoacidosis Type 1 DM Pregnancy Gemfibrozil used with repaglinide
Biguanides Metformin (Glucophage, Glucophage XR)	Decreases hepatic production of glucose Enhances glucose uptake by muscle	Monotherapy (especially with obese patients) or in combination with insulin or other OHAs	May cause gastric distress or diarrhea, but these decrease with time Stop drug 48hr before surgery or any test with iodine contrast dye

13

Decreases LDL and triglyceride levels Not associated with hypoglycemia and weight gain	Give with meals; the extended release tablets are taken once daily, regardless of how many are taken	Monitor for symptoms of lactic acidosis (e.g., malaise, myalgias, respiratory distress, increased somnolence, nonspecific abdominal distress) Can lower vitamin B_{12} levels; check with anemia or if symptoms of peripheral neuropathy develop *Contraindications* Type 1 DM Renal dysfunction (creatinine level >1.5 mg/dl in males or >1.4 mg/dl in females) Pregnancy and lactation Alcohol abuse Acute or chronic metabolic acidosis
α-Glucosidase Inhibitors Acarbose (Precose) Miglitol (Glyset)		
Inhibits small intestine enzymes that break down complex carbohydrates into monosaccharides Prevents the postprandial glucose peak No hypoglycemia because there is no systemic absorption	Monotherapy or in combination with sulfonylureas, metformin, or insulin Take with the *first bite* of the meal	High incidence of GI side effects (e.g., bloating, flatulence, cramping) especially if meal is high in carbohydrates or drug started at comparatively high dose Monitor LFTs q3mo for first year, then periodically Delays absorption of sucrose but not glucose; if patient is also taking insulin or sulfonylureas and experiences hypoglycemia symptoms, give glucose tabs or gel; candy, soda, or sugar-sweetened juices will *not* help

Continued

13

Table 13-9 Oral Hypoglycemic Agents—cont'd

MEDICATION	ACTION	ADMINISTRATION	CAUTIONS
Glitazones Pioglitazone (Actos)	Decreases insulin levels and insulin resistance Enhances glucose transport into cells Decreases triglycerides and increases HDL levels	Monotherapy or in combination with sulfonylureas, metformin, or insulin (rosiglitazone ≤4 mg qd with insulin) Increase dose after 4 wk if necessary	*Contraindications* Ketoacidosis Inflammatory bowel disease Intestinal obstruction Cirrhosis Renal dysfunction (creatinine level >2 mg/dl) Monitor LFTs q2mo for 12mo, then periodically; stop drug if ALT levels are 3 times the upper limit of normal Increased risk of hypoglycemia if used with insulin or sulfonylureas Monitor for signs of edema or CHF and stop the drug at the first signs *Contraindications* Active liver disease History of CHF Type 1 DM

Combination Medications (see individual drugs for actions, dosing, and cautions)
Metformin and glyburide (Glucovance)
Metformin and glipizide (Metaglip)

13

Table 13–10 Pharmacokinetics of Insulin

TYPE OF INSULIN	ONSET	PEAK EFFECT	DURATION
Short-Acting			
Insulin lispro (Humalog)	5–15 min	1–2 hr	4–5 hr
Insulin aspart (Novolog)	5–15 min	1–2 hr	4–5 hr
Regular (Humulin R, Novolin R)	30–60 min	2–4 hr	6–8 hr
Intermediate-Acting			
NPH (Humulin N, Novolin N)	1–3 hr	4 hr	12–14 hr
Lente (Humulin L, Novolin L)	1–3 hr	4–8 hr	13–20 hr
Basal			
Ultralente (Humulin U)	2–4 hr	8–14 hr	18–24 hr
Insulin glargine (Lantus)	2 hr	None	~24 hr

There are also combination insulins available; their pharmacokinetics depend on the individual components:

  70/30 (NPH and Humulin regular)
  75/25 (lispro protamine and insulin lispro)
  70/30 (aspart protamine and insulin aspart)

Table 13–11 Pharmacokinetics of Split or Mixed Injections

TYPE OF INSULIN	PEAK TIME	BLOOD GLUCOSE AFFECTED
Morning short-acting	Between breakfast and lunch	Prelunch
Morning intermediate-acting	Between lunch and supper	Presupper
Evening short-acting	Between supper and bedtime	Bedtime
Evening intermediate-acting	Overnight	Fasting AM

Insulin Dosing and Distribution

- Type 1 DM
  - Total daily dose (TDD) is 0.3 to 1 units/kg/day (start with 0.3 units/kg)
  - 40% to 50% of the TDD is the basal requirement; it should be NPH, Lente, Ultralente, or insulin glargine (Lantus)
  - The rest of the TDD is divided among mealtimes; the individual doses will depend on the calories consumed at each meal and the type of insulin used
  - When adjusting the insulin dose, start conservatively (e.g., 1 unit for every 50 mg/dl glucose above/below desired and titrate as needed); on average, 1 unit of short-acting insulin will lower blood glucose level 20 to 70 mg/dl
- Type 2 DM
  - Assess lifestyle, willingness to start insulin, and blood sugar data
  - A common combination is bedtime insulin added to an existing regimen of an OHA; use intermediate-acting or basal insulin; the starting dose should be 10 units/day and adjust according to self-monitored FBS; the goal is FBS level lower than 100 mg/dl, but none lower than 72 mg/dl; for titration, see chart on p. 389

Insulin Regimens

- Once daily dose of insulin glargine (Lantus) rarely will control hyperglycemia in type 1 DM
- Split or mixed (two injections per day)
  - □ Mixture of rapid or short-acting and NPH insulins before breakfast and supper

    Fasting hyperglycemia is often a problem; this can often be corrected by giving evening NPH or Lente at bedtime rather than with presupper rapid or short-acting insulin (this means more than two injections/day)

    Requires strict timing of meal and snack schedule to avoid hypoglycemia
  - □ Recommended dosing

    Start with two thirds of total daily dose in AM and one third in evening

    AM dose: one third of total dose as rapid or short-acting insulin and two thirds as NPH or Lente

    Evening dose: one half of total dose as rapid or short-acting insulin and one half as NPH or Lente; some clinicians use the same ratio as the morning dose

    Children: often closer to 20% rapid or short-acting insulin and 80% intermediate-acting insulin for both morning and evening doses
- More-than-twice-daily regimens
  - □ Indicated in type 1 DM and in severely insulin-deficient type 2 DM (when once or twice daily injections have not been successful)
  - □ Three times daily: two thirds of total dose in AM; remaining one third split between presupper and bedtime doses

    AM dose is rapid-acting or regular insulin and NPH or Lente

    Presupper dose is rapid-acting or regular insulin

    Bedtime dose is NPH or Lente
- Multiple daily injections
  - □ Regular or rapid-acting insulin, preceding each meal to correct postprandial excursions; regular insulin is taken 30 minutes ac and rapid-acting insulin is taken immediately ac (allows for more flexibility with meal times)
  - □ Basal insulin may be NPH, insulin glargine (Lantus), or insulin detemir (Levemir) at bedtime
- Continuous subcutaneous insulin infusion (CSII)
  - □ "Pump" therapy provides insulin through tubing connected to a subcutaneous catheter; refillable cartridge holds enough insulin for about 2 days
  - □ A basal insulin dose (in units per hour) is infused continuously, and bolus doses are provided for meals and snacks
  - □ Patients should be instructed by a health care team experienced in the use of pumps
  - □ Advantages of multiple daily injections or CSII:

    Increased flexibility in timing of meals

    Adjustments for size of meals are readily made

Easy-to-understand regimen for patients as each component covers a specific time

Intensive regimens have been shown to improve metabolic control to near-normal levels and have been demonstrated to significantly reduce the occurrence and severity of chronic complications of DM

□ Disadvantages of multiple daily injections or CSII:

Both require frequent SMBG

CSII also requires an expert diabetes management team and availability of 24-hour support

Infection at injection site is not uncommon

- Adjusting insulin
  □ The goals of insulin therapy are:

  Fasting glucose of 80 to 110 mg/dl

  Preprandial glucose of 80 to 120 mg/dl

  Bedtime glucose level of 100 to 140 mg/dl

  HbA_{1c} <6.5%

  □ Before changing the insulin dose, determine cause of hypoglycemia or hyperglycemia if possible
  □ Short-term adjustments of insulin dose consist of changes in the short-acting insulin component (see Table 13–7)
  □ Consistent elevations of blood glucose level at the same time each day for 2 to 3 consecutive days that cannot be explained by changes in diet or activity, or by illness or stress can be addressed by changes in the insulin component relevant to that time period (see Table 13–11)
  □ Change the basal dose by only 1 to 2 units at a time and wait at least 3 days before changing it again; a suggested titration schedule follows:

Self-monitored FBS level (mg/dl) for 2 consecutive days with no episodes of severe hypoglycemia	Increase in insulin dose (units/day)
100–120	2
120–140	4
140–180	6
>180	8

Decrease the insulin dose by 2 to 4 units qd per adjustment when self-monitored FBS level <56 mg/dl or severe hypoglycemia occurs.

HYPOGLYCEMIA IN TYPE I DM

251.11

Definition
Blood glucose level <50 to 60 mg/dl

13

TYPE OF HYPOGLYCEMIA	SYMPTOMS	TREATMENT
Mild	Hunger Tremors and palpitations Sweating	Give 10–15 g of simple carbohydrate* Should respond in 10–15 min

Moderate	As above plus:
	  H/A
	  Mood changes, irritability
	  Drowsiness, decreased
	    attentiveness
		May require second dose of simple
		  carbohydrate
		Patient may have more difficulty treating
		  hypoglycemia independently

Severe	Unresponsiveness
	Unconsciousness
	Convulsions
		No oral carbohydrate
		Glucagon 1 mg (0.5 mg if younger that
		  5 yr) IM or SC in deltoid or anterior
		  thigh
		Refer after emergency treatment

*Each of the following foods gives ~10–15 g carbohydrate:
- 4 oz (120 ml) fruit juice
- 8 Life Saver candies
- 1 tbsp honey or Karo syrup
- 2 tsp sugar or raisins
- 3 glucose tablets or gels

Do *not* use chocolate, ice cream, or other fatty foods that delay glucose absorption and contribute to weight gain.

Possible Causes

- Relative insulin excess inhibits hepatic glucose production and stimulates glucose utilization by muscle and fat tissue
- Increase in insulin dose
- Decrease or delay in food intake
- Increase in exercise level
- Alcohol ingestion (inhibits hepatic gluconeogenesis)

Prevention of Hypoglycemia

- Eat meals and snacks on time
- Take insulin as directed at appropriate times
- Make adjustments for decreased or delayed food intake
- Sleeping late
  □ May need to decrease previous evening's NPH or Lente insulin dose by 10% to 15% if sleeping more than 45 minutes later than usual
  □ May require advancing entire day's schedule
- Make adjustments for increased activity or exercise
  □ SMBG essential: refer to Table 13–7 for specifics
  □ If symptomatic hypoglycemia occurs during exercise, stop and eat a snack
  □ Avoid exercising alone

13

Special Problems Related to Hypoglycemia

- Unawareness of hypoglycemia
  - □ Severe hypoglycemia without warning; patients with low HbA_{1c} and repeated episodes of recent hypoglycemia are most vulnerable
  - □ Inability to recognize blood glucose levels lower than 55 mg/dl; refer to diabetes specialist experienced in managing unawareness of hypoglycemia
- Somogyi effect (hypoglycemia with subsequent hyperglycemia)
  - □ Counterregulatory hormone surge during hypoglycemic episode plus decreasing insulin levels and stimulation of hepatic glucose production lead to hyperglycemia and insulin resistance for as long as 12 to 48 hours
  - □ May be partially related to excessive carbohydrate intake
  - □ Increase in insulin dosage merely exacerbates the problem
  - □ Nocturnal rebound hyperglycemia: if the patient has elevated fasting blood glucose level, verify that 2 to 4 AM blood glucose level is higher than 70 mg/dl before increasing evening NPH or Lente; giving NPH or Lente at bedtime rather than before supper should prevent most cases of nocturnal hypoglycemia
- Dawn and predawn phenomena
  - □ Increase in plasma glucose between 5 and 8 AM (increased insulin resistance because of cortisol and growth hormone surge) is the dawn phenomenon
  - □ Insulin requirements generally are at lowest level in predawn period: 1 to 3 AM
  - □ As a result of the previous two points, attempts to normalize fasting blood glucose level can result in nocturnal hypoglycemia
  - □ Identification and prevention

    Measure SMBG at bedtime, 2 to 3 AM, and 7 AM

    Take bedtime snack

    Give evening dose of NPH or Lente at bedtime

    Consider using an insulin pump with variable programmable basal rate

HYPERGLYCEMIA

| 790.6 |

See Table 13–12

SICK DAY MANAGEMENT GUIDELINES FOR DIABETIC PATIENTS
Monitoring

- Check blood glucose level every 4 hours and check urine ketones if glucose level is higher than 250 mg/dl or if patient cannot keep food down or is losing weight
- Patient should call health care provider when preprandial blood glucose levels remain higher than 250 mg/dl or urine has moderate to large ketones

Insulin and Diet

- Do *not* stop insulin, despite N/V or inability to eat

13

Table 13–12 Comparison of Hyperglycemias

Diabetic Ketoacidosis (DKA) **250.1**			
Hyperosmolar Hyperglycemic Nonketotic Syndrome (HHNK) **250.2**			

DEFINITION	SIGNS AND SYMPTOMS	RISK FACTORS	TREATMENT
Diabetic Ketoacidosis (DKA)			
Characterized by metabolic acidosis, ketosis, and hyperglycemia due to insulin deficiency	Polyuria Polydipsia Kussmaul's respirations Dehydration Fruity odor to breath Altered LOC Abdominal pain *Laboratory Values* pH <7.30 Serum bicarbonate ≤15 mmol/L Glucose >250 mg/dl May have increased WBC count, potassium, and amylase	Infection Trauma Acute MI Stroke Omission of insulin (especially during illness)	Consult or refer to physician or emergency department; DKA is a medical emergency requiring immediate interventions in an acute care setting
Hyperosmolar Hyperglycemic State (HHS)			
Severe hyperglycemia in absence of ketosis	Polyuria Polydipsia Dehydration Weakness Hypotension Altered LOC, possible coma *Laboratory Values* Glucose >600 mg/dl Osmolality > 320 mOsm Acidosis may be present (often lactic acidosis)	Older than 50 yr Type 2 DM (over 35% previously undiagnosed) Accompanying infection Diuretic therapy Nursing home residents	Refer immediately; mortality is 12%–42%

- If no N/V and normal activity
  - □ Usual dose of intermediate-acting insulin or insulin glargine (Lantus)
  - □ For blood glucose level higher than 240 mg/dl, increase morning short-acting insulin by 20%
  - □ For blood glucose level higher than 400 mg/dl, increase morning short-acting insulin by 30%
  - □ If urine ketones are moderate to large, increase by an additional 10%

Table 13-13	Foods Allowed on Sick Days

Choose one of these foods for every **fruit** on your meal plan (10 g of carbohydrate each):	Choose one of these foods for every **milk** on your meal plan (12 g of carbohydrate each):	Choose one of these foods for every **starch** on your meal plan (15 g of carbohydrate each):
$^1/_2$ c regular ginger ale	$^1/_2$ c regular cocoa	$^1/_2$ c cooked cereal
$^1/_2$ c Kool-Aid	$^3/_4$ c cream soup	$^1/_4$ c regular pudding
1 c Gatorade	1 c whole milk	$^1/_2$ c ice cream
$^1/_2$ c regular lemonade	$^1/_3$ c tapioca pudding	1 c cream soup
1 Popsicle	$^1/_4$ c vanilla pudding	1 c chicken-noodle soup
$^1/_2$ c soft drink, 7-Up	$^1/_4$ c custard	$^1/_4$ c sherbet
$^1/_4$ c regular gelatin	1 tbsp sugar	$^1/_3$ c regular gelatin
$^1/_4$ c grape juice		1 tbsp jelly
$^1/_3$ c apple juice	Remember, you are taking	$^1/_2$ c instant breakfast
$^1/_4$ c cranberry juice	sweetened drinks and	5 vanilla wafers
2 tsp syrup, sugar	foods because you	6 saltine crackers
	cannot eat other foods!	1 c milk

- If no N/V and decreased activity (e.g., bed rest)
  □ Decrease calorie intake by one third
  □ Adjust insulin as previously mentioned
- If patient is having N/V
  □ Short-acting insulin only (may use NPH or Lente at bedtime per "sliding scale")
  □ Meal plan

  Sweetened liquids such as soft drinks, fruit juices, sweetened tea—4 to 6 oz (180 ml)/hr for adults, 2 to 4 oz (60 to 120 ml)/hr for children

  When tolerated, add soft carbohydrate foods

  Some clinicians teach patients to replace usual carbohydrate calories with "sick day" foods (Table 13–13)

Patient with Type 1 DM Should Seek Medical Attention Immediately When

- Fever is greater than 100° F (37.8° C)
- Diarrhea persists beyond 4 hours
- Patient is vomiting and unable to take fluids for more than 2 to 4 hours
- Blood glucose levels remain higher than 250 mg/dl despite insulin adjustments
- Moderate to large ketones appear in urine
- Patient experiences severe abdominal pain or other unexplained symptoms or has mental clouding
- The illness persists longer than 24 hours

CHRONIC COMPLICATIONS OF DM

See Table 13–14

Table 13–14 Chronic Complications of DM: Detection and Treatment

Accelerated Macrovascular Disease	459.9
Diabetic Retinopathy	250.5
Diabetic Nephropathy	250.4
Neuropathy	355.9

COMPLICATIONS	SCREENING/EVALUATION	TREATMENT
Accelerated Macrovascular Disease Affects coronary, cerebrovascular, and peripheral vessels Occurs at earlier age and with greater frequency than in nondiabetic persons (men 2–4 times as likely to have cardiovascular disease, women 3–4 times) Responsible for 80% of the mortality in adults with DM	Fasting lipid profile ECG Graded exercise treadmill Patients may not have usual symptoms; may have atypical or no chest pain	Weight reduction in obese patients Exercise (e.g., walking 30 min 5 times a week) Low-dose ASA 81–160 mg qd if patient has known macrovascular disease; consider it for primary prevention in patients 40 yr or older with DM and one or more CV risk factors Vigorous treatment of HTN Goal is <120/80 mm Hg Initial therapy may be with ACE inhibitors or ARBs (see Table 6–15) Diuretics and beta blockers may be used in addition, or if patient doesn't tolerate ACE or ARB Treat lipids (see p. 179) Stop smoking (imperative)
Retinopathy Leading cause of new blindness in adults Present in >80% of all patients with DM 15 years after diagnosis	Yearly dilated eye examination with ophthalmologist or optometrist: All patients with type 1 DM of 5 yr or more duration	Treatment usually laser surgery Lowering BP has been shown to decrease progression of retinopathy Optimal glycemic control

13

Much visual loss can be prevented by timely identification and treatment	All type 2 DM patients Early in first trimester for any woman with known DM who becomes pregnant	
Nephropathy Leading cause of end-stage renal disease Occurs in 20%–40% of patients with DM	Yearly urine for microalbuminuria; if positive, repeat test twice in a 3–6 mo period; if two or three tests positive, begin treatment Also see p. 297 for formula to calculate creatinine clearance Sudden decrease in insulin requirements can indicate renal compromise	At time of initial diagnosis, R/O other causes of renal disease (e.g., obstructive uropathy, infection) Refer to nephrologist or diabetes specialist if serum creatinine level >2 mg/dl *or* GFR <70 ml/min (see formula, p. 297) Aggressively monitor and treat HTN For treatment of macroalbuminuria, begin ACE inhibitor or ARB at usual doses (see Table 6–15); HTN does *not* need to be present Limit protein intake to 0.8 g/kg qd Aggressive glycemic control Treat hyperlipidemia (see p. 179) Promptly treat UTIs; repeat UA after treatment

Continued

13

Table 13–14 Chronic Complications of DM: Detection and Treatment—cont'd

COMPLICATIONS	SCREENING/EVALUATION	TREATMENT
Neuropathy ***Peripheral*** Insidious onset, symmetric distribution, progressive course May affect cranial or peripheral nerves (often in the feet first) May present as nerve or skin pain, paresthesias, or muscle pain ***Autonomic*** GI (may have gastroparesis, diarrhea, constipation, or incontinence) GU (may have neurogenic bladder, sexual dysfunction) CV (may have tachycardia, exercise intolerance, orthostatic hypotension)	Yearly examinations for sensation using a Semmes-Weinstein 5.07 (10-g) monofilament EMG, if indicated Ankle-brachial index to check degree of vascular disease, if experiencing claudication (see p. 198) Assess skin integrity of feet, especially between toes and under metatarsal heads, at least annually; note presence of redness, increased warmth or callus formation R/O conditions that may mimic diabetic neuropathy: heavy ETOH use, uremia, pernicious anemia, and exposure to chemical toxins	***Painful Neuropathy*** Improve glycemic control ***Pain/Paresthesia*** Nortriptyline 10–25 mg hs; increase dose q2wk to 75 mg or until dose is not tolerated Gabapentin 300–1800 mg qd in 3 divided doses May try pregabalin (Lyrica) 75 mg, up to 300 mg qd Narcotics should only be used for a short time until therapies effectively reduce pain ***Muscle Pain*** NSAIDs (use cautiously with renal disease) Physical therapy Muscle relaxants Foot care education (see p. 397) Avoid alcohol (may aggravate the development of neuropathy) ***GI Problems*** Small, frequent meals Avoid fat Metoclopramide 10 mg 30 min ac and hs or erythromycin 250 mg 30 min ac may help gastroparesis

13

FOOT CARE INSTRUCTIONS FOR PERSONS WITH DIABETES

These guidelines assume that the person has risk factors for foot problems: neuropathy, vascular disease, or a combination of these (see Appendix D for patient handout).

Footwear

- Wear shoes that fit properly; look for a wide toe box rather than pointed toes; avoid high heels; leather or canvas shoes are best; buy shoes at the end of the day (when your feet are larger) for the best fit
- Change your shoes once or twice during the day to relieve areas of pressure
- Never go barefoot, even at home; especially avoid walking on hot concrete or sand
- Avoid thongs, sandals, or open-toed shoes
- Break shoes in slowly; wear them for only a few hours a day at first, then gradually build up the wearing time
- Before wearing shoes, *always* check the insides for nail points, worn areas, foreign objects, or other rough areas that might cause blisters or rubbing
- Wear appropriate shoes for the weather; avoid wearing wet shoes

Foot Care

- Look at your feet (tops, bottoms, sides, between toes) *daily* for blisters, cuts, scratches, changes in color or discoloration, or changes in temperature; use a mirror if necessary or have someone check your feet for you
- Wash feet daily with mild soap and warm (not hot) water; dry thoroughly and carefully, especially between the toes
- Use creams or petroleum jelly to moisturize skin daily; do not place creams or lotions between the toes
- Wear clean socks daily; be sure that socks are appropriate for the type of shoes worn; do not wear darned or mended socks or socks with holes; avoid socks with seams
- Avoid soaking feet
- Avoid temperature extremes: check water temperature with your elbow before putting feet in
- Avoid all OTC treatments for corns, calluses, and nails; do not use strong antiseptics, astringents, or alcohol on your feet
- Trim nails "to the shape of the end of your toe" (i.e., straight across with slightly rounded edges); do not cut into the corners
- No "bathroom surgery": do not cut corns and calluses yourself; they should be managed by an experienced health care provider
- Avoid using adhesive tape on your feet
- Wear socks if your feet are cold; do not put heating pads or hot water bottles on your feet
- Avoid garters, tight elastic bands on socks, or anything that decreases circulation to your feet (including crossing your legs)

13

- Contact your health care provider when
  - You notice cuts, blisters, or breaks in the skin of your feet
  - You have ingrown nails
  - You notice changes in the color of your feet
  - You have pain or changes in the sensation in your feet
  - You notice a change in the shape or architecture of your foot
- Other things you can do to prevent foot problem
  - Stop smoking!
  - Control your weight, BP, and blood glucose
  - Get regular exercise
  - Have your health care provider check your feet at each visit
  - Special shoes or inserts may be necessary, especially if there are skin changes, calluses, or foot-shape changes

NOTES

NOTES

14

Psychiatric Disorders

Initial Office Visit

It is not uncommon for a nurse practitioner to feel uncomfortable with a patient displaying psychiatric symptoms. Several reasons might account for this discomfort: (1) spending an additional 30 to 45 minutes over the time allotted for a patient who is severely anxious can upset the flow of patients for the day; (2) the nurse practitioner may not feel competent dealing with psychosocial disorders, family secrets, or other sensitive information; (3) medication questions centered around drug selection, abuse potential, and efficacy complicate the care of the patient with a psychiatric disorder; and (4) concurrent medical illnesses may mimic psychiatric symptoms and pose significant problems with drug clearance. Because laboratory tests cannot diagnose the type of mental disorder with certainty or whether a medication is at therapeutic range, the diagnostic skills of the nurse practitioner are extremely valuable.

Nurse practitioners must be constantly aware that 50% of patients who are seen in a primary care setting have psychiatric symptoms and that the possibility of a comorbid condition is high; therefore a complete history and physical examination of patients are essential. Many patients are unable to accurately describe physical symptoms, so family interviews are necessary to determine the symptoms and behavior changes.

HISTORY

In addition to the typical questions asked during a routine history, questions may need to be asked of a patient with a psychiatric disorder that at times seem too personal but provide essential information. Patients and families are often guarded in their answers because of fears of judgment or embarrassment. Confidentiality should be stressed. After the patient is reassured of confidentiality and of the importance of the questions, special note should be made of the following regarding the CNS to rule out organic disease:
- Headache: recent onset or change
- Vision: recent deterioration, blurring, or spots in vision
- Hearing: recent deterioration, other sensations, or changes (e.g., tinnitus, hearing voices)
- Speech: any recent difficulty or change (e.g., muffled, garbled, uncontrollable speech; does the patient ramble on or get focused on the topic? Does the patient swear, mock, joke, or mimic another's words or actions?)

- Writing: any recent difficulty or change from previous functioning
- Memory: recent change of both long-term and short-term memory
- Gait: recent change or deterioration (e.g., shuffling, ataxia, waddling, dragging a limb, limping)
- Dexterity: inability to grab objects, clumsiness
- Sensation: any unusual sensations (e.g., things crawling on patient, fleeting burning pain, pins and needles)
- Strength: weakness recently in any limb, asymmetric grip strength
- Consciousness: history of blackouts or periods of time that cannot be accounted for
- Body movements: uncontrollable body movements (e.g., tongue biting, seizures)
- Substance use: use of drugs or alcohol for anxiety, nervousness, relief of symptoms, or other reasons; use of OTC or herbal products

MENTAL STATUS INTERVIEW

Be alert for cues that something is not quite right (e.g., inappropriate clothes, facial expression, verbal utterances, body language). Is the patient's affect inappropriate (e.g., laughing at sad events, weeping when others are happy)? After the history and physical examination, including CNS questions, a mental status interview should be conducted to determine if the patient has delusions or a psychotic process; suggested questions include the following:

- What brought you to the office today?
- How are you feeling right now? How have you been feeling lately?
- Have you noticed anything unusual in your thinking or behavior?
- Have you experienced rapid mood swings (e.g., highs, lows)?
- Are you troubled by any thoughts or feelings that pop up in your mind and hang around?
- Do you feel others are talking about you or judging you? Do you think anyone is out to harm you?
- Do you feel guilty for anything in your past or are you excessively bothered by past events?
- Have you felt bad enough to think of killing yourself or do you hear voices that tell you that you deserve to die?
- Have you thought of a plan for your suicide?
- Are there others you would like to harm or get revenge on? Do you have a plan?
- Do you feel the desire or need to harm yourself?

RELEVANT LABORATORY AND OTHER TESTS

Relevant tests for a patient with a psychiatric disorder should include the following:

- CBC with differential and ESR
- Full chemistry panel
- Thyroid function in depressive disorders
- EEG for those who are having seizures or sleep apnea
- ECG for patients taking heart medications and for elderly patients

A primary consideration when assessing elderly patients is to distinguish depression from other physical and mental diseases, especially Alzheimer's dementia and delirium.

Depression

311.

Definition

Depression is an illness with many subtypes, each of which is characterized by distinct neurotransmitter abnormalities; there is no one cause

Occurrence

- About 15% to 30% of patients who go to primary care offices have depression
- Onset is highest between the ages of 20 and 40 years
- Twice as many women as men experience depression
- 15% of depressed persons attempt suicide, with elderly persons having twice the rate of completed suicides; risk increases with the following:
  □ Multiple losses (e.g., spouse, friends)
  □ No social network for support
  □ Previous suicide attempts
  □ Chronic medical illness, especially dyspneic conditions and pain
  □ Higher socioeconomic class
  □ History of major depression at a later age of onset, with coexisting anxiety or substance abuse

MAJOR DEPRESSIVE DISORDER: SINGLE EPISODE
Diagnosis (Adults)

This is defined as persistent depression that must last at least two weeks and include at least five of the nine following symptoms, with one symptom being either the first or second one:

- Depressed mood most of the day nearly every day (patient appears sad and reports feelings of emptiness; may be tearful or anxious or totally withdrawn)
- Loss of interest or pleasure in usual activities (anhedonia)
- Significant weight loss or gain (>5%)
- Insomnia or increased need for sleep
- Psychomotor agitation or retardation, *not merely feeling slowed down or restless and unable to sit still*
- Fatigue or loss of energy nearly every day
- Feelings of worthlessness or excessive inappropriate guilt
- Diminished ability to think or concentrate
- Recurrent thoughts of death or suicide

14

Common Physical Symptoms

- Exhaustion
- Vague pain
- Headaches
- Lump in throat
- Sexual complaints
- Nausea

Patient and Family Education

- Duration of depression (6 months to 2 years)
- Chronicity and recurrences
- Disability and intensity associated with depression
- That the patient does not choose to be depressed
- Expected side effects of the prescribed medications (also that particular side effects for each patient cannot be predicted but will be treated)

Clinical Considerations

- Discuss with patient medication therapy and encourage cognitive therapy (counseling)
- Follow-up in 2 to 4 weeks, then in another 2 to 4 weeks, then in 1 to 2 months, then as indicated
- Referral with:
  - No improvement on high-dose SSRI
  - Suicidal/homicidal ideations
  - Comorbidities (e.g., psychosis, bipolar disorder, severe depression, or dysthymia plus acute depressive episode)
- Recurrent depression may result from inappropriate prescription of medications at a dose that is too low for an inadequate trial period, coupled with poor follow-up
- Consider referral for counseling or possible hospitalization

Treatment Guidelines (Adults)

See Table 14–1

- Cognitive therapy (counseling) can work as well as medications, even for severe depression, and is more effective for preventing relapse
- Medications should be started slowly, and the dose should be titrated up to the therapeutic level that resolves the symptoms. Titrate the dose until the patient answers "yes" to the following questions: Are you 100% better? Are you again doing the activities and hobbies you enjoy (i.e., enjoying life again)?
- The dose should be maintained at the therapeutic level for at least 1 year; patients with recurrent depression may require medications throughout their lives
- There is considerable variation in the amount of time required for antidepressants to reach a therapeutic level; traditional agents take around 3 to 6 weeks, whereas some of the newer SSRIs may begin easing depressive symptoms in 3 to 4 days

- St. John's wort 2 to 4 g qd in divided doses; take for 4 to 6 weeks to see benefits; if changing from SSRI or monoamine oxidase inhibitor (MAOI) wait 2 weeks before starting St. John's wort; may cause photosensitivity reaction, hypokalemia, and decreased effectiveness of OCs; never give with grapefruit juice

Practice Pearls

- SSRIs are easy to use and have fewer side effects; they are used most often in less complicated and less advanced cases of depression
  - □ SSRIs may cause hyponatremia, especially in the elderly; check serum sodium before starting and recheck in 1 month
  - □ Paroxetine (Paxil) can decrease cognition in the elderly and cause sedation; it is better for the anxious, younger person
  - □ Fluoxetine (Prozac) is not recommended in the elderly because of its long half-life
  - □ Patients taking fluoxetine or paroxetine who also take OTC cough syrup containing dextromethorphan may experience mental status changes or hallucinations
  - □ SSRIs cause sexual dysfunction in approximately 60% of patients
- Venlafaxine (Effexor) is an SSRI-plus; it has a rapid onset of action and is helpful in patients who need an immediate boost (e.g., no energy or interest in activities)
- Fluoxetine (Prozac) and clomipramine (Anafranil) are particularly effective in patients whose depression has obsessive-compulsive features or predominantly aggressive or violent themes; fluvoxamine (Luvox) can also be used for patients with obsessive-compulsive disorder
- Tricyclic antidepressants (TCAs)
  - □ Use TCAs cautiously in the elderly because of anticholinergic side effects (e.g., dry mouth, constipation, pupil dilation [worsens glaucoma], increased heart rate, urinary retention); nortriptyline (Pamelor) works for depression without anticholinergic effects
  - □ TCAs tend to cause weight gain
  - □ Amitriptyline (Elavil) has potent alpha-blocking properties, which can result in orthostatic hypotension; it may be beneficial in hypertensive, depressed patients
- Amitriptyline and trazodone (Desyrel) are the most sedating antidepressants and are the most beneficial in patients with insomnia; administer the drug in the evening; usual starting dose is amitriptyline 25 mg and trazodone 50 mg
- With anxiety also, try SSRI; if no benefit after 6 weeks, try the other; if still no benefit, refer the patient for psychiatric consultation
- With resistant depression, try an SSRI plus bupropion (Wellbutrin) or an SSRI plus mirtazapine (Remeron)
- Never give fluoxetine (Prozac) and amitriptyline in the same patient; amitriptyline is not metabolized and can become toxic

14

Table 14-1 Antidepressant Therapy

DRUG	STARTING DOSE	MAINTENANCE DOSE (mg qd)	SEDATION
Selective Serotonin Reuptake Inhibitors (SSRIs)			
Citalopram (Celexa)	20 mg qd	20–40	0
Escitalopram (Lexapro)	10 mg qd	10–20	0
Fluoxetine (Prozac, Prozac Weekly)	20 mg AM 90 mg weekly	10–80 90 mg/wk	0/+
Fluvoxamine (Luvox)	50 mg hs	100–300	++
Paroxetine (Paxil)	20 mg qd 10 mg qd (panic)	10–50 10–60	++
(Paxil CR)	25 mg qd 12.5 mg qd (panic)	12.5–62.5	
Sertraline (Zoloft)	50 mg qd 25 mg qd (panic and PTSD)	50–200	0
Tricyclic Antidepressants (TCAs)			
Amitriptyline (Elavil, Endep)	25 mg hs to 25 mg tid	40–150	++++
Clomipramine (Anafranil)	25 mg qd	100–250	+++
Desipramine (Norpramin)	25 mg hs to 25 mg tid	50–300	+
Doxepin (Adapin, Sinequan)	75 mg hs or 25 mg tid	75–300	+++
Imipramine (Tofranil)	75 mg hs 25 mg hs (enuresis)	50–200 50–75	++
Nortriptyline (Aventyl, Pamelor)	25 mg hs to 25 mg tid	50–100	++

*The following can be taken to help with sexual dysfunction, especially when it is a side effect of antidepressants: ginkgo biloba 60 to 240 mg qd; Wellbutrin SR 150 mg qd; Viagra 50 to 100 mg taken 1 hour before intercourse.

†With OCD in pediatric patients, consider strep throat as a precursor.

ADD, Attention deficit disorder; *IBS*, irritable bowel syndrome; *OCD*, obsessive-compulsive disorder; *PMDD*, premenstrual dysphoric disorder; *PTSD*, posttraumatic stress disorder; 0, none; +, slight; ++, moderate; +++, high; ++++, very high.

SEXUAL DYSFUNCTION*	ANTICHOLINERGIC EFFECT	USES	
		APPROVED	NON-FDA APPROVED
0/+	0	Depression	Alcoholism treatment Panic disorder Social phobia Trichotillomania
0/+	0	Depression	Anxiety
0/+	0	Depression Eating disorder OCD†	Panic disorder/PTSD ADHD/ADD
+/++	++	OCD†	Depression Panic disorder/PTSD
++++	0/+	Depression OCD† Panic disorder Social anxiety disorder Generalized anxiety disorder	PTSD Eating disorder
++++	0	Depression OCD† Panic disorder PTSD	Eating disorder
++	++++	Depression	Chronic pain Sleep disorders
+++	+++	OCD†	
+	+	Depression	
++	++	Depression	Chronic pain IBS Sleep disorder
++	++	Depression Enuresis	
++	++	Depression	

Continued

14

Table 14–1	Antidepressant Therapy—cont'd		
DRUG	**STARTING DOSE**	**MAINTENANCE DOSE** (mg qd)	**SEDATION**
Monoamine Oxidase Inhibitors (MAOIs)			
Phenelzine sulfate (Nardil)	15 mg tid	15–90	+
Tranylcypromine sulfate (Parnate)	10 mg tid	10–60	0
Miscellaneous			
Amoxapine (Asendin)	50 mg bid–tid	100–600	++
Bupropion (Wellbutrin, Wellbutrin SR)	100 mg bid 150 mg bid	300 mg	++
Maprotiline (Ludiomil)	75 mg hs or 25 mg tid	75–225	++
Mirtazapine (Remeron, Remeron Soltab)	15 mg hs	15–45	+++
Nefazodone (Serzone)	100 mg bid	200–600	++
Trazodone (Desyrel)	50 mg tid	50–400	++++
Serotonin Norepinephrine Reuptake Inhibitors (SNRIs)			
Duloxetine (Cymbalta)	20 mg qd	40–60	0
Venlafaxine (Effexor, Effexor XR)	37.5 mg bid 37.5 mg qd	75–225	0

*The following can be taken to help with sexual dysfunction, especially when it is a side effect of antidepressants: ginkgo biloba 60 to 240 mg qd; Wellbutrin SR 150 mg qd; Viagra 50 to 100 mg taken 1 hour before intercourse.

ADD, Attention deficit disorder; *IBS*, irritable bowel syndrome; *OCD*, obsessive-compulsive disorder; *PMDD*, premenstrual dysphoric disorder; *PTSD*, posttraumatic stress disorder; 0, none; +, slight; ++, moderate; +++, high; ++++, very high.

- Mirtazapine (Remeron) can cause weight gain; this may be an advantage in elderly patients with weight loss or poor appetite
- Be aware of the *many* other medications that can cause depression (e.g., propranolol [Inderal], cimetidine [Tagamet], methyldopa [Aldomet], OCs, corticosteroids); also, ETOH or marijuana used for a long time and cocaine or methamphetamine withdrawal are depressants
- SSRIs, bupropion, and venlafaxine may worsen sleep, at least at the start of therapy

MAJOR DEPRESSION IN PEDIATRIC PATIENTS

| Major Depression Disorder: Single Episode | 296.20 |

Possible Causes
- Sexual abuse
- Substance abuse

SEXUAL DYSFUNCTION*	ANTICHOLINERGIC EFFECT	USES	
		APPROVED	NON-FDA APPROVED
	0	Depression	Panic disorder Phobia
	0	Depression	Panic disorder Phobia
	++	Depression	
	++	Depression	Smoking cessation
++	++	Depression Anxiety with depression	
0	++	Depression	Appetite enhancer
		Depression	
+		Depression	Sleep disorders Chronic pain
+++	0	Depression Generalized anxiety disorder	

- Metabolic problem (obtain FBS level and thyroid and chemistry profiles)
- Psychomotor seizures; associated with anger outbursts (obtain EEG)

Diagnosis
- Difficulty concentrating
- Hyperirritability (not getting along with others)
- Not doing well in school

Treatment (for Children <12 Years)
- Counseling and consultation with pediatric psychiatrist

ANTIDEPRESSANT WITHDRAWAL
292.0

TCAs
- Occurs from 24 to 48 hours up to 2 weeks after discontinuation
- Symptoms
  □ GI complaints with or without anxiety
  □ Sleep disturbances

- Movement disorders
- Paradoxical mania

SSRIs

- Timing depends on which one used (half-life varies)
- Symptoms
  - Dizziness
  - Paresthesias
  - Anxiety
  - Nausea
  - Insomnia, nightmares

MAOIs

- Comparable to opiate and amphetamine withdrawal
- Symptoms
  - Anxiety
  - H/A
  - Muscle weakness, shivering
  - Paresthesias
  - Psychosis, delirium, hallucinations

Treatment

- Withhold medicine with mild symptoms, since they are temporary, *or*
- Restart medicine and taper off over 2 to 4 weeks or longer

SEROTONIN SYNDROME

333.99

Associated with alterations in cognition and behavior, in autonomic nervous system function, and in neuromuscular activity

The risk may be greater in patients with hepatic problems (including long-term alcohol abuse/use), hypertension, and atherosclerosis

Thought to be caused by increased or excessive serotonin activity and may be related to taking more than one of the following:

Medications	Herbs/Supplements
SSRIs	St. John's wort
Venlafaxine (Effexor)	L-tryptophan
Trazodone (Desyrel)	SAMe
Nefazodone (Serzone)	Dextromethorphan
"Triptans"	
Ergotamine	
Tramadol (Ultram/Ultracet)	
MAOIs	
TCAs	
Meperidine (Demerol)	
Propoxyphene (Darvon, Darvocet)	

Medications	Herbs/Supplements
Buspirone (BuSpar)	
Lithium	

	"Street Drugs"
	Amphetamines
	Cocaine
	MDMA (Ecstasy)
	LSD

Attacks are generally mild but can progress to coma and can be fatal; symptoms usually develop from 2 to 24 hours after adding a new medication or increasing the dose of a current medication

Symptoms

Symptoms include sudden onset and rapid progression of some or all of the following (at least four are needed for a diagnosis):
- Cognitive/behavioral: confusion, agitation, unresponsiveness, drowsiness, insomnia, hallucinations, hyperactivity
- Autonomic dysfunction: tremor, shivering, hyperreflexia, myoclonus, seizures, muscle rigidity, positive Babinski's reflex
- Neuromuscular dysfunction: fever, diaphoresis, diarrhea, sinus tachycardia, hypertension/hypotension, tachypnea, dilated pupils, flushed skin, drooling

Treatment

- Mild cases: stop potential offending medications—usually self-limited with complete recovery within a few days
- More severe cases: immediate referral to emergency department; treatment focuses on supporting respiratory and cardiovascular systems

Dysthymic Disorder

300.4

Clinical Findings

- Depressed mood for most of the day, for more days than not, for at least 2 years (never symptom free)
- During the depression, at least two of the following are present:
  - Poor appetite or overeating
  - Insomnia or hypersomnia
  - Low energy or fatigue
  - Low self-esteem
  - Poor concentration
  - Feelings of hopelessness

14

- May have heightened anger and brood about the past
- Patient describes life as stressful or boring
- Little satisfaction with job or personal relationships

Treatment

- Often has an early and insidious onset and is a chronic disorder
- Antidepressants have been effective in a majority of patients (see Table 14–1)
- Counseling to deal with some of the issues has also been very helpful for some patients
- Group therapy is an effective adjunct to help interpersonal relationships

Bipolar Disorder: Single Manic Episode

296.60

Clinical Findings

- Cannot sit still and is intensely overactive in both body and mind
- Speech pressure (often loud, inappropriate; often jumps from one subject to another)
- Mood liability
  - Irritability
  - Euphoria
  - Suspiciousness
- Cognitive abnormalities
  - Poor concentration
  - Grandiosity
  - Manipulativeness
  - Delusions
- Hypersexuality
- Assaultiveness
- Sleeplessness
- May be too hyperactive to eat and drink, causing fluid depletion and weight loss

Treatment

- Refer to psychiatrist
- May need inpatient treatment, especially initially
- When interviewing the patient, talk in a calm nonjudgmental fashion
- Do not take the patient's comments personally, no matter how personal they seem (e.g., "you are an alcoholic, and I'm not talking to you")

Suicide Assessment and Prevention in Primary Care

Associated Factors

- Living alone
- Unemployment

- Recent loss
- Physical illness or impairment
- Insomnia
- Lack of future plans
- Male gender
- Bisexual or homosexual
- Divorced
- Family history of suicide or severe family disease
- Sexual abuse
- Low self-esteem
- Recent childbirth
- High risk
  - Major psychiatric disorders
  - Patient's belief that he or she has a fatal illness (when the patient really does not)

Determine Risk (Questions to Ask the Patient)

- Have you ever thought of suicide or considered suicide as a serious option?
- Do you find that you have urges to harm yourself that are hard to control?
- Have you ever attempted suicide?

If the patient answers "yes" to any of these questions, an assessment of suicide risk must be made. The family or significant others can frequently become involved and be instrumental in preventing the patient from acting on impulse. At times it may be necessary to hospitalize the patient for a brief period (e.g., overnight) to ensure safety and allow time for crisis intervention and pooling of resources. The nurse practitioner must understand that it is not always possible to prevent suicide, but every effort must be made to minimize the risk.

Treatment

- Refer for treatment and possible hospitalization
- Medication is used to raise the serotonin level in the brain; if the patient is an immediate suicide risk, prescribe *no more than 5 days' worth of medicine*
- The family or significant others must be made aware of the danger of death in these patients

Anxiety Disorders

300.00

Anxiety is a normal reaction if it is aroused by realistic danger, if the reaction is appropriate to the threat, and if the anxiety disappears when the threat ceases. Anxiety that exceeds this definition is outside the patient's voluntary control and often renders the patient unable to function. Anxiety is among the most disabling of diseases and frequently is a comorbid illness with depression, substance abuse, psychiatric disorders, and medical conditions.

Classification of Anxiety Disorders

- Social phobia
- Generalized anxiety disorder (GAD)
- Acute stress disorder
- Panic disorder
- Agoraphobia
- Obsessive-compulsive disorder (OCD)
- Posttraumatic stress disorder (PTSD)

Signs/Symptoms

The frequency and intensity determine if the anxiety meets the *DSM-IV** criteria
- Adults
  - Extreme fear (may be specific or vague)
  - Tachycardia, palpitations, chest pain
  - SOB
  - Sweating
  - Muscle tension
  - Blushing
  - Nausea, diarrhea
  - Tremulousness and leg weakness
- Pediatrics
  - Ritualistic behavior
  - "Magical" stuff

Treatment

- Individualized plan combining the following:
  - Education
  - Reassurance
  - Behavior therapy
  - Medications
  - Long-term follow-up
- Often referred to a psychiatric nurse practitioner, psychologist, or psychiatrist for management
- Need for counseling and drug therapy for long-term success
- Adults
  - See Table 14–2 for medications
  - For panic disorder, consider benzodiazepine for first few weeks until SSRI starts working; taper benzodiazepine 10% per week to limit withdrawal symptoms and recurrent panic
  - Propranolol (Inderal) 10 mg before anxiety-producing events
- Pediatrics
  - Try imipramine (Tofranil) first for 6 to 8 weeks
  - If not very effective, decrease dose and add an SSRI (SSRIs increase TCA levels)

Diagnostic and Statistical Manual of Mental Disorders (4th ed.).

14

Table 14–2 Anxiolytics

DRUG	DOSAGE RANGE (mg qd)	HALF-LIFE OF PARENT DRUG (hr)
Benzodiazepines*		
Alprazolam (Xanax)	General: 0.25–4	12–15
	Panic: 1.5–10	
Chlordiazepoxide (Librium, Mitran)	15–100	5–30
Clonazepam (Klonopin)	1.5–20	18–50
Clorazepate (Tranxene)	15–60	n/a
Diazepam (Valium, Zetran)	4–40	20–80
Lorazepam (Ativan)	2–4	10–20
Oxazepam (Serax)	30–120	5–20
Selective Serotonin Reuptake Inhibitors (SSRIs)		
Fluoxetine (Prozac)	10–60	24–72
Fluvoxamine (Luvox)	100–300	16
Paroxetine (Paxil)	20–50	21
Sertraline (Zoloft)	25–50	26
Miscellaneous		
Buspirone (BuSpar)	15–60 (not for prn use)	48–72
Hydroxyzine (Atarax, Vistaril, others)	50–400	n/a

*Benzodiazepines have the potential for addiction. Consult with physician before initiating therapy.

Extrapyramidal Symptoms (EPSs)

333.90

May be seen with use of antipsychotic agents (Table 14–3)

Consult with the physician if EPSs are suspected

PSEUDOPARKINSONISM (4% TO 40% OCCURRENCE)

332.0

Symptoms
- Masklike facies
- Drooling
- Tremors
- Pin rolling
- Cogwheel rigidity or shuffling gait

Treatment
- Control with an antiparkinsonism agent for a few weeks to 2 to 3 months; after this, evaluate whether the patient requires further treatment
- Occasionally, reduction in the dose of the antipsychotic agent or discontinuation of the agent is necessary

Table 14–3 Antipsychotic Agents*

DRUG	DOSAGE RANGE (ADULT; mg qd)	SEDATION	EXTRAPYRAMIDAL EFFECTS	ORTHOSTATIC HYPOTENSION	ANTICHOLINERGIC EFFECTS
Aripiprazole (Abilify)	2–30	+	0	+	0/+
Chlorpromazine (Thorazine)	50–200	+++	++	+++	++
Clozapine† (Clozaril)	75–900	+++	+	++	+++
Fluphenazine (Prolixin)	0.5–40	+	+++	+	+
Haloperidol (Haldol)	2–100 IM	0/+	+++	+	+
Loxapine (Loxitane)	20–250	+	++	+	+
Mesoridazine (Serentil)	30–400	+++	+	++	+++
Molindone (Moban)	15–225	++	++	+	+
Olanzapine (Zyprexa)	5–20	+++	+	++	+++
Quetiapine fumarate (Seroquel)	50–750	++	+	++	0
Risperidone (Risperdal)	4–16	+	+	+	0/+
Thioridazine (Mellaril)	150–800	+++	+	+++	+++
Thiothixene (Navane)	6–60	+	+++	++	+
Trifluoperazine (Stelazine)	2–40	+	+++	+	+

0, None; +, slight; ++, moderate; +++, high.

*Many of these medications can cause weight gain, diabetes (monitor FBS level at least yearly), and hyperlipidemia (monitor periodically).

†Monitor WBC count with differential weekly while patient is undergoing therapy and for 4 weeks after discontinuation.

DYSTONIAS (2% TO 50% OCCURRENCE)

333.6

Symptoms

- Neck muscle spasms
- Extensor rigidity of back muscles
- Hyperreflexia
- Carpopedal spasm
- Trismus
- Torticollis or opisthotonos
- Oculogyric crises
- Aching or numbness of limbs
- Protrusion, discoloration, aching, and rounding of tongue
- Tonic spasm of masticatory muscles
- Tight feeling in throat or dysphagia

Acute Treatment

- Diphenhydramine (Benadryl) 50 mg (2 mg/kg, up to 50 mg, for children) IV or IM; refer immediately
- Discontinue use of antipsychotic agent; symptoms subside within 24 to 48 hours

AKATHISIA (7% TO 20% OCCURRENCE)

781.0

Symptoms
- Constant motor restlessness
- Possibly feelings of muscle quivering, an inability to sit still, and an urge to constantly move about

Occurrence
- Can occur early or after several months of treatment
- 30- to 60-year-olds are more susceptible

Treatment
- Benzodiazepines, propranolol, and clonidine (Catapres) have been used for treatment
- Anticholinergic agents are ineffective

SUGGESTED EVALUATION FOR EXTRAPYRAMIDAL SYMPTOMS
- Evaluate upon initiation of antipsychotic agents and every 6 months thereafter
- Use the same format for evaluation each time for consistency (suggested format follows)
- There is no "right" score; comparison of scores provides information on the development of involuntary movements (i.e., tardive dyskinesia)

Tardive Dyskinesia Rating Scale
Face

1. Blinking of eyes	—	Score:
2. Tremor of eyelids	—	1 = absent
3. Tremor of upper lip (rabbit syndrome)	—	2 = questionable
4. Pouting of the (lower) lip	—	3 = mild
5. Puckering of lips	—	4 = moderate
6. Sucking movements	—	5 = moderately severe
7. Chewing movements	—	6 = very severe
8. Smacking of lips	—	
9. Bonbon sign	—	
10. Tongue protrusion	—	
11. Tongue tremor	—	
12. Choreoathetoid movements of tongue	—	
13. Facial tics	—	
14. Grimacing	—	
15. Other (describe)	—	
16. Other (describe)	—	

Neck and Trunk

17. Head nodding	—
18. Retrocollis	—

14

Continued

19. Spasmodic torticollis   —
20. Torsion movements (trunk)   —
21. Axial hyperkinesia   —
22. Rocking movement   —
23. Other (describe)   —
24. Other (describe)   —

Extremities (Upper)
25. Ballistic movements   —
26. Choreoathetoid movements—fingers   —
27. Choreoathetoid movements—wrists   —
28. Pill-rolling movements   —
29. Caressing or rubbing face and hair   —
30. Rubbing of thighs   —
31. Other (describe)   —
32. Other (describe)   —

Extremities (Lower)
33. Rotation and/or flexion of ankles   —
34. Toe movements   —
35. Stamping movements—standing   —
36. Stamping movements—sitting   —
37. Restless legs   —
38. Crossing/uncrossing legs—sitting   —
39. Other (describe)   —
40. Other (describe)   —

Entire Body
41. Holokinetic movements   —
42. Akathisia   —
43. Other (describe)   —

Dementia

294.8

Definition

Dementia is defined as memory problems, especially with learning new things plus at least one of the following:

- Apraxia: difficulty with voluntary movements even though motor systems are intact
- Agnosia: difficulty recognizing previously known item (e.g., pencil)
- Executive functioning: decision-making abilities and the ability to carry out the plan
- Aphasia

14

Dementia Disorders

Alzheimer's Disease	331.0
Delirium	780.09
Confusion	298.9
Hydrocephalus	331.4
Vascular Dementia	290.40

DISORDERS	SYMPTOMS
Alzheimer's disease	Insidious onset; slowly progressive
	Impairment of memory
	More common in elderly
Confusion	Acute onset
	Normal alertness but abnormal thought content
	Unable to process information, inattention
Delirium	Abrupt onset
	Inattention and clouding of sensorium
	Perceptual disturbances, hallucinations
	Anxiety, drowsiness
Hydrocephalus	Slowly progressive over weeks to months
	Dementia
	Gait disturbances
	Urinary incontinence
Vascular dementia	Rarely insidious onset; stepwise deterioration with improvement after each downward step
	Neurologic examination with focal findings
	Stroke risk factors

Evaluation

An evaluation is performed to rule out reversible causes of dementia.*

- Laboratory tests: CBC, ESR, vitamin B_{12} and folic acid levels, thyroid function tests, chemistry panel, and serum ammonia
- Consider RPR or VDRL (neurosyphilis), HIV (as indicated)
- Probable CT or MRI of brain (subdural hematoma, brain tumor, cryptococcosis)
- Carotid Doppler studies; possibly echocardiogram
- Clock drawing test (screening tool to differentiate normal elderly from Alzheimer's disease)
  □ Ask patient to draw a clock, putting numbers in correct positions
  □ Have patient draw hands indicating either 10 minutes after 11 or 20 minutes after 8
  □ Score 0 to 5; score <5 indicates need for further evaluation

---

*Also includes depression, ETOH intoxication, and drug toxicity.

14

Draws closed circle	1 point
Places numbers in sequence	1 point
Correct spatial arrangement	1 point
Includes clock hands	1 point
Places hands in correct positions	1 point

- Mental status examination—sample questions for testing (with MMSE form)
  - Question 3: use apple–table–penny
  - Question 4: If patient has a mathematical background, use serial 7s; otherwise, ask patient to spell "world" backwards
- Consider neuropsychologic testing

Treatment
- Alzheimer's disease
  - Cholinesterase inhibitors: donepezil (Aricept), rivastigmine (Exelon), galantamine (Reminyl)
  - Vitamin E 400 IU bid
  - Treat sleep disturbances, depression, hallucinations, etc., as needed
- Vascular dementia
  - Control risk factors (e.g., HTN, DM, hyperlipidemia)
  - Stop smoking
  - Ginkgo biloba 120 mg bid
  - Vitamin E 400 IU bid
  - Treat sleep disturbances, depression, hallucinations, etc., as needed
  - Cholinesterase inhibitors may be of benefit (see above)
- Both types
  - Family education and support
  - Use memory aids and cues (e.g., handwritten daily schedule, labeling rooms and drawer contents, medication organizers)
  - Continued involvement in social activities (e.g., church, senior citizen activities) is important
  - Ensuring a safe environment (e.g., turn water heater to 120°F, provide good lighting and night lights, place locks on windows and doors, "unclutter" the house)
  - When independent living is no longer safe, options other than nursing home placement include live-in assistance (family or hired caregivers), adult daycare, respite care, residential care
  - Be sure the patient gets the recommended daily allowance of folic acid and vitamins B_6 and B_{12} (to decrease homocysteine levels)
  - If serum ammonia level is high, treat with Chronulac; start with 2 oz (60 ml) daily; monitor stools (the goal is three or four soft, formed stools daily) and serum ammonia levels; if constipation occurs, increase Chronulac by 1 tbsp (15 ml) per day every 4 days; if diarrhea occurs, decrease by 1 tbsp per day every 4 days; dementia may or may not improve

NOTES

NOTES

15

Pediatric Disorders

For complete history and physical exam, see Chapter 2.

MANAGING FEVER IN INFANTS AND CHILDREN
Fever
- Any core body temperature greater than 98° F (37° C)
- Can result from:
  □ Bacterial and viral infections
  □ Dehydration
  □ Overly warm rooms, overdressing
  □ As a response to some medications
- Investigate when an infant's fever is low grade and any of these symptoms are present:
  □ Flushing
  □ Seizure
  □ Inconsolable crying
  □ Restlessness
  □ Anorexia
  □ Tachycardia
  □ Lethargy
  □ Tachypnea
- Treatment includes:
  □ Fever control
  □ Managing the underlying condition or cause of the fever
  □ Managing any dehydration (see Table 15–1 for clinical signs of dehydration)
  □ Making the infant or child comfortable
- Initial treatment includes:
  □ Removing any excess clothing and using a lightweight sheet to cover the child
  □ Tepid sponge baths with both the parent and the child sitting in tub (caution the parent *not* to leave any infant or child alone in the bath)
  □ Give antipyretics to reduce temperature; there are three common antipyretics that can be used (Tables 15–2 and 15–3):
    1. Acetaminophen (Tylenol): Dose is 10 to 15 mg/kg q4h; not to exceed 5 doses in 24 hours; monitor liver function if doses are exceeded or if child is

Table 15–1 Clinical Signs of Dehydration in Children

SIGNS	MILD	MODERATE	SEVERE
Activity	Normal	Lethargic, irritable	Listlessness to coma state
Color	Pale	Pale–grayish	Mottled and cool extremities, cyanosis
Urine output	Decreased (<1–2 diapers per day or <2–3 ml/kg/hr)	Oliguric (1 diaper per day or <1 ml/kg/hr) Specific gravity >1.030	Anuria
Fontanelle	Flat	Depressed	Sunken fontanelle and sunken eyes
Mucous membrane	Dry with few tears noticed and decreased, thickened saliva	Very dry with diminished or no tear production and very little saliva	Cracked
Skin turgor and elasticity	Slight decrease	Marked decrease	Tenting
Pulse	Normal to increased	Increased	Tachycardic at rest
Capillary refill	<1.5 sec	1.5–3 sec	>3 sec
Blood pressure	Normal	Normal to slightly decreased	Decreased
Weight loss	5%	10%	15%
Treatment	Rehydrate at 10 ml/kg of appropriate formula, liquids, or foods Replace each fluid loss or give 1–2 tbsp of fluids q30min Avoid fluids and foods high in fat, simple sugars, and whole milk	Be aggressive with rehydration; if infant or child will not or cannot cooperate or tolerate fluids, refer to nearest hospital for IV fluids	*Refer* immediately *or* call for ambulance Initiate IV fluids if possible Start oxygen

Table 15–2 Acetaminophen Fever Control Chart

AGE	WEIGHT	INFANTS DROPS (80 mg/0.8 ml dropper q4h)	CHEWABLE TABLET (80 mg per tablet q4h)	ELIXIR (160 mg/5 ml q4h)	JUNIOR STRENGTH CHEWABLE TABLETS AND CAPLETS (160 mg per tablet q4h)
0–3 mo	6–11 lb (2–5 kg)	$\frac{1}{2}$ dropper (40 mg)	N/A	N/A	N/A
4–11 mo	12–17 lb (6–7 kg)	1 dropper (80 mg)	N/A	$\frac{1}{2}$ tsp (80 mg)	N/A
12–23 mo	18–23 lb (8–10 kg)	$1\frac{1}{2}$ dropper (120 mg)	N/A	$\frac{3}{4}$ tsp (120 mg)	N/A
2–3 yr	24–35 lb (11–15 kg)	2 dropper (160 mg)	2 tab (160 mg)	1 tsp (160 mg)	N/A
4–5 yr	36–47 lb (16–21 kg)	N/A	3 tab (240 mg)	$1\frac{1}{2}$ tsp (240 mg)	N/A
6–8 yr	48–59 lb (22–26 kg)	N/A	4 tab (320 mg)	2 tsp (320 mg)	2 cap or tab (320 mg)
9–10 yr	60–71 lb (27–32 kg)	N/A	5 tab (400 mg)	$2\frac{1}{2}$ tsp (400 mg)	$2\frac{1}{2}$ cap or tab (400 mg)
≥11 yr	>72 lb (>33 kg)	Can use adult dosing schedule			

Table 15–3	Ibuprofen 100 mg/5 ml Fever Control Chart		
AGE	WEIGHT (approx kg)	LOW FEVER (≤102.5° F [39.2° C]) 5 mg/kg q6-8h	HIGH FEVER (≥102.5° F [39.2° C]) 10 mg/kg q6-8h
6–11 mo	13–17 lb (6–7 kg)	¼ tsp (25 mg)	½ tsp (50 mg)
12–23 mo	18–23 lb (8–10 kg)	½ tsp (50 mg)	1 tsp (100 mg)
2–3 yr	24–35 lb (11–15 kg)	¾ tsp (75 mg)	1½ tsp (150 mg)
4–5 yr	36–47 lb (16–21 kg)	1 tsp (100 mg)	2 tsp (200 mg)
6–8 yr	48–59 lb (22–26 kg)	1¼ tsp (125 mg)	2½ tsp (250 mg)
9–10 yr	60–71 lb (27–32 kg)	1½ tsp (150 mg)	3 tsp (300 mg)
11–12 yr	72–95 lb (33–43 kg)	2 tsp (200 mg)	4 tsp (400 mg)

taking barbiturates, carbamazepine, isoniazid, rifampin, or sulfinpyrazone; some acetaminophen preparations contain aspartame; infants and children with phenylketonuria cannot take these preparations

2. Ibuprofen 100 mg/5 ml (Motrin); dose is based on patient's fever: fever <102.5° F (39.2° C) = 5 mg/kg q6–8h; >102.5° F (39.2° C) = 10 mg/kg q6–8h; maximum dose is 40 mg/kg/24 hr

3. Aspirin is not the drug of choice because of association with Reye's syndrome; aspirin is contraindicated with viral illnesses, bleeding disorders, and hypersensitivity

• Febrile seizures
  □ Most common in infants between the ages of 6 months and 5 years
  □ Usually occur when temperature is rapidly rising or falling
  □ All infants should be evaluated when febrile seizures occur

SCOLIOSIS SCREENING

Scoliosis is a lateral curvature of the spine that is painless initially and usually does not cause disability if slight; the child may not think anything is wrong and may only notice that clothing does not fit right. Scoliosis in girls usually progresses more frequently than that in boys, requiring correction. Early screening physical exams should start in the fifth to seventh grades. The examiner should have good lighting, maintain privacy for the exam, and for optimal results use an inclinometer to determine the amount of angle present.

• Begin by having child stand in front of you with minimal clothing and observe posture and physical proportions. Child's head should be aligned over sacrum: Observe shoulder height, scapula position and prominence, waistline symmetry, and levelness of pelvis
  □ Deviation represents curvature especially if asymmetrical elevation of scapula, uneven waistline or rib humps

- □ Tall, thin person may have Marfan syndrome (see p. 193); abnormally long metacarpals/metatarsals, idiopathic scoliosis with long sweeping right thoracic curve and left lumbar curve, pectus excavatum, and arm span greater than height
- □ Cutaneous changes such as hair patches, dermal sinuses or clefts, or >5 café-au-lait spots may indicate neurofibromatosis
- Forward-bending test with child standing is a good test to determine vertebral rotation: Have child stand with feet together and knees straight; straighten elbows and put palms together while bending forward at the waist; observe child while moving
  - □ View back of child with head down, laterally, and from behind child
  - □ Visible hump is caused by convexity of ribs and suggests vertebral rotation
  - □ An inclinometer can measure rotational deformity and approximate lateral curvature
  - □ The smaller the curve, the longer the follow-up; a 5-degree rotation in an immature child should be followed closely during the growth spurt
- Leg-length discrepancy can be tested by having the person stand with both feet together; examiner places index fingers on iliac crest area, fingers should be same height; asymmetry indicates one hip is higher than the other
- Assess fine and gross motor skills, balance, and reflexes of upper and lower extremities
- Inspect chest for deformity in rib cage or sternum
- Radiographic evaluation is needed to confirm scoliosis and to denote where the curvature(s) is located (most common is right thoracic curve)
- Early referral for evaluation, correction, or both is important for person's well-being

REMOVAL OF CERUMEN IMPACTION

Cerumen impaction can occur because of smaller ear canals, overproduction of cerumen, or improper cleaning of ear canals with cotton swabs, thus causing wax to be packed into canal.

Usual complaints of decreased hearing, fullness, or pressure are noticed first; pain may occur later.

Ear wax removal:
- Use Cerumenex 4 drops qd for 1 week *or* Colace liquid 2 to 3 drops every night for 1 week *or* Debrox drops bid for 1 to 2 weeks then
- Have person return to office and attempt to irrigate wax out with warm water squirted into ear canal gently (can use 20-cc syringe with 20-g IV catheter cut off midway) until wax is floated out; if unable to remove, retry wax softener for another week
- If ear canal is irritated or reddened after removal of wax, instill antibiotic/steroid drops tid for 24 to 48 hours and then reevaluate
- Follow-up every 3 months if indicated to reirrigate

REMOVAL OF FOREIGN OBJECT IN EAR CANAL

Foreign objects in the ear canal are common in children because children are curious about body orifices and what they will hold; always question parent about child's habits.

Common complaints are fullness, purulent drainage, foul odor, pain, "funny sounds," decreased hearing.

Gently examine canal, do not forcefully insert speculum; this may push object in farther.

If the object is visible in the outer two thirds of the ear canal, use topical anesthetic and try to remove object:
- If object is vegetable matter, do not use water because this will cause the vegetable to expand; use alligator forceps to grasp object and remove
- If object is an insect, use mineral oil to suffocate insect, then either flush it out or use alligator forceps to remove it
- If object is a small, round, hard object like a BB, seeds, or popcorn, use small wire loop/curette to scoop out
- If object is a watch battery, send to emergency department or ENT immediately

After removal of object, prophylactic antibiotic ear drops may be indicated for 1 week.

IRON REPLACEMENT THERAPY

The following chart can be used for iron replacement therapy. There are many different types of iron replacement preparations; these are only a few. When iron replacement therapy is selected, elemental (ferrous) iron is the drug of choice, and the dosage is 4 to 6 mg/kg qd. Read the label to identify the actual amount of elemental iron contained in each preparation because this may differ from product to product.

INFANTS (FERROUS SULFATE DROPS [FER-IN-SOL]): 75 mg (15 mg elemental iron)/0.6 ml			
WEIGHT	FERROUS SULFATE DROPS (ml)	NO. OF DROPPERS	FREQUENCY
5–7 kg (11–15 lb)	0.6	1	qd
7–10 kg (15–22 lb)	0.9	1.5	qd
10–13 kg (22–28 lb)	1.2	2	qd
13–16 kg (28–45 lb)	1.2*	2*	qd

From U.S. Department of Health and Human Services, Primary Care and Family Health Division, Children's Medical Services Branch, 2002.
*13–16 kg, may give 2 droppers qd or change to Ferrous Sulfate Elixir.

TODDLERS AND OLDER CHILDREN (FERROUS SULFATE ELIXIR [FEOSOL]): 220 mg (44 mg elemental iron)/5 ml		
WEIGHT	FERROUS SULFATE ELIXIR (ml)	FREQUENCY
10–11 kg (22–24 lb)	3.0	qd
11–13 kg (24–29 lb)	4.0	qd
13–17 kg (29–38 lb)	5.0	qd
17–24 kg (38–53 lb)	3.0 *or*	bid
	5.0	qd
24–31 kg (53–68 lb)	4.0 *or*	bid
	5.0	qd
>32 kg (>68 lb)	4.0 *or*	bid
	5.0†	qd

From U.S. Department of Health and Human Services, Primary Care and Family Health Division, Children's Medical Services Branch, 2002.

*13–16 kg, may give 2 droppers qd or change to Ferrous Sulfate Elixir.

†>32 kg, give as noted as elixir, or change to Ferrous Sulfate Tablets, 195 mg (39 mg elemental iron)/tablet twice daily, or 325 mg (60 mg elemental iron)/tablet once daily.

Practice Pearls

- Iron absorption is increased when given on an empty stomach; iron should be given 3 times a day between meals; avoid giving milk with iron preparations
- Giving iron in or with fruit juices will enhance absorption of iron and make the preparation more palatable
- Because iron preparations may cause gastric upset, it may be necessary to give iron shortly after meals to decrease upset stomach and poor compliance
- Iron preparations can also stain teeth; oral iron preparations should be taken with a straw, or place the dropper on the back of the child's tongue and have the child rinse the mouth or brush teeth immediately after swallowing the drops
- Warn the parents that stools may turn black or green, and stool consistency may change to either diarrhea or constipation
- Tell the parents that therapy may take as long as 6 months to complete and that follow-up may be required yearly if the problem persists
- Teach the parents how to give medications safely
- Advise the parents on the child's greater dietary needs for vitamin C and for foods rich in iron (see Appendix B)
- Caution parents to keep iron preparations out of reach of child because iron is the most commonly overingested pediatric drug

PRIMARY CARE DISORDERS

Table 15–4 provides an overview of selected pediatric disorders encountered in primary care.

Text continued on p. 458

Table 15–4 Primary Care Disorders

DISORDER	SIGNS AND SYMPTOMS	DIAGNOSIS
Attention-Deficit Hyperactivity Disorder (ADHD) and Attention Deficit Disorder (ADD)		
Attention-Deficit Hyperactivity Disorder (ADHD) 314.01		
Defined by developmentally inappropriate degrees of inattention, impulsiveness, and hyperactivity	Parental reports of child's behavior Symptom duration of at least 6 mo Onset before age 7 yr *Must Exhibit at Least Eight of the Following* Often fails to finish things he or she starts Often does not seem to listen Easily distracted Has difficulty concentrating on tasks Is always on the "go" Often acts before thinking Goes from one activity to another rapidly Needs a lot of supervision Frequently calls out in class Has difficulty waiting turn in games or groups Runs about or climbs on things excessively Has difficulty sitting still or fidgets a lot Cannot stay seated Excessive movement during sleep	Assess behavior while in exam room Screening lab: TSH, lead screen, CBC *Not to Be Missed* Refer for assessment of learning disabilities, IQ, hand-eye coordination, auditory and visual perception, comprehension, and memory (resources include school and private psychologists) Neoplasms causing hyperactivity Other intracranial assaults or abnormalities causing hyperactivity Psychosocial maladjustment Pervasive developmental disorders
Upper Respiratory Tract Disorders		
Otitis Media 382.9 Otitis Externa 380.10 Allergic Rhinitis 477.9 Sinusitis 473.9 Pharyngitis (Pharyngotonsillitis) 465.8 Common Cold 460. Influenza 487.1		
Otitis Media Inflammation or infection of middle ear; purulent vs. serous effusion	Fever, malaise, ear pain, irritability, ear drainage (indicates perforation), N/V	Abnormal results from tympanometry Positive results from tympanocentesis and culture

*Often cease to be effective after 9 to 18 months and require change to another class of antidepressant.

TREATMENT	EDUCATION
Consider Medication *Amphetamine stimulant* Dextroamphetamine/amphetamine (Adderall) *Methylphenidate stimulant* Ritalin, Concerta *Non-stimulants* Atomoxetine (Strattera) <70 kg: 0.5 mg/kg day; 70 kg: 40–80 mg day Guanfacine (Intuniv) 6–17 yr: 1–4 mg/day; adjust dose based on age and size *Antidepressants* Bupropion (Wellbutrin) 1.4–6 mg/kg/day Paroxetine (unlabeled use) 10–20 mg/day Sertraline (unlabeled use) 50 mg bid *Miscellaneous* Clonidine; dose dependent on age and weight	Review monitoring routines for medications and appointments Absorption of stimulants is significantly impaired by citric acid and vitamin C; *do not* take these products 1 hr before or after medication. (e.g., citrus fruit and juice, toaster pastries, most carbonated beverages, granola/breakfast bars, high vitamin cereals, oral suspension medicines) Teach parents behavioral modification techniques and to provide firm, realistic, and environmental limits Educate parents regarding the best way to assist their child to learn Refer for special education, if needed
Uncomplicated AOM: Consider 5-day course of antibiotics; if complicated, use 10 days	Hydration Finish all the antibiotics as prescribed Proper feeding methods to prevent fluid reflux

Continued

Table 15–4 Primary Care Disorders—cont'd

DISORDER	SIGNS AND SYMPTOMS	DIAGNOSIS
Common Causes	*Acute Otitis Media (AOM)*	Abnormal results from
Bacteria	Inflammation, erythema,	hearing and language
Streptococcus pneumoniae	distorted landmarks, diffuse	screenings
Haemophilus influenzae	light reflex, decreased	*Not to Be Missed*
Moraxella catarrhalis	tympanic membrane (TM)	Unresponsive to
β-Hemolytic streptococcus	mobility, more acute onset	treatment
Viruses	*Otitis Media with Effusion*	AOM: 3 recurrences in
RSV	*(OME)*	6 mo
Adenoviruses	Usually occurs after AOM	Chronic OME: more
Influenza A	TM pink or orange, opaque,	than 12 wk duration
	slightly bulging, or retracted	Evidence of hearing loss
	Will see fluid level or bubbles	or speech delay
	Usually associated with	R/O mastoiditis,
	symptoms of URI	cholesteatoma, and
		meningitis
		Do not confuse with red
		TM due to crying
Otitis Externa		
External ear infection or	Pruritus, tinnitus	Diagnostic findings
inflammation	Pain associated with	nonspecific
Common Causes	movement of pinna,	*Not to Be Missed*
Pseudomonas	pressure on tragus, or ear	Unresponsive to
Staphylococcus epidermidis	examination	treatment
Aspergillus	Full or clogged feeling	Serious systemic
If furuncles noted in	Hearing loss in affected ear	symptoms
external acoustic meatus,	Otorrhea (white or green	Mastoiditis
cause is probably	discharge)	
Staphylococcus aureus or	History of swimming in lake	
Streptococcus pyogenes	or pool	
Commonly associated with	History of frequent swimmer's	
eczema and seborrheic	ear	
dermatitis	Ear canal edema	
	Preauricular and postauricular	
	adenopathy	
Allergic Rhinitis		
IgE-mediated allergic	Itching, burning eyes with	Eosinophil count elevated
response to pollens,	mild conjunctivitis	either in nasal

TREATMENT	EDUCATION
Antibiotic Choices Amoxicillin (still first choice); if no improvement in 72 hr, increase dose to 80–90 mg/kg qd or use alternative antibiotic Azithromycin (second choice) 10 mg/kg/ qd × 3 days or 30 mg/kg once; if no improvement in 72 hr, use alternative antibiotic **Alternative Antibiotics** Amoxicillin/clavulanate ES 600 mg/5 ml bid or Cefuroxime 20 mg/kg qd in bid dosing Ceftriaxone 50 mg/kg IM up to 1 g (single dose) **Pain Relief** Auralgan 2–4 gtts prn pain Acetaminophen, ibuprofen on routine basis for 48 hr Heat or cold application Otikon Otic solution Analgesia with codeine	Avoid exposure to cigarette smoking Follow-up in 2 wk–1 mo to determine if otitis media has resolved Eustachian tube autoinflation to build up positive pressure in nasopharynx: have child chew gum, or blow up balloon, or hold nose and puff cheeks and swallow Consider pneumococcal vaccine for children >2 yr with recurrent AOM Refer to ENT specialist with persistent AOM or 4 cases in 6 mo Persistent OME can occur but does not require antibiotic treatment Prophylactic therapy for recurrent AOM may be used with each URI instead of daily at lower doses because of increased resistance
If possible, irrigation to remove debris Ear wick first 24–48 hr (aids with distributing medication to ear canal) **Topical Antibiotic × 5–7 days** Cortisporin otic solution or suspension 3–4 drops tid Vasocidin ophthalmic solution 1–2 drops tid Ciprofloxin Otic suspension 3 drops bid Ofloxacin Otic suspension 5 drops bid × 10 days If persistent, suspect *Aspergillus*; use acetic acid (VoSol) 4 drops tid	Prevention: instill a few drops of a 1:1 solution of white vinegar and rubbing alcohol after swimming or "swimmer's ear" solution or use cotton or tissue wick after swimming or showering to remove excess water in ear canal Keep all water out of ear, using small cotton ball impregnated with petrolatum (Vaseline) during shampoo Follow-up in 5–10 days, if not improved Can consider routine use of ear plugs with water exposure, but this can cause irritation and return of symptoms Treat eczema and seborrheic dermatitis if this is cause
Decongestants OTC of choice	Avoid known allergens Air conditioning and air purifiers at home

Continued

Table 15–4	Primary Care Disorders—cont'd		
DISORDER	**SIGNS AND SYMPTOMS**	**DIAGNOSIS**
grasses, weeds, dust, mold, animal dander or saliva, or something in the child's environment	Allergic "shiners," allergic "salute," and allergic expression (gaping mouth) Sneezing, coughing, nasal congestion, or rhinorrhea with clear discharge Irritable, short tempered, and cranky Mouth breathing and snoring Boggy, bluish discoloration to nasal mucosa	secretions or serum Positive results from skin testing for allergens
Sinusitis Responsible organisms: *H. influenzae* *S. pneumoniae* *M. catarrhalis* GABHS *S. aureus*	Fever H/A Coughing attacks, usually from postnasal drip and usually occur at night Purulent rhinorrhea that lasts beyond common cold symptoms Pain in upper teeth (maxillary sinus) or pain when bending forward (frontal sinus) Facial pain Halitosis Tenderness over forehead or below eyes with percussion Inflamed nasal mucosa	CT sinuses for persistent infection

TREATMENT	EDUCATION
Antihistamines OTC of choice *or* Hydroxyzine 2–4 mg/kg qd q6h Cetirizine (Zyrtec) 2.5–10 mg qd; adjust for age >2 yr Fexofenadine (Allegra) 30 mg bid for age >6 yr Desloratadine (Clarinex) 5 mg qd for age >12 yr *Leukotriene Antagonist* Montelukast (Singulair) 4 or 5 mg qd hs *Intranasal Steroids* Beclomethasone (Beconase AQ) 1–2 sprays bid Flunisolide (Nasalide) 1–2 sprays bid Mometasone furoate (Nasonex) for children 2–12 yr, 1 spray qd Fluticasone (Flonase) for children >4 yr, 1 spray qd *Other Intranasal Spray* Cromolyn sodium 1 spray q4h (onset takes ~2–4 wk) not a steroid; start before known exposure *Topical Medications* OTC of choice	Watch child for hearing loss from chronic otitis media May have nosebleeds from dryness; apply nonpetrolatum product at night to anterior nares Follow-up 2 wk to monitor progress

Antibiotics
Usually given for a minimum of 10 days because of the difficulty of penetrating the sinus cavities:
Amoxicillin 400 mg/5 ml, 40 mg/kg qd in 2 doses
Amoxicillin/clavulanate 400 mg/5 ml, 25 mg/kg qd in 2 doses
Cefuroxime axetil 250 mg/5 ml, 30 mg/kg qd in 2 doses
Cefdinir (Omnicef) 250 mg/5 ml 14 mg/kg/day q12–24h
 	
Topical Steroids
Usually recommended for children >6 yr:
Beclomethasone (Beconase AQ) 1–2 sprays each nostril bid
Flunisolide (Nasalide) 1–2 sprays each nostril bid
	Humidification
	Saline nose spray
	Analgesics:
	  Acetaminophen
	  Ibuprofen
	Epistaxis may occur with dryness or increased blowing of nose and inflammation; have parents or child use a nonpetrolatum jelly for insertion into anterior nares
	Showering in the morning and before bedtime will help humidify respiratory system

Continued

Table 15–4 Primary Care Disorders—cont'd

DISORDER	SIGNS AND SYMPTOMS	DIAGNOSIS
Pharyngitis (Pharyngotonsillitis)		
Bacteria	*Bacterial*	Throat culture
GABHS is the most common bacterium	Usually occurs in a child >3 yr	Rapid streptococci screen
	Sudden onset	CBC
Viruses	Moderately ill appearing	
Viruses are the most common cause	Sore throat, abdominal pain, and N/V	
	Petechial pattern on soft palate	
	Fine sandpaper-like red rash on face and torso	
	Fever >102° F (38.8° C)†	
	Tender, enlarged cervical lymph nodes†	
	Tonsils are enlarged and inflamed with varying degrees of purulent exudate†	
	No cough†	
	Viral	
	Can occur at any age	
	Gradual onset	
	Appears mildly to moderately ill	
Common Cold	Mucoid rhinorrhea	None indicated
Rhinovirus most common	Scratchy throat	Diagnosis based on symptoms
	Nonproductive cough	
	Loss of taste and smell	
	Sneezing	
	Feeling "stuffed up"	

†With all four criteria, treat for strep. With two or three criteria, get a rapid strep test and treat if results are positive. With less than two criteria, do not treat for strep, but treat symptoms.

TREATMENT	EDUCATION

Decongestants
Topical for short-term use and older children
Oral antihistamines may worsen and prolong congestion
 	
Follow-up
At the completion of antibiotics or if symptoms worsen
 	
Bacterial
Penicillin VK 250 mg/5 ml (25–50 mg/kg qd) tid × 10 days
Azithromycin 12 mg/kg (maximum 500 mg) qd × 5 days
Cefaclor 250 mg/5 ml (20–40 mg/kg qd) in 2–3 doses × 7–10 days
Cefdinir (Omnicef) 14 mg/kg/day bid
Bicillin CR, single dose
  <30 lb, 600,000 U
  30–60 lb, 900,000 to 1.2 million U
  >60 lb, 1.2 million to 2.4 million U
 	
Viral
Usually supportive care
 	
Follow-up
In 24–48 hr
	Symptomatic Treatment for Bacterial and Viral Infections
	Warm saline gargles
	Isolation until 24 hr after antibiotic therapy was started
	Child may return to school when temperature has been normal for 24 hr
	Push fluids, either cold or warm
	Throat lozenges or hard candy may help pain
	Acetaminophen for fever or pain q4h for 48 hr
	Humidification
	Discard toothbrush; buy 2 new ones; use 1 for first 48 hr; then use the second one

No antibiotics unless secondary infection occurs **Decongestants/Antihistamines** *OTC of Choice* *Prescription* (see package for dosing) Rynatan Pediatric suspension Nalex A liquid Palgic D syrup **Other Treatment** Analgesics	Symptoms should last ~7–10 days; if longer, follow-up is needed

Continued

Table 15–4 Primary Care Disorders—cont'd

DISORDER	SIGNS AND SYMPTOMS	DIAGNOSIS
Influenza Viral strains vary on an annual basis	Sudden onset of: Malaise Fever H/A Myalgia Coryza Cough Sore throat	Usually none Rapid influenza testing is available depending on viral strain

Lower Respiratory Tract Disorders

> Bronchiolitis **466.19**
> Croup **464.4**
> Epiglottitis **464.30**
> Respiratory Syncytial Virus (RSV) **079.6**
> Pneumonia **486.**

Bronchiolitis and Other Croup Syndromes		
Inflammation of the airways Causative agents: usually viral	Barky cough, especially sporadic at night Temperature low to normal Abrupt onset stridor, hoarseness, and coryza Lungs: diffuse rales, wheezes, and decreased breath sounds	"Steeple sign" of epiglottis on lateral neck x-ray film WBCs: normal to low CXR may show hyperinflation and mild infiltrates
		Not to Be Missed Respiratory distress Bacterial infection Pertussis or diphtheria Aspiration of foreign body Epiglottitis
Epiglottitis Severe, rapidly progressive infection of the epiglottis Leads to airway obstruction *H. influenzae* is most common cause	Acute, severe sore throat and drooling ***Do not* inspect pharynx until ready to intubate; inspection may cause laryngospasm and airway obstruction** Acute high fever >105° F (40.5° C)	CBC: increased WBCs Lateral neck x-ray film shows thickened mass

TREATMENT	EDUCATION
Rest Increase fluid intake Humidifier or vaporizer	

No antibiotics unless secondary infection
  occurs
Analgesics
Cough or cold preparations
Rest
Push fluids
	Symptoms should last ~7–10 days; if
	  longer, follow-up is needed

Humidified air
O$_2$ if child is hypoxic
Prevention of dehydration
Antibiotics only if secondary infection is
  present
Consider nebulized bronchodilator and
  budesonide (Pulmicort) 0.25% bid
Consider systemic steroids if severe (see
  Table 4–3)
Dexamethasone suspension 0.6 mg/kg
  IV/IM for severe croup or 12.5 ml in
  50 ml cherry-flavored syrup × 1 for mild
  croup
	Methods of humidifying home
	S/S of complications
	Optimal hydration

Refer immediately to emergency department	Prevention: Hib vaccine

Continued

Table 15–4 Primary Care Disorders—cont'd		
DISORDER	**SIGNS AND SYMPTOMS**	**DIAGNOSIS**
	Froglike voice	
	Respiratory distress	
	Anxiety, irritability, restlessness, and fear	
	Tripod position with hyperextended neck	
Respiratory Syncytial Virus (RSV)		
Acute viral illness	Very contagious	RSV throat culture or sputum culture: results are positive
Most severe in infancy	Respiratory distress	
Most common in winter–spring	Rhinorrhea	
	Pharyngitis	***Not to Be Missed***
	Cough	Severe respiratory distress, hypoxia, or tachypnea
	Sneezing	
	Wheezing	Bacterial superinfection such as pneumonia
	Sternal retractions	
Pneumonia		
Common in the winter	Usual history of URI	WBCs: 18,000–40,000 with shift to left if bacterial
Common to all age groups	Sudden rise in temperature up to 104° F (40° C) with chills	
Bacterial pneumonia has an abrupt onset	Cough	CXR: patchy infiltrates with lobar consolidation
Viral pneumonia has a more insidious onset	Tachypnea	
	Inspiratory rales that do not resolve with cough	***Not to Be Missed***
	Intercostal retractions	Signs of increasing respiratory distress such as cyanosis, grunting respirations, flaccid appearance, and respirations >60 with severe intercostal retraction
	Hyperresonance over areas of consolidation	
	Decreased breath sounds	
	May be unilateral or bilateral lung involvement	
	Symptoms not present at birth	

TREATMENT	EDUCATION
Consider referral or consultation Hospitalize if severe respiratory distress Ribavirin by nebulizer may be indicated in hospital Humidification (cold) Rehydration with oral or IV therapy Control fever (if present) with acetaminophen NOTE: Consider SYNAGIS for prophylaxis for premature infants or those with bronchopulmonary dysplasia; do not use if infection is present	Special care to prevent spread of infection Methods to humidify room/house Review possible complications and when to return to office or go to hospital Optimal hydration therapy
Suspected Bacterial Origins Antibiotics: Amoxicillin/clavulanate 400 mg/5 ml, 60 mg/kg qd in 2 doses × 10 days Cefuroxime axetil 250 mg/5 ml, 20 mg/kg qd in 2 doses × 10 days Azithromycin 200 mg/5 ml, 10 mg/kg on day 1, then 5 mg/kg qd on days 2–5 (max. 250 mg)	Discuss methods of hydration and types of fluids to use Place humidifier or vaporizer at bedside Teach how to use and read a thermometer Teach how to give medications to the child
Suspected Viral Origin Supportive care with humidifier or vaporizer Push fluids Acetaminophen for fever q4h Cough suppressants at night with dextromethorphan If wheezing, may need albuterol liquid 0.1–0.2 mg/kg per dose q6–8h	

Continued

15

Table 15-4	Primary Care Disorders—cont'd	
DISORDER	SIGNS AND SYMPTOMS	DIAGNOSIS

Abdominal Disorders

Pyloric Stenosis	537.0
Intussusception	560.0
Gastroenteritis	558.9
Encopresis	307.7
Acute Diarrhea	787.91
Gastroesophageal Reflux Disease (GERD)	530.81

Pyloric Stenosis

DISORDER	SIGNS AND SYMPTOMS	DIAGNOSIS
Pyloric sphincter is hypertrophied, leading to obstruction	Symptoms not present at birth Nonbilious emesis, usually starts at 2–4 wk Vomiting after feeding; progressively worsens and becomes projectile May lead to complete obstruction by 4–6 wk Poor weight gain Hungry infant after emesis Constipation Dehydration Visible peristaltic waves traversing epigastrium left to right Palpable pyloric "olive" (to right of umbilicus below liver edge) more prominent after vomiting Lethargy and irritability	Upper GI tract radiographic studies reveal delayed gastric emptying and an elongated, threadlike pyloric channel ("string sign") Blood work may show metabolic alkalosis, decreased Na^+, decreased K^+, and other fluid and electrolyte imbalances *Not to Be Missed* Complete obstruction is an acute emergency
Intussusception Telescoping of one bowel segment into another, most commonly at the ileocecal valve	Sudden, acute abdominal pain, vomiting (especially after viral illness) Colicky, abdominal pain characterized by drawing up knees and stiffening legs Bloody or "currant jelly" stools several hours after onset of pain Sausage-shaped mass in right upper quadrant Fever, lethargy Shocklike state if not reduced	Barium enema is definitive but dangerous to perform if bowel is already perforated; so obtain an abdominal x-ray film to detect intraperitoneal air first 10% resolve spontaneously, but 90% worsen, and child will die without treatment *Not to Be Missed* Rule out incarcerated hernia Malrotation of colon

TREATMENT	EDUCATION
Refer to surgeon for surgery as soon as possible Restoration of fluid and electrolyte balance	Some vomiting in first 24–48 hr postoperatively is normal Analgesics for pain after surgery
Refer to surgeon	Watch for passage of normal brown stool as indication that the intussusception has resolved First 3 days after reduction are greatest risk for recurrence

Continued

Table 15–4	Primary Care Disorders—cont'd	

DISORDER	SIGNS AND SYMPTOMS	DIAGNOSIS
Gastroenteritis May be viral (often in winter), bacterial (often in summer), or parasitic Recent history of antibiotic use Recent history of travel, especially internationally Recent history of playing in or drinking from streams or rivers	Anorexia, N/V, diarrhea of varying severity Weight loss and dehydration (see Table 15–1) Assess for other diagnosis that causes N/V such as otitis media, streptococcal pharyngitis, or pneumonia, UTI Hyperactive bowel sounds and abdominal tenderness (diffuse) Splenomegaly with bacterial agents Fever (worsens dehydration)	Assess: Dehydration status (see Table 15–1); BUN, electrolytes, pH, HCO_3^-, etc. Stool for O&P, WBC, culture UA and C&S if indicated *Not to Be Missed* Reye's syndrome Food allergy Metabolic disease (DM) Severe dehydration (see Table 15–1) Gastroenteritis not relieved with treatment
Encopresis Syndrome with repeated incontinence of stools usually secondary to constipation without an organic problem Cycle of constipation: pain with bowel movement, withholding stool, colon enlarges, larger stool holding capacity, constipation Decreased sensation to defecate Seen more often in boys, usually older than 4 years	Stool leakage with or without knowledge of event Abdominal pain and distention Stools are hard, dry, and small May have increased straining when defecating May have decreased anal tone with large rectal vault and hard stool Fissures around anus May palpate soft, nontender mass in left lower quadrant Anorexia	Abdominal x-ray examination for fecal volume UA *Not to Be Missed* Hirschsprung's disease Irritable bowel syndrome Hypothyroidism Neuromuscular dysfunction Cerebral palsy Obstruction in urinary tract system Sexual abuse Anal fissures
Acute Diarrhea Usually a self-limited disorder that consists of an increased number of liquid stools Many different causes (see p. 232), but diet is the most common cause	Dehydration (see Table 15–1) May have fever Abdominal distention with hyperactive bowel sounds and increased tympany May have some abdominal tenderness	May do stool for O&P, C&S Stool for occult blood (results should be negative) CBC with differential UA

TREATMENT	EDUCATION
Most diarrhea and vomiting is self-limited Correct dehydration, fluid and electrolyte imbalance, and acid-base imbalance Oral rehydration fluids such as Infalyte oral solution or Pedialyte Begin offering liquids in small amounts for first 24 hr; try 1 tbsp q10–15 min; increase as liquids are better tolerated Antimicrobials or antiparasitics as indicated No antimotility drugs Probiotics bid for 1 mo No whole milk for 48 hr; may use diluted skim milk or lactose-free formula Follow-up in 24 hr If symptoms unresolved, may need IV fluids	Review proper sanitation, hand washing, and food preparation Within 24 hours of onset reintroduce feedings such as breast milk, dilute formula, or BRATY diet (see Appendix B) Advance to regular diet as soon as possible to avoid "starvation diarrhea" Jell-O, Gatorade, and soda contain too much carbohydrate and too little sodium to be used as proper rehydration solutions May need lactose- or sucrose-free formula for a short period for the 20% of infants who develop intolerance to their usual formula after infectious diarrhea
Bowel Training Program (to Break the Hard Stool–Pain Cycle) FLEETS enema for initial visit Use mineral oil (not near meals) 1–3 tsp tid or qid until results are achieved; decrease amount until ~2 stools a day Establish regular schedule to defecate Do not put "pressure" on child to defecate After stools are established, increase fiber in diet, push fluids and water-soluble vitamins B complex and C Docusate sodium (Colace) 5–10 mg/kg qd for maintenance after stools are established Chronulac 15–30 cc qd	Discourage laxatives and enemas Reinforce that bowel habits are individualized Advise to make bathroom time quiet and pleasant and have appropriate size toilet stool Discuss dietary changes Follow-up q2wk
Rehydrate (see Gastroenteritis for hydration tips) Rest bowel Begin feeding slowly; if breast-feeding, continue nursing Isomil DF for 7–10 days in infants to toddlers	Teach signs of dehydration Discuss types of foods to use and foods to avoid such as milk, high-sugar juices, and meats until diarrhea begins to resolve Use protective ointment or gels for diaper area to prevent irritation

Continued

Table 15–4 Primary Care Disorders—cont'd

DISORDER	SIGNS AND SYMPTOMS	DIAGNOSIS
Diarrhea can be caused by infection, inflammation, antibiotics, anatomic diseases, protozoa and parasites (i.e., giardia, cryptosporidium), and various other parasites (e.g., roundworms, pinworms) Common condition during infancy and early childhood	Get an estimate of number of stools per day, color, odor, amount, and any associated vomiting Is child acting ill with diarrhea and is child eating well? When was last meal and where? Any worms noted in stools?	*Not to Be Missed* Starvation Food intolerance Otitis media UTI Pneumonia GABHS Pharyngitis Pseudomembranous colitis Inflammatory bowel disease Malabsorption syndromes Necrotizing enterocolitis
Gastroesophageal Reflux Disease (GERD) Reflux of gastric secretions into esophagus and oropharynx Common in premature infants up to the age 6 mo but usually resolves by age 1 yr Symptoms may persist into adulthood Chronic reflux may lead to remodeling of distal esophageal mucosa with metaplastic intestinal-like epithelium (e.g., Barrett's esophagus, adenocarcinoma) Increased risk in all patients with neurologic impairments (e.g., cerebral palsy, seizures, growth retardation)	Chronic cough Sore throat, failure to nurse/suck Hoarseness Wheezing, asthma Apnea Bradycardia Dental erosions Halitosis Laryngitis Sinusitis Otitis media Frequent spitting up *Warning Signs* Recurrent vomiting Weight loss, failure to thrive Hematemesis Constipation Diarrhea Fever Lethargy Abdominal distention/pain	Complete blood count Electrolytes BUN/creatinine Swallowing studies Endoscopy Biopsy Esophageal pH monitor Upper GI studies to detect structural abnormalities: Strictures Intestinal malrotation Hiatal hernia

TREATMENT	EDUCATION

If worms noted in stool or at anal opening:
   Vermox 100 mg bid for 3 days for
     roundworms, 100 mg × 1 for pinworms
Evaluate entire household
No whole milk for 48 hr; may use skim milk
   or lactose-free formulas
Follow-up in 24 hr
	Careful hand washing
	Check weight daily
	Follow-up in 24 hr
	Explain necessity to return to office or
	   emergency department if child stops
	   taking fluids, starts vomiting, or appears
	   dehydrated

If baby is formula fed, switch to
   hypoallergenic formula
Add rice cereal to formula one or two times
   daily
Elevate head of bed or put infant in
   portable carrier after meals (if placing
   baby in carrier, put small pillow under
   buttocks to keep hips extended to prevent
   undue increase in gastric pressure)
Have older child sleep on left side; position
   with pillows
 	
Pharmacotherapy Includes
Antacids of Choice
Sucralfate (Carafate) 1 g/10 ml
   Infants >1 mo: 0.25 g–0.5 g orally qid
Children >6 yr: 0.5 g–1 g qid
Caution if patient has renal failure
 	
Metoclopramide (Reglan) 5 mg/5 ml
   Infants >1 mo: 0.1–0.2 mg/kg po, may use
     up to qid, not to exceed 0.5 mg/kg qd
 	
H_2 Blocker
Famotidine (Pepcid) 40 mg/5 ml
   <3 mo: 0.5 mg/kg qd
   3–11 mo: 0.5 mg–1 mg/kg bid
   1–16 yr: 1 mg/kg/d bid
   Not to exceed 40 mg bid
Ranitidine (Zantac) 15 mg/ml
   1 mo–16 yr: 5–10 mg/kg in 2 divided
   doses
	Counsel family to abstain from cigarette
	   smoking
	Minimize intake of any foods that might
	   worsen reflux (e.g., caffeine, chocolate,
	   and fried, fatty, or spicy foods)
	Encourage weight loss if child is obese
	Encourage physical activity
	Encourage small, frequent meals

Continued

Table 15–4 Primary Care Disorders—cont'd		
DISORDER	**SIGNS AND SYMPTOMS**	**DIAGNOSIS**

Genitourinary Tract Disorders

Hypospadias   752.61
Cryptorchidism (Undescended Testicles)   752.51
Enuresis   788.30
Urinary Tract Infection   599.0

Hypospadias

Urinary meatus located on ventral side of penis, most often on glans	Abnormal urinary stream Chordee causing a ventral curve	*If Severe* X-ray examination, U/S or excretory urography to R/O associated anomalies *If Mild* No pertinent diagnostic studies ***Not to Be Missed*** Associated GU tract abnormalities and meatal stenosis

Cryptorchidism (Undescended Testicles)

Incidence is 3%–6% in general population, 30% in preterm boys 20% chance of testicular cancer later in life Increased incidence of hypogonadism even after repair	Differentiate between cryptorchidism and retractile testes by having child sit with crossed legs (tailor sit) and examine on several occasions to document true cryptorchidism	If bilateral, chromosomal study for gender genotype may be indicated

TREATMENT	EDUCATION

Cimetidine (Tagamet) 200 mg/20 ml; 300 mg/5 ml
  Infants: 10 20 mg/kg in 2 divided doses
  Children: 20–40 mg/kg qd divided every 6 hr
 	
PPI
Omeprazole (Prilosec)
  No oral solution available; capsule can be opened and sprinkled on applesauce: may be given to children as young as 2 yr
  <20 kg: 10 mg qd
  ≥20 kg: 20 mg qd
Lansoprazole (Prevacid) 15 mg and 30 mg granule packets; may be given to children as young as 1 yr
  ≤30 kg: 15 mg qd
  >30 kg: 30 mg qd	

Refer to urologist for corrective surgery for cosmetic, functional, or psychologic reasons	Repair should be done early for psychologic reasons
Refer to urologist by 10 mo Assess often in infancy and yearly thereafter Surgical correction Timing of corrective measures varies from before 3 yr to adolescence in hope that testicle will descend	Educate about the disorder, treatment options, and complications Stress the need for yearly testicular examinations even after correction

Continued

15

Table 15–4 Primary Care Disorders—cont'd

DISORDER	SIGNS AND SYMPTOMS	DIAGNOSIS
Increased incidence of infertility	Usually unilateral but may be bilateral	
Enuresis Inability to control urination *Primary enuresis:* child was never dry *Secondary enuresis:* child was dry and now is incontinent of urine Daytime continence is usually achieved by 18–24 mo; in 80% of children by age 28 mo Nighttime continence is usually achieved by age 6 years	Family history of UTI Usual urinary habits (does child go to bathroom at school, does child wait until the last minute and then cannot make the toilet) Family history of enuresis History of sexual abuse, encopresis Physical examination is usually normal, but thoroughly examine the genitalia for abnormality, anal area for sphincter control and trauma Observe growth of legs and feet, gait Assess neurologic reflexes in lower abdomen for perianal sensation and cremasteric reflex Observe gait Observe for abnormal curvature of spine, clefts, or hair tufts at base of spine Assess interaction with parents and environment	UA *Not to Be Missed* UTI Gait abnormalities Urinary meatal malformation
Urinary Tract Infection Commonly caused by *Escherichia coli* secondary to fecal contamination and poor hygiene	Consider UTI in any infant with unexplained fever May be insidious; infants cannot tell you it hurts Fever Crankiness, fussy Decrease in appetite Weight loss Decrease in urine output; darkening of urine or strong odor Vomiting or diarrhea or both Behavior change	UA with microscopy (see p. 290) and culture if indicated CBC if indicated KUB or renal ultrasound if patient does not respond to medications *Not to Be Missed* Pinworm infestation Hypercalciuria Sexual abuse Topical irritants (e.g., bubble baths)

TREATMENT	EDUCATION
Imipramine (Tofranil) will increase bladder capacity and sphincter tone; if child is >6 yr, start with lowest dose 10–25 mg about 1 hr before bedtime; may increase if needed; monitor ECG for heart block DDAVP acts as antidiuretic; expensive but effective; start with 20 mcg (1 puff each nare) at bedtime; may adjust up to 40 mcg; if child responds to 20 mcg, consider decreasing to 10 mcg; can use this on prn basis if child is going to spend night at someone's house; will be less effective if child has "cold" symptoms due to nasal congestion; monitor Na, K, Cl Oxybutynin (Ditropan) >5 yr 0.2 mg/kg/day bid – qid Try to wean off therapies q6–12 mo	Supportive attitude for parents and child Usually child will outgrow the condition May need to educate parents and child on ways to strengthen bladder muscle by urinating on schedule during the day and gradually lengthening period between urination times Nighttime alarms may be helpful; many commercial products are available Decrease liquid intake after 6 PM and voiding before sleep No caffeine Refer if suspect underlying neurologic, genitourinary, or psychologic condition
Antibiotic treatment for 7–14 days (short regimen may not be sufficient in infants and children) TMP-SMZ suspension 8 mg/kg qd in 2 doses Amoxicillin/clavulanate 125 mg/5 ml, 30 mg/kg qd in 2 doses Cefuroxime axetil 250 mg/5 ml, 20–30 mg/kg qd in 2 doses Nitrofurantoin 5–7 mg/kg/day divided q6h × 7 days	Increase fluid intake Decrease carbonated and caffeine drinks and juices Drink cranberry juice before bedtime; may prevent future UTI Discourage bubble baths Encourage all-cotton underwear and removal of wet clothing and swimsuits immediately after use Good perineal hygiene Refer to urologist with first UTI in boys and second UTI in girls

Continued

Table 15–4	Primary Care Disorders—cont'd	
DISORDER	SIGNS AND SYMPTOMS	DIAGNOSIS
	In older children, symptoms are urgency, dysuria, frequency, hesitancy, dribbling of urine, or incontinence (in previously continent child); occasionally fever; sometimes suprapubic pain or tenderness	Candidiasis Pyelonephritis

Musculoskeletal System Disorders

Congenital Hip Dysplasia or Dislocation	754.30
Congenital Talipes Equinovarus (Club Foot)	754.51
Osgood-Schlatter Disease (Tibial Tubercle Apophysitis)	732.4

Congenital Hip Dysplasia or Dislocation

| Imperfect development of hip joint affecting the femoral head and the acetabulum, or both; may be partially or completely dislocated; femoral head dysplasia may cause flattening of the acetabulum; untreated, this will lead to immobility of the affected joint; may be hereditary or related to breech birth (14 times greater incidence) or to capsular laxity
Most often left hip
Most often in girls | ***Birth–3 Mo***
Barlow maneuver causes hip to dislocate
Ortolani maneuver reduces the joint and a "clunk" or "click" is felt
Older Infant
Limited abduction of hip
Thigh fold asymmetry
Leg length asymmetry
Unequal knee heights when supine and knees flexed
Lax hamstrings
Walking Child
Scoliosis
Leg length discrepancy | AP pelvic x-ray examination after 3 mo of age
Positive Barlow or Ortolani test for an infant <3 mo of age
U/S or MRI scan is diagnostic from birth throughout infancy for diagnosis and monitoring
Not to Be Missed
Septic arthritis
Benign clicks of hip |

Congenital Talipes Equinovarus (Club Foot)

| Forefoot abduction and inversion and ankle plantar flexion | Malformed foot
Toe-in gait
Physical appearance; inability to straighten the deformity with manipulation | Metatarsus varus is inversion of forefoot without ankle involvement
Differentiated from metatarsus varus (pigeon toe) by ankle involvement |

TREATMENT	EDUCATION
Identify early and refer to orthopedist	Stress compliance with treatments and careful follow-up
Refer to orthopedist for early treatment	Stress the need to comply with the special shoe usage, serial casting, postoperative care

Continued

| Table 15–4 | Primary Care Disorders—cont'd |

DISORDER	SIGNS AND SYMPTOMS	DIAGNOSIS
Osgood-Schlatter Disease (Tibial Tubercle Apophysitis)		
Painful, self-limiting tibial tubercle swelling caused by overuse activity	Keep pain especially during periods of rapid growth Extension of knee against resistance with application of pressure over tibial tubercle aggravates the pain Pain worsens with activity and lessens with rest Prominent tibial tuberosity	*Not to Be Missed* X-ray examination for: Osteosarcoma Patellar tendinitis Osteomyelitis Hip diseases

Hematopoietic System Disorders

Iron Deficiency Anemia	280.9
Labial Agglutination	752.49
Vulvovaginitis	616.10

Iron Deficiency Anemia		
Microcytic, hypochromic anemia Most common anemia found in infants and children *Causes* Inadequate diet, especially between the ages of 9 and 24 mo, if milk is primary food Low birth weight babies Rapid growth Blood loss from the GI tract	Anemia may develop slowly with initial symptoms of PICA and irritability *Symptoms May Progress to* Pallor, listlessness, fatigue Headache Anorexia, poor feeding, and refusing solid foods May be obese with poor muscle tone or underweight Delayed development Increased number of infections, tachycardia, and cardiac problems (e.g., murmurs, failure) Blue sclera Koilonychias Angular stomatitis	CBC with RBC indices will show: Low Hgb, Hct microcytic, hypochromic red cells MCV <80 fl Reticulocyte count may be decreased Serum iron <30 μg TIBC >350 μg/dl Stool guaiac after 2 yr; 20% of results may be positive Lead level *Not to Be Missed* Any type of blood dyscrasia (e.g., leukemia) Hereditary blood anomalies (e.g., thalassemia) Lead poisoning Anemia of chronic disease Diet deficient in table foods

TREATMENT	EDUCATION
Decrease activity during painful episodes Ice application 20 min qid NSAIDs (see Appendix E) Quadriceps stretching and strengthening program Knee pads may help control symptoms Refer to sports medicine clinic if symptoms persist	Teach about the disorder and treatment regimen Stress that the disorder is not permanent
Screening Hgb and Hct at 9 mo, between 12 and 15 mo, at 24 mo, between 11 and 15 yr, and follow-up in 6 mo if anemia present Iron replacement therapy (see p. 428) Follow-up in 1 mo and 3 mo after therapy Give multivitamin with iron daily after anemia has resolved until diet has improved	*Diet Therapy* Encourage iron-fortified formula for infants until 12 mo old Educate parents on foods high in iron (see Appendix B) Limit whole milk intake after 12 mo of age to 24 oz/d Offer foods high in vitamin C to enhance ingestion of dietary Fe (e.g., citrus fruits, strawberries, cantaloupe)

Continued

Table 15-4 Primary Care Disorders—cont'd

DISORDER	SIGNS AND SYMPTOMS	DIAGNOSIS
Labial Adhesions		
Most common in female infants 13–23 mos	Adhesion of the labia minora	If absent uterus or ambiguous sexual organs are suspected, send for U/S of pelvis
Caused by chronic irritation from bubble baths, harsh soaps, overcleaning after diaper changes	Skin may be pale and dry Urethra opening should be present Adhesion starts below clitoris and extends to posterior fourchette; unable to visualize vaginal opening	
May cause local inflammation, recurrent vulvovaginitis, or recurrent UTI		
Not seen in newborn due to circulating maternal estrogen		
Vulvovaginitis		
Inflammation of the vulva and vagina due to lack of protection from normal labial fat pads and pubic hair	Burning, itching, discharge, bleeding, dysuria	If suspicious of sexually transmitted disease, culture and refer to child advocacy center for examination and documentation
Commons causes:	Labia may be excoriated, red, have rash or bruising	
Poor perineal hygiene	Vaginal discharge: if foul odor, suspect foreign object; yellow color, suspect skin infection from scratching; white discharge without odor, suspect *Candida*	Can obtain culture and sensitivity of any drainage
Irritation from bubble baths, improper wiping after stooling		
Tight clothing		
Sand from sandbox	Labial thickening, suspect foreign object	
Hypoestrogenic state		
Bacterial infections caused by *Streptococcus, H. influenzae, E. coli, Staphylococcus*		

TREATMENT	EDUCATION
DO NOT forcefully separate labia Apply topical estrogen cream to labia minora daily for 2 wk up to 6–8 wk; when resolved, continue with use of A&D ointment Use A&D ointment or Vaseline routinely to maintain opening If patient becomes symptomatic or adhesions do not resolve, refer to pediatrician	This usually resolves by puberty

Remove irritant
Sitz bath with clear water 20 min bid
If *Candida* is suspected, use OTC cream topically
If bacteria suspected, start antibiotics for 7–10 days:
  Cephalexin 250 mg/5 ml, 25–50 mg/kg qd in 3 doses
  Amoxicillin 400 mg/5 cc, 25–50 mg/kg qd in 2 doses
For recurrent vulvovaginitis, consider nightly dose of cephalexin or amoxicillin for 30 days (after 7- to 10-day course of antibiotics)
	Educate on perineal hygiene activities
	Discourage tight clothing
	Avoid bubble baths and perfumed products
	Encourage all-cotton underwear
	Encourage thorough perineal hygiene

HYPERBILIRUBINEMIA

Jaundice is the most common condition of the newborn. This is usually benign, requiring no treatment, and usually resolves within a week of birth. In a minority of cases jaundice is an indicator of a more serious condition.

The cause of physiologic jaundice is a developmental delay in the body's ability to conjugate and excrete bilirubin. Bilirubin levels may be elevated between 6 and 8 mg/dl in the first few days after birth. Levels should decrease to normal by the end of the first week after birth. Increased levels are usually more marked in premature infants initially but should follow the same pattern as full-term infants for return to normal levels.

Close monitoring and follow-up are essential to prevent any complications and neurologic damage that could occur with sustained elevated bilirubin levels.

Hyperbilirubinemia in the Healthy Term Infant

Hyperbilirubinemia 782.4	

AGE	TREATMENT OPTIONS
<24 hr	Pathologic jaundice should be considered Thorough evaluation and treatment may be indicated Continue breast-feeding up to 12 feedings per 24 hr
25–48 hr	Discontinue breast-feeding and use formula Monitor bilirubin levels daily Consider phototherapy when total serum bilirubin ≤12 mg/dl; phototherapy should be started when bilirubin is 15 mg/dl
49–72 hr	Phototherapy indicated if bilirubin is 18 mg/dl Monitor bilirubin levels daily Consider stopping breast-feeding and using formula
>72 hr	Start phototherapy if bilirubin ≥20 mg/dl Monitor bilirubin levels daily
>14 days	Suggestive of liver or metabolic disease Evaluate thoroughly Refer to pediatrician

NOTES

NOTES

APPENDIXES

A. BODY MASS INDEX TABLES

Body Mass Index Table

Calculation of body mass index (BMI) is recommended by the National Heart, Lung, and Blood Institute as a practical means of assessing body fat. Persons with a BMI of 18.5 to 24.9 are considered to be of normal weight. Those with a BMI of 25.0 to 29.9 are overweight. Patients with a BMI of 30.0 to 34.9 or 35.0 to 39.9 are in obesity class I or II, respectively; and those with a BMI of 40 and over are considered extremely obese (obesity class III).

BMI	19	20	21	22	23	24	25	26	27	28	29	30	31	32	33	34	35	36
Height (inches)								Body weight (pounds)										
58	91	96	100	105	110	115	119	124	129	134	138	143	148	153	158	162	167	172
59	94	99	104	109	114	119	124	128	133	138	143	148	153	158	163	168	173	178
60	97	102	107	112	118	123	128	133	138	143	148	153	158	163	168	174	179	184
61	100	106	111	116	122	127	132	137	143	148	153	158	164	169	174	180	185	190
62	104	109	115	120	126	131	136	142	147	153	158	164	169	175	180	186	191	196
63	107	113	118	124	130	135	141	146	152	158	163	169	175	180	186	191	197	203
64	110	116	122	128	134	140	145	151	157	163	169	174	180	186	192	197	204	209
65	114	120	126	132	138	144	150	156	162	168	174	180	186	192	198	204	210	216
66	118	124	130	136	142	148	155	161	167	173	179	186	192	198	204	210	216	223
67	121	127	134	140	146	153	159	166	172	178	185	191	198	204	211	217	223	230
68	125	131	138	144	151	158	164	171	177	184	190	197	203	210	216	223	230	236
69	128	135	142	149	155	162	169	176	182	189	196	203	209	216	223	230	236	243
70	132	139	146	153	160	167	174	181	188	195	202	209	216	222	229	236	243	250
71	136	143	150	157	165	172	179	186	193	200	208	215	222	229	236	243	250	257
72	140	147	154	162	169	177	184	191	199	206	213	221	228	235	242	250	258	265
73	144	151	159	166	174	182	189	197	204	212	219	227	235	242	250	257	265	272
74	148	155	163	171	179	186	194	202	210	218	225	233	241	249	256	264	272	280
75	152	160	168	176	184	192	200	208	216	224	232	240	248	256	264	272	279	287
76	156	164	172	180	189	197	205	213	221	230	238	246	254	263	271	279	287	295

BMI	37	38	39	40	41	42	43	44	45	46	47	48	49	50	51	52	53	54
58	177	181	186	191	196	201	205	210	215	220	224	229	234	239	244	248	253	258
59	183	188	193	198	203	208	212	217	222	227	232	237	242	247	252	257	262	267
60	189	194	199	204	209	215	220	225	230	235	240	245	250	255	261	266	271	276
61	195	201	206	211	217	222	227	232	238	243	248	254	259	264	269	275	280	285
62	202	207	213	218	224	229	235	240	246	251	256	262	267	273	278	284	289	295
63	208	214	220	225	231	237	242	248	254	259	265	270	278	282	287	293	299	304
64	215	221	227	232	238	244	250	256	262	267	273	279	285	291	296	302	308	314
65	222	228	234	240	246	252	258	264	270	276	282	288	294	300	306	312	318	324
66	229	235	241	247	253	260	266	272	278	284	291	297	303	309	315	322	328	334
67	236	242	249	255	261	268	274	280	287	293	299	306	312	319	325	331	338	344
68	243	249	256	262	269	276	282	289	295	302	308	315	322	328	335	341	348	354
69	250	257	263	270	277	284	291	297	304	311	318	324	331	338	345	351	358	365
70	257	264	271	278	285	292	299	306	313	320	327	334	341	348	355	362	369	376
71	265	272	279	286	293	301	308	315	322	329	338	343	351	358	365	372	379	386
72	272	279	287	294	302	309	316	324	331	338	346	353	361	368	375	383	390	397
73	280	288	295	302	310	318	325	333	340	348	355	363	371	378	386	393	401	408
74	287	295	303	311	319	326	334	342	350	358	365	373	381	389	396	404	412	420
75	295	303	311	319	327	335	343	351	359	367	375	383	391	399	407	415	423	431
76	304	312	320	328	336	344	353	361	369	377	385	394	402	410	418	426	435	443

From the National Heart, Lung, and Blood Institute. (1998). *Clinical guidelines on the identification, evaluation, and treatment of overweight and obesity in adults: The evidence report.* Bethesda, MD: National Institutes of Health.

2 to 20 years: Girls
Body mass index-for-age percentiles

NAME _____

RECORD # _____

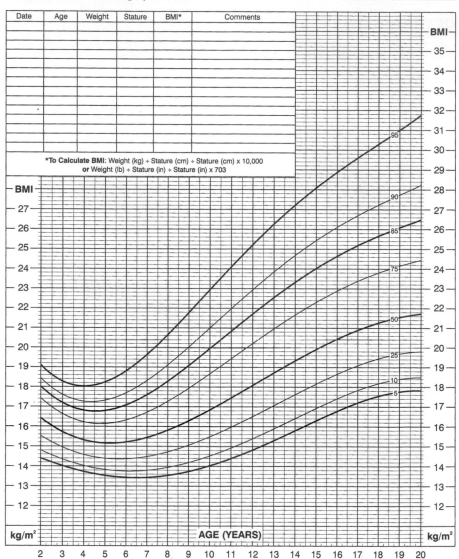

United States Centers for Disease Control and Prevention growth chart for girls, aged 2 to 20 years, BMI for age, 5th to 95th percentiles. (Developed by the National Center for Health Statistics in collaboration with the National Center for Chronic Disease Prevention and Health Promotion [2000]. Available at http://www.cdc/gov/growthcharts)

2 to 20 years: Boys
Body mass index-for-age percentiles

NAME _____

RECORD # _____

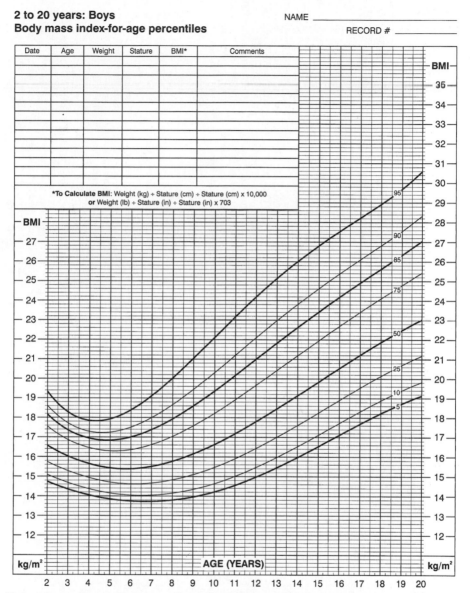

*To Calculate BMI: Weight (kg) ÷ Stature (cm) ÷ Stature (cm) x 10,000
or Weight (lb) ÷ Stature (in) ÷ Stature (in) x 703

United States Centers for Disease Control and Prevention growth chart for boys, aged 2 to 20 years, BMI for age, 5th to 95th percentiles. (Developed by the National Center for Health Statistics in collaboration with the National Center for Chronic Disease Prevention and Health Promotion [2000]. Available at http://www.cdc/gov/growthcharts)

B. FOOD SOURCES FOR SELECTED NUTRIENTS

VITAMIN K	IRON	FOLIC ACID	POTASSIUM	SODIUM	CALCIUM
GREEN, LEAFY VEGETABLES	**MEATS AND MEAT SUBSTITUTES**	**GREEN LEAFY VEGETABLES**	**CEREALS**	**FOODS TO AVOID ON A SODIUM-RESTRICTED DIET**	**DAIRY PRODUCTS** (providing at least 200 mg per serving)
Broccoli	Organ meats	Asparagus	Kellogg's All Bran	**MILK AND DAIRY PRODUCTS**	Yogurt
Brussels sprouts	All meats and poultry	Broccoli	Nabisco 100% Bran	Buttermilk	Milk (whole, 2%, or skim)
Cabbage	Shellfish	**CEREALS**	Bran flakes	Malted milk	Ice cream
Collard greens	Egg yolk	Wheat bran	Shredded wheat	Many cheeses	Milk shakes
Cucumber peel	Tofu, soybeans	Oatmeal	**FRUITS**	**MEATS AND MEAT SUBSTITUTES**	Cheese: hard cheese, ricotta, and cottage cheese
Endive	**FRUITS**	**MISCELLANEOUS**	Orange, grapefruit, or tomato (fruit or juice)	Any meat, fish, or poultry that is smoked, cured, salted, or canned (e.g., bacon, dried beef, corned beef, cold cuts, ham, turkey ham, hot dogs, sausages, sardines, anchovies, pickled herring)	**MEATS AND MEAT SUBSTITUTES** (providing at least 100 mg per serving)
Green scallions	Apricots, prunes	Red beans	Apricots, dates, or peaches (dried or fresh)	Pickled eggs	Sardines and salmon (with bones)
Kale	Raisins	Liver	Cantaloupe	**BREAD AND GRAINS**	Tofu
Lettuce	Grapes	Fish	Watermelon	Breads and rolls with salted tops	Clams
Mustard greens	**VEGETABLES**	Bananas	Prunes and raisins	Quick breads	Oysters
Parsley	Green, leafy vegetables	Peanut butter	Banana	Instant hot cereals	Shrimp
Spinach	Broccoli		Avocado	Dry cereals with added salt	**VEGETABLES AND FRUITS** (providing at least 90 mg per serving)
Turnip greens	Brussels sprouts		**VEGETABLES**	Crackers with salted tops	Spinach
Watercress	Collard greens		Baked potato or sweet potato	Pancakes, waffles, muffins, biscuits, and corn bread with salt, baking powder, or self-rising flour or as instant mixes	Kale, turnip greens
FATS	Celery		Baked winter squash	Regular bread crumbs or cracker crumbs	Okra
Canola, salad, soybean, and olive oils	Lettuce		Beet greens	Instant rice and pasta mixes	Broccoli
Mayonnaise	**MISCELLANEOUS**		Chard		Orange juice (calcium fortified)
Margarine	Dried peas, beans		Peas, cooked		**BREADS, GRAINS, LEGUMES** (providing at least 90 mg per serving)
MISCELLANEOUS	Grains, legumes		Spinach, fresh		English muffin
Beans	Fortified cereals, including baby cereals		Lima beans		
Pickles	Potatoes		Asparagus		
Sauerkraut			Broccoli		
Soybeans			Carrots		
			Mushrooms		
			MISCELLANEOUS		
			Cooked white beans		
			Canned tomato sauce		
			Blackstrap molasses		
			Sardines canned in oil		
			Chocolate, unsweetened		

Sunflower seeds
Peanuts

Commercial stuffing
Commercial casserole mixes

VEGETABLES AND FRUITS

Regular canned vegetables (over one half cup qd), vegetable juices
Sauerkraut and pickled vegetables, pickles, olives
Potato casserole mixes
Frozen vegetables in sauce, frozen lima beans or peas
Salted prunes

MISCELLANEOUS

Salt in seasonings (e.g., garlic salt)
Seasonings containing sodium or monosodium glutamate (MSG, Accent)
Regular catsup, chili sauce, mustard, horseradish, Kitchen Bouquet, barbecue sauce, soy and teriyaki sauce, Worcestershire sauce and steak sauces
Salted snack foods (e.g., chips, pretzels, nuts, seeds, popcorn)
Regular canned or dried soups, bouillon

Waffle
Beans
Fortified, ready-to-eat cereal
Fortifed bread

BRATY Diet.
The BRATY diet can be used for children or adults experiencing gastroenteritis, particularly nausea and vomiting. The consistency of the food item depends on the age of the patient and personal preference; for example, bananas can be fresh fruit, mashed, or from a baby food jar. The diet can be used up to 24 hours.
B: bananas
R: rice or rice cereal
A: apples, applesauce
T: toast, crackers (preferably dry)
Y: yogurt (preferably plain); live culture

C. PEAK EXPIRATORY FLOW RATE

How to calculate predicted expiratory peak flow:
• Have the patient blow into peak flow meter 3 times; then calculate average exhalations.
• Divide the patient's peak flow into the predicted peak flow; answer equals percentage of normal expected peak flow rate.
Example: patient is 10-year-old male and 52″ tall. Expected normal peak flow would be 234. Patient's average peak flow today is 100. 100 ÷ 234 = 0.427 (43% of normal). After treatment with nebulizer with albuterol, patient's peak flow is 200. 200 ÷ 234 = 0.85 (85% of normal). An improvement is noted.
• Can be used as a guide to patient's condition at time of examination and after nebulizer treatment has been given to determine if beta$_2$ inhalers would be beneficial as treatment to relax bronchopulmonary tree.

Predicted Peak Expiratory Flow Rate

Child and Adolescent Female: Age 6–20 yr

Height (in)	42	46	50	54	57	60	64	68	72
Age 6	134	164	193	223	245	268	297	327	357
8	153	182	212	242	264	287	316	346	376
10	171	201	231	261	283	305	335	365	395
12	190	220	250	280	302	324	354	384	414
14	209	239	269	298	321	342	373	403	432
16	228	258	288	317	340	362	392	421	451
18	247	277	306	336	358	381	411	440	470
20	266	295	325	355	377	400	429	459	489

Child and Adolescent Male: Age 6–20 yr

Height (in)	44	48	52	56	60	64	68	72	76
Age 6	99	146	194	241	289	336	384	431	479
8	119	166	214	261	309	356	404	451	499
10	139	186	234	281	329	376	424	471	519
12	159	206	254	301	349	396	444	491	539
14	178	226	274	321	369	416	464	511	559
16	198	246	293	341	389	436	484	531	579
18	218	266	313	361	408	456	503	551	599
20	238	286	333	381	428	476	523	571	618

Adult Female: Age 25–80 yr

Height (in)	58	60	62	64	66	68	70
Age 25	350	365	379	394	409	424	439
30	342	357	372	387	402	417	431
35	335	350	364	379	394	409	424
40	327	342	357	372	387	402	416
45	320	335	349	364	379	394	409
50	312	327	342	357	372	387	401
55	305	320	334	349	364	379	394
60	297	312	327	342	357	372	386
65	290	305	319	334	349	364	379
70	282	297	312	327	342	357	371
75	275	290	304	319	334	349	364
80	267	282	297	312	327	342	356

Adult Male: Age 25–80 yr

Height (in)	63	65	67	69	71	73	75	77
Age 25	492	520	549	578	606	635	664	692
30	481	510	538	567	596	624	653	682
35	471	499	528	557	585	614	643	671
40	460	489	517	546	575	603	632	661
45	450	478	507	536	564	593	622	650
50	439	468	496	525	554	582	611	640
55	429	457	486	515	543	572	601	629
60	418	447	475	504	533	561	590	619
65	408	436	465	494	522	551	580	608
70	397	426	454	483	512	540	569	598
75	387	415	444	473	501	530	559	587
80	376	405	433	462	491	519	548	577

▊D. PATIENT INSTRUCTION SHEETS

These sheets may be photocopied for patient use.

1. Peak flow monitoring and patient self-management
2. Diabetic foot care
3. Allergen control measures
4. HSV/HPV symptomatic relief measures
5. Oral contraceptive information

Peak Flow Monitoring and Patient Self-Management

1. Patient must know his or her average peak flow.
2. Provider calculates the values for the instruction sheet (e.g., the initial blank is usually the patient's predicted peak flow: the green zone is usually >80% of the predicted value; the yellow zone is usually 60% to 80% of the predicted value; and the red zone is usually <60%).
3. Provider completes the blanks in the instruction sheet with appropriate numbers (not percentages). For example, if the patient's average peak flow was 275 ml, the value for the green zone would be >220; the yellow zone value would be 165 to 220; and the red zone value would be <165.
4. The provider also completes the prednisone instructions and gives a prescription for the medicine so it can be started without a phone call.

Continued

If your peak flow is less than _____, note any signs or symptoms of distress you may be having (e.g., increased cough, breathlessness, wheeze, chest tightness, or use of your chest or neck muscles for breathing). Follow these instructions for treatment:

- Use up to 3 treatments of 2 puffs of albuterol or pirbuterol at 20-minute intervals *or* a single nebulizer treatment.
- Then recheck peak flow; results determine the next step(s).

GREEN	YELLOW	RED
Peak flow _____	Peak flow _____	Peak flow _____
No wheeze or shortness of breath	Persistent wheezing and shortness of breath	Marked wheeze and shortness of breath
Effects of albuterol or pirbuterol last at least 4 hr	1. Continue taking albuterol or pirbuterol every 3–4 hr for 24–48 hr (until peak flow stabilizes)	1. Repeat albuterol or pirbuterol immediately
1. May continue to use albuterol or pirbuterol every 3–4 hr for 24–48 hr (until peak flow stabilizes)	2. Take prednisone as directed below: _____ _____ _____	2. Take prednisone as directed below: _____ _____ _____
2. For patients taking inhaled steroids, double dose for 7–10 days	Contact our office urgently (this day) for further instructions	3. If distress is severe and nonresponsive, call our office or proceed to the emergency department; consider calling 911
Contact our office for follow-up instructions		

Foot Care Instructions for Persons with Diabetes

These guidelines assume that the person has risk factors for foot problems: neuropathy, vascular disease, or a combination of these.

FOOTWEAR

- Wear shoes that fit properly; look for a wide toe box rather than pointed toes; avoid high heels; leather or canvas shoes are best; buy shoes at the end of the day (when your feet are larger) for the best fit
- Change your shoes once or twice during the day to relieve areas of pressure
- Never go barefoot, even at home; especially avoid walking on hot concrete or sand
- Avoid thongs, sandals, or open-toed shoes
- Break shoes in slowly; wear them for only a few hours a day at first, then gradually build up the wearing time
- Before wearing shoes, *always* check the insides for nail points, worn areas, foreign objects, or other rough areas that might cause blisters or rubbing
- Wear appropriate shoes for the weather; avoid wearing wet shoes

FOOT CARE

- Look at your feet (tops, bottoms, sides, between toes) *daily* for blisters, cuts, scratches, changes in color or discoloration, or changes in temperature; use a mirror if necessary or have someone check your feet for you
- Wash feet daily with mild soap and warm (not hot) water; dry thoroughly and carefully, especially between the toes
- Use creams to moisturize skin daily; do not place creams or lotions between the toes
- Wear clean socks daily; be sure that socks are appropriate for the type of shoes worn; do not wear darned or mended socks or socks with holes; avoid socks with seams
- Avoid soaking feet
- Avoid temperature extremes: check water temperature with your elbow before putting feet in
- Avoid all OTC treatments for corns, calluses, and nails; do not use strong antiseptics, astringents, or alcohol on your feet
- Trim nails "to the shape of the end of your toe" (i.e., straight across with slightly rounded edges); do not cut into the corners
- No "bathroom surgery": do not cut corns and calluses yourself; they should be managed by an experienced health care provider
- Avoid using adhesive tape on your feet
- Wear socks if your feet are cold; do not put heating pads or hot water bottles on your feet

Continued

- Avoid garters, tight elastic bands on socks, or anything that decreases circulation to your feet (including crossing your legs)

Contact your health care provider when
- You notice cuts, blisters, or breaks in the skin of your feet
- You have ingrown nails
- You notice changes in the color or discoloration of your feet
- You have pain or changes in the sensation in your feet
- You notice a change in the shape or architecture of your foot

Other things you can do to prevent foot problems
- Stop smoking!
- Control your weight, BP, and blood sugar
- Get regular exercise
- Have your health care provider check your feet at each visit
- Wear special shoes or inserts that may be necessary, especially if there are skin changes, calluses, or foot-shape changes

Allergen Control Measures

Because many people with asthma have environmental stimuli that exacerbate their symptoms, allergen control is important. These are measures that must be instituted in the home and other places where you spend a lot of time. It is important that you carry out these measures daily to get the best results.

Allergens usually fall into two categories: outdoor and indoor.

OUTDOOR ALLERGENS

- Determine if there is a particular season that aggravates your asthma or allergies
- Keep your windows closed and use air-conditioning with ultrasensitive filters
- When out driving, keep your windows up and use air-conditioning in car
- Limit your outdoor activity to early morning or late evening
- Limit number of house plants in your house
- Wear mask when outdoors if you are going to mow the yard or rake leaves

INDOOR ALLERGENS

- Wear mask when vacuuming or cleaning draperies or curtains
- Remove carpeting wherever possible
- Dust mite control should include:
  - Covering or encasing mattresses and pillows with plastic covers
  - Wash bedding weekly in hot water
  - Replace bedroom carpets with hardwood floors or linoleum
  - Vacuum bedroom carpets frequently using HEPA ultrasensitive filters
  - Remove any upholstered pieces of furniture and other dust collectors
  - Decrease humidity in house and especially in bedroom
- Limit exposure to cockroaches and to the feces from cockroaches by:
  - Prompt cleanup after meals and wash dishes
  - Seal all food sources and dishes tightly
  - Seal gaps around kitchen and bathroom pipes
  - Either use some brand of roach bait stations or have cockroaches in house professionally exterminated
- Cat and dog allergens are another possible source of stimuli for people with asthma:
  - If possible remove cat and dog from your environment
  - If you cannot remove your pet from your environment, keep your pet out of your bedroom
  - Minimize contacts with animals whenever possible
  - Wash your pet weekly in water to decrease dander and loose hairs
  - Keep pets off your furniture, especially chairs that you use frequently
  - Vacuuming to remove dander and loose hairs is important and must be done weekly
  - Make sure your pet has no fleas or ticks

Tips for Symptomatic Relief of Human Papillomavirus (HPV) and Herpes Simplex Virus (HSV) Infections

- Warm, wet soaks
- Bathing vs. showering
- Dry well after a shower or urinating; do not rub area vigorously; pat dry
- Perform genital hygiene no more than once a day using a gentle nondeodorant soap
- No feminine hygiene products or douching
- Sleep "bare bottomed"
- Wear only 100% cotton underwear
- Wear loose, natural fiber clothing
- Wear thigh-high or knee-high hose or cut the crotch out of panty hose
- No minipads; for increased vaginal discharge carry extra underwear
- Use only unscented laundry detergent
- Use unscented white toilet tissue
- Change coital positions to decrease constant contact to the same area
- Sit on a donut pillow to increase ventilation to the area
- Use hydrocortisone cream 0.25% to 0.5% for irritation

Tips on Taking Oral Contraceptives

The following are a few helpful comments on pill use:

- Start the pills on the first day of menstrual bleeding or on the Sunday after your period starts, even if you are still menstruating; use a backup contraceptive method for the first cycle or month of your pills
- Take the pill at the same time every day; if you get nauseated, take it with food or at bedtime
- Use a backup method of birth control for 1 week if you are spotting during any of your cycles
- If a pill is missed, take that pill as soon as remembered and take the next pill as scheduled; use a backup method for birth control for the next 7 days
- If 2 pills are missed in the first 2 weeks, take 2 pills for 2 days; if 2 pills are missed in the last 2 weeks of the monthly cycle, take 1 pill every day until the active pills are finished and then start a new pack; use backup contraception for rest of cycle
- If 3 or more pills are missed, you will probably start a normal menstrual cycle; you can take 1 pill every day until the active pills are finished and then start a new pack; use a backup method for 7 days after the new pack is started
- Notify the practitioner immediately if any of these warning signs occur:
  A—abdominal pain
  C—chest pain
  H—headaches (unlike any you have had before)
  E—eye changes (like blurred or double vision)
  S—swelling or severe leg pain
- If you miss one period while taking the pill, there is no reason for concern; if you miss two periods while taking the pill, perform a pregnancy test
- Pregnancy is more likely to occur when pills are missed just before or just after the hormone-free pills are taken

▬ E. NONSTEROIDAL ANTIINFLAMMATORY DRUGS (NSAIDs)

AGENT	USUAL DOSE (MAXIMUM DOSE)	COMMENTS
Salicylates		
Acetylsalicylic acid (ASA, Ascriptin, Bufferin, Ecotrin)	325–1000 mg q4–6h (5.4 g)	Available in rectal suppository; #1 cause of gastropathy in elderly patients
Choline magnesium trisalicylate (Trilisate)	1–1.5 g q12h (4 g)	Available in liquid; lower level of GI tract side effects
Diflunisal (Dolobid)	500–1000 mg q8–12h (1.5 g)	
Salsalate (Disalcid, Salsitab)	1–1.5 g q8–12h (4 g)	
Propionic Acids		
Ibuprofen (Advil, Motrin, Motrin IB, Rufen)	200–800 mg q4–6h (3.2 g)	Available in liquid
Fenoprofen calcium (Nalfon)	200 mg q4–6h (3.2 g)	
Flurbiprofen (Ansaid)	50–100 mg q6–8h (300 mg)	
Ketoprofen (Orudis, Orudis KT)	25–50 mg q6–8h (300 mg)	Available in rectal suppository
(Oruvail, extended release)	100–200 mg qd (200 mg)	
Naproxen (Naprosyn)	250–500 mg bid–tid (1.5 g)	Available in liquid; increased incidence of gastropathy in elderly patients
Naproxen sodium (Aleve [OTC])	220 mg q8h (660 mg)	
(Anaprox)	275–550 mg q6–8h (1650 mg)	
(Naprelan [controlled release])	750–1000 mg qd (1000 mg)	
Oxaprozin (Daypro)	1200 mg qd (1800 mg)	
Oxicams		
Meloxicam (Mobic)	7.5–15 mg qd (15 mg)	
Piroxicam (Feldene)	10–20 mg qd (20 mg)	
Fenamates		
Meclofenamate sodium (Meclomen)	50–100 mg q4–6h (400 mg)	
Mefenamic acid (Ponstel)	250–500 mg q6h (1 g)	
Acetic Acids		
Diclofenac potassium (Cataflam)	50–75 mg q6–12h (200 mg)	
Diclofenac sodium (Voltaren)	50–75 mg q6–12h (200 mg)	
Diclofenac sodium/misoprostol (Arthrotec)	OA: 50 mg tid (150 mg) RA: 50–75 mg tid or qid (225 mg)	
Etodolac (Lodine)	200–400 mg q6–12h (1.2 g)	
Indomethacin (Indocin)	25–50 mg q8–12h (200 mg)	Available in rectal suppository; high risk for gastropathy in elderly patients
Nabumetone (Relafen)	500–750 mg q12h (2000 mg)	
Sulindac (Clinoril)	150–200 mg q12h (400 mg)	
Tolmetin sodium (Tolectin)	400–600 mg q8–12h (2000 mg)	
COX-2 Inhibitors		
Celecoxib (Celebrex)	OA: 100 mg bid (200 mg) RA: 100–200 mg bid (400 mg)	Caution with sulfa allergy

OA, Osteoarthritis; *RA*, rheumatoid arthritis.

■ F. DIETARY SUPPLEMENTS

SUPPLEMENT	COST PER SERVING	CALORIES	PROTEIN (g)	FAT (g)	SODIUM/POTASSIUM (mg)
Milk shake, 1 c; no vitamins and minerals added		250	9	7	215/415
Carnation Hot Cocoa Mix, 1 envelope with 1 c whole milk	50¢	260	10	9	250/590
Ultra SlimFast, 1 can (11 oz); no added sugars; contains 5 g fiber + vitamins and minerals	89¢ to $1.19	250	10	3	220/530
Ironman Protein shake, 1 scoop in 4 oz skim milk	50¢	130	24	1.5	95/—
Carnation Instant Breakfast with 1 c whole milk; no fiber but has added vitamins and minerals	40¢ to 52¢	290	12	9	220/350
Ensure Plus, 1 c; added vitamins and minerals	$1.45	360	14	12	260/477
Ensure, 1 c; no fiber but added vitamins and minerals	$1.35	250	9	9	200/370
Ensure Light, 1 c; lactose free added vitamins and minerals	$1	200	10	3	200/370
Sustacal, 1 c; no lactose or fiber but added vitamins and minerals	$1.10	240	15	6	225/495
Equate Dietary Supplement, 1 c no fiber added vitamins and minerals	85¢	250	9	6	200/370
Sport Shake, 7.5 oz; no fiber; added vitamins and minerals	88¢	290	9	9	240/570
Boost, 1 c; no fiber; added vitamins and minerals	$1.00	240	10	4	130/400
Enlive (clear liquid supplement), 8 oz.; fat and lactose free; in apple and peach flavors		300	10	0	65/40

G. PAIN MANAGEMENT GUIDELINES

ACUTE PAIN

Associated with recent trauma, surgery, or illness

Expected to be self-limiting

CHRONIC PAIN

Pain persisting longer than 3 to 6 months

May be continuous, intermittent, or a combination of both

Often associated with sleep or appetite disturbances, irritability, social withdrawal, depression

Types—any of these may be malignant or nonmalignant
- Neuropathic
  - Injury or dysfunction of the CNS; onset usually weeks to months after acute nerve injury
  - May be central or peripheral; follows nerve distribution
  - May be intermittent or constant
  - Described as "on fire," lancinating, burning, numbness, tingling, shooting
  - Causes:

    Heat or cold injury (e.g., burns, frostbite)

    Ischemic injury

    Diabetic neuropathy

    Phantom pain

    Microbiologic injury (e.g., postherpetic neuralgia, AIDS neuropathy)

    Nerve damage from surgery or trauma
- Nociceptive
  - Intact CNS
  - Somatic:

    Well-localized, constant, aching, throbbing

    Associated with bone, joint, connective tissue, muscle
  - Visceral:

    Poorly localized, noxious

    Dull, aching, deep, cramping, squeezing, possibly referred

    Associated with organs, pancreas, GI tract

With chronic pain, do not just address pain relief, but also try to improve function; patient may also have insomnia, depression/anxiety, fatigue, N/V, constipation, H/A

PAIN ASSESSMENT

First and most important step in pain management

Evaluate using a rating scale (e.g., 0 to 10 with 0 being no pain and 10 being the worst pain ever)

TREATMENT

When developing a treatment plan, consider the ultimate goal of therapy (e.g., comfort or restoration of function)

See below for suggested therapies; also see the other tables in Appendix G

PAIN LEVEL	NOCICEPTIVE PAIN	NEUROPATHIC PAIN
Mild-to-moderate pain (1–4 out of 10)	Nonopioid analgesic +/– adjuvant therapy	Adjuvant therapy +/– nonopioid analgesic
Moderate pain (4–7 out of 10)	Weak opioid analgesic +/– adjuvant therapy	Adjuvant therapy +/– weak opioid analgesic
Severe pain (7–10 out of 10)	Strong opioid analgesic +/– adjuvant therapy	Adjuvant therapy +/– strong opioid analgesic

Adjuvant therapies may include:
- Tricyclic antidepressants
  - Amitriptyline (Elavil) 10 to 25 mg hs, up to 100 mg
  - Desipramine (Norpramin) 10 to 25 mg bid–tid, slowly titrated up to 200 mg qd
- Anticonvulsants
  - Gabapentin (Neurontin) 300 to 1800 mg qd in 3 divided doses
  - Carbamazepine (Tegretol) 100 mg bid with food, increasing gradually in increments of 100 mg bid, up to 1200 mg qd
- Topical preparations
  - Lidocaine patch (Lidoderm): apply up to three patches in a single application, and may leave in place for up to 12 hours in any 24-hour time period
  - Capsaicin (e.g., Zostrix OTC cream): apply to affected areas at least tid–qid (less often decreases efficacy)
- Prednisolone or prednisone for inflammatory pain (dose individualized)
- To help sleep:
  - Trazodone 25 to 50 mg hs, up to 200 mg
  - Diphenhydramine (Benadryl) 50 mg hs
- Anxiolytics to decrease stress and anxiety
  - Alprazolam (Xanax) 0.25 to 0.5 mg tid; titrate up to maximum of 4 mg qd
  - Lorazepam (Ativan) 2 to 6 mg qd in divided doses
  - Clorazepate (Tranxene) 7.5 to 15 mg bid–qid

PRACTICE PEARLS

In patients with a history of substance addiction, short-acting opioids may cause craving for drugs because of cycling of pain during the day; long-acting opioids can be better because the pain can be better controlled

Chronic pain is best treated with round-the-clock dosing (with a long-term medication) with as needed medications available for breakthrough pain

"Rescue" medication (short-acting) should be available for use between scheduled doses of long-acting medication; it can also be offered preemptively before physical therapy, bath, etc; use of the short-acting form of the medication used for long-term pain relief is recommended; suggested rescue dosing (usually equivalent to 15% to 20% of the total scheduled dose of long-acting agent):

- Oxycodone immediate release, 5 mg 1 to 2 tablets po q4h prn
- Morphine sulfate immediate release, 15 to 30 mg q4h prn
- Hydromorphone immediate release, 2 to 4 mg q4h prn

Titrate the long-acting medicine as necessary every 24 to 48 hours for severe pain; an easy way to figure a new dose is to add the total mg of long-acting and short-acting given in a 24 hour period and this becomes the new long-acting dose for 24 hours

NSAIDs use

- Cautious use in the elderly patient or in persons with DM or renal or lung disease
- With long-term NSAID use, periodically check stools for occult blood for GI blood loss; consider PPI to decrease GI risk
- Check for developing renal insufficiency and monitor closely for any drug interactions

When prescribing opioid analgesics, initiate a prophylactic bowel regimen to prevent constipation (e.g., Senokot or frozen Vaseline balls [freeze ½ tsp–size Vaseline balls, coat with powdered sugar, and then store in freezer; have patient swallow one "ball" 1 to 3 times qd between meals, for constipation])

To ensure patient compliance with therapeutic regimen, obtain unscheduled urine drug screens; this checks:

- To see if patient is taking the medications prescribed and
- To see if any other drugs are being taken

Precautions with urine drug screens:

- Medications taken in a patch form will not show up in urine
- When checking for oxycodone, ask lab to remove all filters used when checking the urine
- Poppy seeds taken orally (e.g., poppy seed muffin) can give a false-positive test

Nonpharmacologic therapies are often helpful in giving patients some control over their pain:

- Relaxation techniques
- Self-hypnosis or psychotherapy
- Exercise programs
- Educational programs (pertinent to diagnosis)
- Physical modalities (e.g., chiropractic, massage, heat therapy, acupuncture, electrical nerve stimulation, and physical therapy)

Herbal products (not exclusive)

- Comfrey topical preparation to bruises, pulled muscles or sprains; do not use on broken skin, for more than 6 weeks, or if pregnant
- Aloe topical gel or spray to burns
- Witch hazel topically to treat skin inflammation; not intended for oral use

Remember that not everyone can verbalize pain; look for confusion or increased irritability, decreased eating and drinking, or frequent falls

Nonnarcotic and Narcotic Treatment for Chronic Pain

DRUG	PAIN LEVEL	INITIAL ADULT DOSE* (ORAL UNLESS OTHERWISE NOTED)	MAXIMUM DOSE* (ORAL UNLESS OTHERWISE NOTED)	ROUTES OF ADMINISTRATION
Nonopioids				
Acetaminophen	Mild	325–650 mg q4–6h, 1 g tid or qid	4 g qd	Oral or rectal
Aspirin	Mild	325–650 mg q4h	5.4 g qd	Oral or rectal
NSAIDs	Mild to moderate	See Appendix E		
Propoxyphene napsylate with acetaminophen (Darvocet)	Mild to moderate	65–100 mg q4–6h	600 mg qd of propoxyphene; 4 g qd of acetaminophen	Oral
Tramadol (Ultram)	Mild to moderate	50–100 mg q4–6h	400 mg qd (300 mg qd if patient >75 yr or with creatinine clearance <30 ml/min or with cirrhosis)	Oral
Tramadol with acetaminophen (Ultracet)	Mild to moderate	37.5 mg/325 mg 2 tabs q4–6h	4 g qd of acetaminophen (with Ultracet)	
Weak Opioids				
Acetaminophen with codeine	Moderate	1–2 tab q4h	4 g qd acetaminophen	Oral
Acetaminophen with oxycodone (Percocet)	Moderate to severe	5–10 mg oxycodone q4–6h	4 g qd acetaminophen	Oral
Acetaminophen with hydrocodone (Lortab, Vicodin)	Moderate to severe	5–10 mg hydrocodone q4–6h	4 g qd acetaminophen	Oral
Butorphanol (Stadol)	Moderate to severe	Nasal: 1 spray q60–90 min, prn		Intranasal, IV, IM
Strong Opioids				
Morphine sulfate	Severe	Controlled release 15–30 mg q8–12h	None	Oral, rectal, IV, IM, PCA
Oxycodone (Oxycontin)	Severe	Controlled release 10 mg q12h	None	Oral
Fentanyl (Duragesic)	Severe	Transdermal 25–300 mcg/h	None	Lozenge, IV, transdermal, transmucosal
Hydromorphone (Dilaudid)	Severe	IM, IV, PO: 1–4 mg q4–6h; rectal: 3 mg q6–8h	None	Oral, rectal, IV, IM

*All drug doses are approximate. Doses must be specific to patients.

Narcotic Equianalgesic Dosing Chart

DRUG	ROUTE	EQUIANALGESIC DOSE (mg)
Morphine	IM	10
	PO	30–60
Hydromorphone (Dilaudid)	IM	2
	PO	8
Hydrocodone (e.g., Lortab)	PO	20
Oxycodone (OxyContin)	PO	20
Codeine	IM	60
	PO	180
Butorphanol (Stadol)	IM	3
	Intranasal	1 spray (1 mg)
Fentanyl (Duragesic)	IM	0.15
	Transdermal	50 mcg/h

H. HERBAL THERAPY

For suggested herbal use, see specific chapter, condition, or disease

Herbs Considered of No Benefit or Unsafe for Human Use

COMMON NAME	PURPORTED USE	COMMENTS
Borage	Diuretic, antidiarrheal	Both safety and efficacy are questionable; contains toxic pyrrolizidine alkaloids
Calamus	Reduce fever, digestive aid	Contains varying amounts of carcinogenic *cis*-isoasarone; Indian type most toxic; North American type nontoxic
Chaparral	Anticancer	No proven efficacy; purported to induce severe liver toxicity, but limited number of cases have been seen in spite of widespread use
Dong quai		Not recommended for use—may stimulate estrogen-sensitive breast tumors and photosensitivity
Ephedra (Ma-huang)	Anorectic, bronchodilator	Not shown safe or effective with weight loss; effective for bronchodilation; misuse has caused deaths
Germander	Anorectic	Unsafe and ineffective; causes hepatotoxicity because of diterpenoid derivatives
Kava Kava	Anxiety	Hepatotoxicity
Licorice	Expectorant, antiulcer	Effective, but safe only in small doses for short periods of time (e.g., <4 wk); high doses for longer periods of time cause pseudoaldosteronism
Life root	Promotes or assists menstrual flow	Hepatotoxic and no proven efficacy
Pau D'Arco	Folk medicine for many different conditions	Active ingredient toxic to human beings
Pokeroot	Tonic (increases muscle tone and strength), antirheumatic, anticancer	Unsafe and ineffective; should not be sold or used; may be fatal in children
Sassafras	Stimulant, antispasmodic, antirheumatic, tonic (increases muscle tone and strength)	Unsafe and ineffective; volatile oil contains carcinogenic safrole

Herbs Considered Unsafe in Specific Conditions

Asthma
Fir needle oil
Pine needle oil

Cardiac Arrhythmias (Fast or Slow)
Belladonna
Henbane leaf
Jimsonweed
Larkspur
Lily-of-the-valley powdered extract
Monkshood
Oleander leaf powdered extract
Pheasant's eye fluid extract
Scopolia root
Squill powdered extract

Diabetes Mellitus
Blackthorn flower
Echinacea purpurea (injectable)
Psyllium seed and seed husk, blonde
Senna leaf

Glaucoma
Belladonna
Ephedra
Henbane leaf
Scopolia root

HIV
Echinacea pallida root
Mistletoe herb
Woody nightshade stem

Hypertension
Eleuthero root
Ephedra
Guarana
Kola nut
Jimsonwed
Yohimbe (*Corynanthe yohimbe*)

Infants and Children
Aloe
Anise oil
Buckthorn bark and berry
Cajeput oil
Camphor
Caraway oil
Cascara sagrada bark
Chamomile flower
Eucalyptus leaf and oil
Fennel oil
Horseradish
Licorice root

Mint oil (externally)
Nasturtium
Pennyroyal
Peppermint oil (externally)
Psyllium seed husk, blonde
Rhubarb root
Senna leaf and pod
Thyme
Turpentine oil
Watercress

Lactation
Aloe
Buckthorn bark and berry
Caraway oil
Cascara Sagrada bark
Coltsfoot leaf
Indian snakeroot
Peppermint oil
Petasites root
Rhubarb root
Senna leaf
Uva Ursi

Liver Disease
Angelica root
Anise seed
Boldo leaf
Caraway oil
Chamomile flower
Eucalyptus leaf and oil
Fennel oil and seed
Gentian root
Haronga bark and leaf
Iceland Moss
Kava kava
Licorice root
Marshmallow root
Mint oil
Niauli oil
Pennyroyal oil or tea
Peppermint oil and leaf
Primrose root
Thyme
Wormwood

Pregnancy
Aloe (internally)
Angelica root
Anise oil and seed
Autumn crocus
Black cohosh
Buckthorn bark and berry

Herbs Considered Unsafe in Specific Conditions—cont'd

Caraway oil and seed
Cascara sagrada bark
Chamomile flower
Chaste tree fruit
Cinchona bark
Cinnamon bark
Coltsfoot leaf
Comfrey herb and leaf
Eucalyptus oil (internally)
Fennel oil and seed
Feverfew
Gentian root
Gingerroot
Ginseng
Goldenseal
Gotu kola
Hawthorn
Indian snakeroot
Juniper berry
Licorice root
Mayapple root and resin
Parsley herb and root
Peppermint leaf
Petasites root
Primrose root
Rhubarb root
Sage leaf
Saw palmetto
Senna leaf
Siberian ginseng
St. John's wort
Uva Ursi leaf

Renal Inflammation or Disease
Anise seed
Asparagus root
German chamomile flower
Horseradish
Juniper berry
Licorice root
Lovage root
Marshmallow root
Peppermint leaf
Primrose root
Sandalwood, white
Watercress
Wormwood

Ulcers (Gastric and Duodenal)
Angelica root
Bitter orange peel
Cola nut
Devil's claw root
Fennel seed
Gentian root
Gingerroot
Horseradish
Indian snakeroot
Nasturtium
Peppermint oil
Pokeweed
Rhubarb root
Watercress
Wormwood

▪ I. SUGGESTED HOSPITAL ADMISSION ORDERS

Admission status (e.g., short-term observation or full admit)

Diagnosis or diagnoses

Activity (e.g., bed rest, up ad lib)

Diet

IV orders—consider:
- IV rate
- With diabetic patient, no dextrose (at least not initially)
- With debilitated and dehydrated patient, consider Aminosyn with electrolytes or ProcalAmine (i.e., amino acid solution with electrolytes)
- Is any additive (KCl) needed?
- Blood transfusions, if needed
- With infants: use 0.225 sodium chloride (¼ NS) and no KCl

Medications
- Antibiotics, if needed; remember with aminoglycosides to obtain peak and trough with fifth dose and with third dose after changes; monitor BUN and creatinine
- Patient's routine medications (including eye drops, hormones, and patches)
- Medications prn for pain, sleep, bowels, N/V, and fever >101° F
- Oxygen, if needed

Laboratory, x-ray, cardiology, respiratory orders
- Tests ordered must have a diagnosis (not "rule out" or "possible") or current symptom(s)
- Consider if recently performed test will suffice (e.g., CXR in past month on a well patient undergoing an elective operation)

Miscellaneous
- Egg crate mattress or special bed
- Other consultations (e.g., dietician, physical therapy, physician specialist)
- Fingerstick blood glucose monitoring (e.g., Accucheck), if needed
- Other equipment, such as NG tube, Foley catheter, telemetry

▉ J. BIOLOGICAL DISEASE AGENTS

Biological agents have caused great concern in our country. These agents are easily created and disseminated and can cause extreme panic when identified. Health care practitioners will need to maintain a high level of suspicion when any groupings of unusual symptoms/diseases appear in specific communities. The CDC has many references available to both the health care community and the general public regarding biological agents and how to mobilize the health care industry quickly and efficiently. Category A pathogens are those that do not originate in the United States and are likely to be used by terrorists because they:

- Can be easily spread or transmitted from person to person
- Can cause numerous deaths
- Can cause general panic and social disruption

The most common Category A biologicals are listed below:

DISEASE	GENERAL INFORMATION	SIGNS AND SYMPTOMS	TREATMENT

Anthrax (*Bacillus anthracis*)	Infectious disease caused by spore-forming bacterium
	Most commonly occurs in hoofed mammals and can also infect human beings
	Three forms:
	  Inhalation
	  Cutaneous
	  Intestinal
	Inhalation most toxic
	Cutaneous most common; spread by skin contact with infected animal or animal products
	Intestinal spread by ingestion of contaminated food
		Incubation ranges from 1–7 days
		Early symptoms do not include a runny nose
		Inhalation form:
		  Sore throat
		  Mild fever
		  Myalgia, malaise
		  Respiratory failure
		  Meningitis
		Cutaneous form:
		  Small papule progress to vesicle to necrotic ulcer that is painless
		  Fever, malaise
		  H/A
		  Regional lymphadenopathy
		Intestinal form:
		  Severe abdominal pain
		  Fever
		  Sepsis
		  Sore throat
		  Lesions at base of tongue
		  Dysphagia
		  Regional lymphadenopathy
		  N/V, bloody diarrhea
		  Anorexia
			Early antibiotic treatment is essential
			Antibiotics for 60 days:
			  Ciprofloxacin 500 mg bid
			  Doxycycline 100 mg bid
			  Amoxicillin 500 mg bid
			No vaccine

Smallpox (variola major)	Virulent infection, sometimes fatal	Incubation ranges from 7–17 days	No specific treatment Vaccine is available

Continued

DISEASE	GENERAL INFORMATION	SIGNS AND SYMPTOMS	TREATMENT
	Transmission occurs with prolonged face-to-face contact and direct contact with infected body fluids or linens, rarely spread via droplets Human beings are natural hosts Not transmitted by insects or animals Last case of smallpox in United States was in 1949 Last case in the world was in 1979	Most contagious when rash appears Contagious until all scabs have fallen off First symptoms last 2–4 days with: Fever, malaise Myalgia, H/A Vomiting Rash starts on tongue and mouth as small red spots then develops into ulcers, followed by rash starting on face and spreading down arms/legs to hands and feet Lesions are raised, fluid filled, and indented in center Lesions change to pustules; pustules form crust and scab; start falling off within 2 wk May leave scars	
Plague (*Yersinia pestis*)	Early treatment is essential Caused by bacterium found in rodents and fleas Highly contagious Found in many areas of world and U.S. Usually destroyed by sunlight and drying, but may be able to survive for up to 1 hr outdoors	Incubation ranges from 2–6 days Transmitted by bite of infected animal Symptoms include: Swollen, tender lymph node called *bubo* Fever, chills, H/A Cough, SOB, bloody sputum Can rapidly progress to death Quarantine any persons exposed to illness	No vaccine Antibiotics for 10 days: Streptomycin 1 g IM bid Gentamycin 5 mg/kg IM/IV once daily Doxycycline 100 mg IV bid or 200 mg IV qd
Viral hemorrhagic fever (VHF) (Ebola, Marbug, Lassa, Hanta)	Group of viruses that cause overall vascular damage with internal bleeding Natural reservoir is animal or insect, not human beings Human beings are infected via infected	Incubation ranges from 1–7 days Specific symptoms vary by virus: Marked fever Fatigue, myalgia Dizziness Loss of strength Exhaustion	No cure or treatment Supportive care only

DISEASE	GENERAL INFORMATION	SIGNS AND SYMPTOMS	TREATMENT
	host either with droplet or cutaneous injury; occasional human-to-human transmission	Bleeding from external orifices Quarantine persons exposed to virus Vector control to slow onslaught of disease	
Botulism (*Clostridium botulinum*)	Toxin made by a bacterium causes muscle paralysis Not spread from person to person Foodborne botulism can occur in any age; severity increases with very young or very old	Incubation ranges from 6 hr to 2 wk after eating toxin-containing food Symptoms include: Double vision Blurred vision Drooping eyelids Slurred speech Difficulty swallowing Dry mouth Muscle weakness that descends down body Can lead to paralysis of respiratory muscles	Botulinum antitoxin (available through CDC) *and* Antibiotics for 10–14 days: Penicillin G 2–4 million units IV q4–6h *or* Clindamycin 600 mg IV q8h *or* Metronidazole 500 mg IV/PO q12h *or* Chloramphenicol 500 mg IV q6h

BIBLIOGRAPHY

American Diabetes Association. (2003). American Diabetes Association: Clinical practice recommendations 2003. *Diabetes Care, 26* (Suppl. 1), S1–S153.

Bartlett, J. G., Dowell, S. F., Mandell, L. A., File, T. M. Jr, Musher, D. M., & Fine, M. J. (2000). Practice guidelines for the management of community-acquired pneumonia in adults. *Clinical Infectious Disease, 2,* 347–382.

Bates, B. (1991). *A guide to physical assessment* (5th ed.). Philadelphia: J.B. Lippincott.

Beck, A. T., Ward, C. H., Mendelson, M., Mock, J., & Erbaugh, J. (1961). An inventory for measuring depression. *Archives of General Psychiatry, 4,* 561–571.

Berman, N. R. (2002). Human papillomavirus and cervical cancer screening. *Advance for Nurse Practitioners, 10,* 26–36.

Burns, A., Lawlor, B., & Craig, S. (1999). *Assessment scales in old age psychiatry.* London: Martin Dunitz.

Callen, J. P., Greer, K. E., Hood, A. F., Paller, A. S., & Swinyer, L. J. (1993). *Color atlas of dermatology.* Philadelphia: W.B. Saunders.

Callen, J. P., Greer, K. E., Hood, A. F., Paller, A. S., & Swinyer, L. J. (2000). *Color atlas of dermatology* (2nd ed.). Philadelphia: W.B. Saunders.

Carcio, H. (2002). Urogenital atrophy: A new approach to vaginitis diagnosis. *Advance for Nurse Practitioners, 10,* 4051.

Carroll, P. (1999). Latex allergy: What you need to know. *RN, 62,* 40–45.

Centers for Disease Control and Prevention. (2001). *Diagnosis and management of foodborne illnesses: A primer for physicians.* Retrieved January 26, 2001, from www.cdc.gov/mmwr/preview/mmwrhtml/rr5002aL.htm

Centers for Disease Control, Special Pathogens Branch. (2002). Retrieved March 4, 2003, from www.cdc.gov/ncidod/dvrd/spb/mnpages/disinfo.htm

Cleeman, J. I. (2001). Second report of the National Cholesterol Program (NCEP) Expert Panel on Detection, Evaluation, and Treatment of High Blood Cholesterol in Adults (ATP III). *Journal of the American Medical Association, 285,* 2486–2497.

Cuzzell, J. (2002). Wound healing: Translating theory into clinical practice. *Dermatology Nursing, 14,* 257–266.

Dickey, P. R. (2002). *Managing contraceptive pill patients* (10th ed.). Durant, OK: Essential Medical Systems, Inc.

Dockery, G. (Ed.). (1997). *Cutaneous disorders of the lower extremity.* Philadelphia: W. B. Saunders.

Fenstermacher, K. (1998). *Dysrhythmia recognition and management* (3rd ed.). Philadelphia: W. B. Saunders.

Fitzpatrick, T. B., Johnson, R. A., Polano, M. K., Suurmond, D., Wolff, K. (1994). *Color atlas and synopsis of clinical dermatology* (2nd ed.). New York: McGraw-Hill.

Freedman, R. R. (2001). Physiology of hot flashes. *American Journal of Human Biology, 13,* 453–464.

Goldsmith, L. A., Lazarus, G. S., Tharp, M. D. (1997). *Adult and pediatric dermatology: A color guide to diagnosis and treatment.* Philadelphia: F. A. Davis.

Goodheart, J. P. (1999). Hyperpigmentation disorders. *Women's Health in Primary Care, 2,* 923–930.

Goodman, A. (2000). Abnormal genital tract bleeding. *Clinical Cornerstone, 3,* 25–35.

Gray, J. A. (2002). Onychomycosis: New treatments are effective. *Clinician Reviews, 12,* 7–8.

Gross, J., Fetto, J., & Rosen, E. (1996). *Musculoskeletal examination.* Cambridge, MA: Blackwell Science.

Hendrix, S. (2002). Implications of the women's health initiative. *The Female Patient, 11,* 4–13.

Hobus, P. (2002). Snaring a silent threat: Chlamydia. *Advance for Nurse Practitioners, 10,* 63–65.

Hunt, S. A., Baker, D. W., Chin, M. H., Cinquegrani, M. P., Feldman, A. M., Francis, G. S., et al. (2001). ACC/AHA guidelines for the evaluation and management of chronic heart failure in the adult: A report of the American College of Cardiology/American Heart Association task force on practice guidelines. *Journal of the American College of Cardiology, 38,* 2101–2113.

Jarvis, C. (2002). *Physical examination and health assessment* (3rd ed.). Philadelphia: W. B. Saunders.

Johnson, P. H. (Ed.). (1997). *Professional guide to signs and symptoms* (2nd ed.). Springhouse, PA: Springhouse.

Katz, P. R., Dube, D. H., & Calkins, E. (1985). Use of a structured functional assessment format in a geriatric consultative service. *Journal of the American Geriatrics Society, 23,* 681–686.

Knesper, P. J., Riba, M. B., & Schwenk, T. L. (1997). *Primary care psychiatry.* Philadelphia: W. B. Saunders.

Krasner, D., & Kane, D. (Eds.). (2001). *Chronic wound care: A clinical source book for healthcare professionals* (3rd ed.). Wayne, PA: Health Management Publications.

Mathias, S., Nayak, U. S., & Isaacs, B. (1986). Balance in elderly patients: The "get-up and go" test. *Archives of Physical Medicine and Rehabilitation, 67,* 387–389.

Mercier, L. (1995). *Practical orthopedics* (4th ed.). St. Louis: Mosby.

O'Donnell, J. A., Gelone, S. P., & Abrutyn, E. (2002). Selecting drug regimens for urinary tract infections: Current recommendations. *Infectious Medicine, 19,* 14–22.

Oprica, C., Emtestam, L., & Nord, C. E. (2002). Overview of treatments for acne. *Dermatology Nursing, 4,* 242–246.

Oski, F. A., DeAngelis, C. O., Feigin, R. D., McMillan, J. A., Warshaw, J. B. (1999). *Principles and practices of pediatrics* (3rd ed.). Philadelphia: Lippincott Williams & Wilkins.

Pannell, M. (2002). Polycystic ovary syndrome: An overview. *Topics in Advanced Practice Nursing eJournal, 2*(3) Retrieved July 30, 2002, from www.medscape.com/viewarticle/438597

Pearson, T. A., Blair, S. N., Daniels, S. R., Eckel, R. H., Fair, J. M., Fortmann, S. P., et al. (2002). AHA guidelines for primary prevention of cardiovascular disease and stroke: 2002 update. Consensus panel guide to comprehensive risk reduction for adult patients without coronary or other atherosclerotic vascular diseases. *Circulation, 106,* 388–391.

Prescriber's Letter, published monthly. Stockton, CA. Phone: 209–472–2240. Web address: www.prescribersletter.com

Rakel, R. E. (Ed.). (2003). *Conn's current therapy 2003: Latest approved methods of treatment for the practicing physician.* Philadelphia: Elsevier Science.

Reeves, J. R. T., Maiback, H. I. (2001). *Clinical dermatology illustrated: A regional approach* (3rd ed.). Philadelphia: F. A. Davis.

Romer, M. (2002). Bioidentical hormone replacement therapy. *Advance for Nurse Practitioners, 11,* 47–54.

Saslow, D., Runowicz, C. D., Solomon, D., Moscicki, A. B., Smith, R. A., Eyre, H. J., et al. (2002). American Cancer Society guidelines for the early detection of cervical neoplasia and cancer. *CA: A Cancer Journal for Clinicians, 52,* 342–362.

Scott, L. W. (2002). Heart-healthy diet for children. *Lipid Disorders Updates, 2,* 1–9.

Store, J. K., Wyman, J. F., & Salisbury, S. A. (1999). *Clinical gerontological nursing: A guide to advanced practice* (2nd ed.). Philadelphia: W. B. Saunders.

Sussman, C., & Bates-Jensen, B. (Eds.). (1998). *Wound care: A collaborative practice manual for physical therapy and nurses.* Gaithersburg, MD: Aspen.

Weston, W. L., Lane, A. T., Morelli, J. G. (2002). *Color textbook of pediatric dermatology* (3rd ed.). Philadelphia: Mosby.

White, G. M., Cox, N. H. (2002). *Diseases of the skin: A color atlas and text* (2nd ed.). Philadelphia: Mosby.

Wright, J. V., & Morgenthaler, J. (1997). *Natural hormone replacement for women over 45.* Petaluma, CA: Smart Publications.

Index

Figures denoted by *f*; tables denoted by *t*.